Arterial Behavior and Blood Circulation in the Brain

Arterial Behavior and Blood Circulation in the Brain

George Mchedlishvili

Beritashvili Institute of Physiology
Georgian Academy of Sciences
Tbilisi, USSR

Edited by

John A. Bevan, M.D.

College of Medicine
University of Vermont
Burlington, Vermont

CONSULTANTS BUREAU • NEW YORK AND LONDON

Library of Congress Cataloging in Publication Data

Mchedlishvili, G. I. (Georgiĭ Iosifovich)
  Arterial behavior and blood circulation in the brain.

  Bibliography: p.
  Includes index.
  1. Brain—Blood-vessels. 2. Regional blood flow—Regulation. 3. Cerebral
arteries. I. Bevan, John A., 1930–   . II. Title. [DNLM: 1. Brain—blood supply.
2. Cerebral Arteries—physiology. 3. Cerebrovascular Circulation. WL 302 M478a]
QP108.5.C4M394 1986   612′.824   86-8953
ISBN 0-306-10985-9

This volume is published under an agreement with the Copyright Agency
of the USSR (VAAP).

© 1986 Plenum Press, New York
A Division of Plenum Publishing Corporation
233 Spring Street, New York, N.Y. 10013

Printed in the United States of America

Foreword

The circulation in the brain, and particularly the cerebral cortex which deals with the highest development of life, would be expected to be the most complex and most effectively adaptable and responsive to local tissue demands in the organism. In this monograph, Professor Mchedlishvili synthesizes his ideas on the control and regulation of the cerebral circulation in relation to the needs of the brain. This is based on a lifetime of thought and reflection, observation and experimentation, argument and discussion, and is particularly important since much of the work of the author and his colleagues is not easily available to many scientists. This book develops the idea of the "effectors" of the brain circulation — their structure, function, and individuality — and presents a convincing attempt to integrate a multiplicity of observations around this idea.

Professor Mchedlishvili feels that the cerebral circulation contains many secrets yet hidden that will be revealed only by a concerted effort of many scientists and clinicians from many disciplines throughout the world using a variety of increasingly complex techniques. The answers will not come to one person, nor to one lab. One senses his frustration at finding so many impediments to progress. He suggests a "systems" approach to the remaining problems: The better these systems are defined, the better we realize what we do not know and the more cohesive, fruitful, and interacting can be the efforts of discovery. In this way, perhaps solutions can be found to the increasingly common problems of disturbances in blood flow. He emphasizes that the history of the discovery of the cerebral circulation tells us that new ideas must precede new discoveries, and that, in most instances, the techniques are awaiting their application. The systems approach to the definition of the whole context of investigation should provide a better setting in which these creative pursuits can flourish.

The phenomena of the regulation of the cerebral circulation by specific vascular effectors is a discovery recorded in the Registry of Discoveries of the USSR in 1981, which refers to the author's original work carried out in 1959 and pursued ever since. Each sequential segment of the arterial arborization to the brain, including the microcirculation, seems to have its own special role to play and unique control to maintain cerebral homeostasis. Seemingly, each aspect can be disturbed.

v

It may be that some feel that such an ordered approach to investigation does not provide the best context for creative study. However, they would surely agree that the conscious elaboration of such a system is a most helpful and major creative act in itself. Many of us probably need to spend more time in this sort of enterprise. Professor Mchedlishvili does not see this approach as restrictive; it allows for new developments, is not an end in itself, and is not a limit to endeavor. It is a device that is sufficiently elastic, and dare we say temporal, to accommodate things in the circulation not yet dreamt of. And in this context we can only applaud it.

This is a book to be read and reread, to have on the shelf and to be frequently taken down and pored over; it represents a lifetime of patient observation and experiment, and is a monument to the laboratory and to the man from Tbilisi.

John A. Bevan, M.D.

Preface

This book gives the present level of knowledge concerning a specific biomedical problem — cerebral arterial behavior under both physiological and pathological conditions, and its role in the phenomena of microcirculation. It is intended for postgraduate students and biomedical personnel — both scientists and medical doctors — who are interested in the cerebral blood flow, as well as in peripheral circulation in general.

Present knowledge of peripheral arterial behavior has gradually increased, thanks to the efforts of many researchers working in the field for more than a century. Within this period every epoch has had its specific points of interest, and only now has it become possible to summarize the subject of this book. This book is thus the fruit of research and development in cardiovascular physiology during the recent decades.

Although physiologists have always agreed that the main function of the circulatory system is to supply blood to particular parts of the body, the focus of their specific interest was initially restricted to heart function and systemic circulation, particularly arterial pressure. Thus, the most intensively studied physiological problems of the nineteenth and the first half of the twentieth centuries were concerned with general circulatory processes pertaining to the whole body. A few decades ago, special interest began to be concentrated on peripheral circulation as such and on the blood flow phenomena of singular organs in particular.

The cerebral blood flow was naturally the paramount concern from the very beginning of that period, due to its great significance not only in neurology and neurosurgery, but also in other medical fields. Therefore, it is not surprising that the investigations were carried out mainly by researchers who were closely associated with medical practice. This, in turn, influenced the trends of the research: the majority of the cerebral blood flow studies, carried out not only on humans but also on animals, had mainly an applied character. Comparatively few professional physiologists were engaged in the investigations. Nevertheless, the fundamental circulatory processes in the brain, specifically the physiological mechanisms operating under conditions of health and disease, gradually became the topic of detailed study. Thus the theoretical and technical approaches of basic science were gradually introduced into cerebral blood flow research. This concerned the trends of microvascular research, which has primarily developed since the first half of the present century as a re-

sult of the classical works of August Krogh, Benjamin Zweifach, and some
other researchers.

The reader will find in this book the first attempt at presenting an
account of the principles underlying the physiological behavior of the
cerebral arteries, which is chiefly, if not uniquely, related to the regulation of cerebral blood flow. This approach is closely associated with
the development of the concept that the brain's vascular mechanisms are
closely linked with the structure and function of specific cerebral arteries. Another topic covered in this book is the pathological behavior of
cerebral arteries, particularly during development of vasospasm and vasoparalysis, which cause disturbances of cerebral blood flow. It has become evident in the last two decades that the pathophysiological mechanisms
that bring about these pathological responses of cerebral arteries are
closely related to their physiological behavior. The present book also attempts to relate the behavior of the arteries, under physiological and
pathological conditions, with the microcirculatory events in the minute
blood vessels determining the coupling of circulation with metabolism of
the tissue.

There are two types of figures in this book. The first type explains
ideas using schematic drawings to provide visual images of the events, as
well as the concepts, considered in the book. The second type of figures
provides experimental evidence related mainly to concepts which have not
yet been widely accepted. The legends for figures are self-explanatory.
Thus, illustrations can be considered independent of the text.

An enormous, and still increasing, amount of experimental and clinical data on cerebral blood flow has been published in the world's scientific literature in recent decades, but this does not always help to clarify
the problems; it sometimes even creates certain difficulties in understanding them. Therefore, it has gradually become more difficult to summarize
the published data. The material presented in this book is related more
to the principles of arterial behavior and microcirculation than to specific topics. Therefore, instead of describing, for example, vasospasm
development under specific conditions, we present such topics only to il-
lustrate the principles of this pathological arterial behavior. This is
probably not very convenient for medical doctors in their everyday consideration of concrete cases of vasospasm in patients, but it is probably
much better to emphasize the principles rather than the great amount of
facts published in the scientific literature.

The book offers mostly theoretical considerations of the physiology
of cerebral blood flow. This does not mean, however, that the new, or different from commonly accepted, concepts are based on pure hypotheses deprived of experimental evidence. I have never tried to be original in
principle, but I have always attempted to make theoretical statements
which seem to be true, whether they are generally accepted or not. All
theoretical considerations presented in this book are based on published
experimental evidence, some of which has been obtained in my laboratory.

Hundreds of references have been utilized in the course of preparation
of this book, although the bibliography is certainly far from complete.
The references which I selected seemed to be most relevant to the topic being considered, especially if they substantiated modern concepts. Many of
the references belong to publications from my laboratory, since they probably deserve more attention than they have generally been given.

The scientific literature contains many repetitions of similar experimental data, and the actual progress of new knowledge is comparatively slow. Many current concepts are dominating scientific theories in published data, although some of them may be more or less incorrect, which may be misleading to further research. But it is sometimes not easy to reject them from general thought. I hope that the book will add sufficient new knowledge to the readers who are interested in these problems.

George Mchedlishvili
Beritashvili Institute of Physiology
Georgian Academy of Sciences
14 Gotua Street, 380060 Tbilisi, USSR

Acknowledgments

The present book summarizes the experimental results accumulated, as
well as the physiological concepts assimilated, by the author in the course
of his scientific work from the middle 1940s. His principal scientific
teacher has been Vladimir Voronin, an outstanding expert and theorist in
the field of normal and pathological physiology of circulation. The
author's research of cerebral circulation has been carried out in the Institute of Physiology, Georgian Academy of Sciences, founded and headed for
several decades by the distinguished Georgian physiologist Ivan Beritashvili (Beritoff). The author has been greatly influenced by the scientific
atmosphere of the Institute. The daily contacts with its collaborators
went a long way toward ensuring the progress in his research and thinking.

The author's investigations have been accomplished in association with
a closely knit research team of the Laboratory of Physiology and Pathology
of Cerebral Circulation, including Leila Ormotsadze, Leah Nikolaishvili,
Dodo Baramidze, Ramin Antia, Nodar Mitagvaria, Valerius Mamisashvili,
Michael Itkis, Natalie Sikharulidze, Manana Varazashvili, and several co-
workers of a younger generation, without whose tremendous efforts the results of the research would never have been obtained. The persistence and
technical competence of this group were indispensable to the successful
completion of studies of questions concerning the regulation and pathology
of the cerebral circulation.

The author wishes to sincerely thank all the scientists, representing
various research fields, with whom he collaborated at various times when
investigating different topics related to the arterial behavior and blood
circulation in the brain. Some of these specialists were representatives
of the Beritashvili Institute of Physiology: Peter Kometiani, biochem-
ist; Alexander Roitbak and Michael Khananashvili, neurophysiologists;
Marina Kuparadze, Elijah Lazriev, and Ada Tsitsishvili, neurohistologists.
The others worked in various scientific institutions of Tbilisi: Vakhtang
Akhobadze, cardiologist; George Amashukeli, surgeon; Medea Devdariani,
physiologist; Vladimir Gabashvili, neurologist; Shalva Toidze, anatomist;
Vladimir Dolidze and Revaz Kolelishvili, electrochemists; and Murtaz
Babunashvili, expert in systems research. Some others were from different
cities of the USSR: Beronice Samvelian, pharmacologist from Erevan;
Catherine Pletchkova, Anatolius Borodulya, and Natalie Lavrentieva, histologists from Moscow; Oleg Kaufman, anatomist from Moscow; Ratmir Orlov,
physiologist from Leningrad; Raisa Reidler, histochemist from Leningrad;

Yuri Levkovitch, optical mechanic from Leningrad. Some of the author's joint investigations have been carried out either in Tbilisi or abroad in collaboration with foreign specialists: Tadeusz Garbuliński, pharmacologist from Wroclaw, Poland; Adam Gosk, physiologist from Wroclaw, Poland; David Ingvar, neurophysiologist from Lund, Sweden; Bengt Falck, histochemist from Lund, Sweden; Christer Owman, histochemist from Lund, Sweden; Rolf Eckberg, neurologist from Lund, Sweden; Miroslaw Mossakowski, neuropathologist from Warsaw, Poland; Andrej Kapuśtiński, radiologist from Warsaw, Poland; Roman Gadamski, histochemist from Warsaw, Poland; Slavomir Januszewski, x-ray technician from Warsaw, Poland.

The people I wish especially to thank for help with reviewing and criticizing the manuscript are my nearest co-workers Drs. Dodo Baramidze, Valerius Mamisashvili, and Michael Itkis, who have shown permanent interest in our common work.

Professor Irina Gannushkina (Moscow, USSR), Prof. Peter Kometiani (Tbilisi, USSR), and Prof. John A. Bevan (Los Angeles, California) have very helpfully criticized the manuscript of individual chapters of this book. Dr. Murtaz Babunashvili (Tbilisi, USSR) trained me to consider the processes of cerebral blood flow regulation from the systems viewpoint. To all of them I owe a debt of gratitude which I cannot easily express.

The text of this book was not translated into English but directly written in the language, which is certainly not native for the author. This created certain difficulties, but at the same time provided definite advantages for the author who finds the English language very precise and adequate for expressing scientific thoughts. Therefore, sincere thanks are due to my teachers of the English language: Nina Gogolashvili and George Bei-Mamikonian, who helped me to become familiar with it and educated me to a degree where I am able to write scientific texts in this foreign language. I am indebted to Miss Ninel Skhirtladze, Mrs. Ada Azo, and Mrs. Lali Bablidze for their kind help in preparing and revising the English manuscript of this book.

I wish to thank those who helped me to prepare the illustrations to make the book more comprehensive. Sixty-nine new illustrations have been prepared by Tinatin Tsiskaridze and Vladimir Gadziacki from raw sketches prepared by the author. Manana Varazashvili, David Lominadze, and Maxim Badojan have given me perfect technical assistance in the preparation of the majority of illustrations for this book.

Several of the original illustrations published in this book first appeared in articles by the author and his associates in the following scientific periodicals: Bulletin of the Georgian Academy of Sciences (USSR), Sechenov Physiological Journal of the USSR, Bulletin of Experimental Biology and Medicine (USSR), Reports of the USSR Academy of Sciences, Pathological Physiology and Experimental Therapy, Korsakov Journal of Neuropathology and Psychiatry (USSR), Acta Physiologica Polonica, Nature (London), Experimental Neurology (USA), Pflügers Archiv (West Germany), Bibliotheca Anatomica (Switzerland), Microvascular Research (USA), Biochemistry and Experimental Biology (Italy), Stroke (USA), Blood Vessels (Switzerland), Biorheology (USA), and others.

A number of illustrations were reproduced or modified from scientific articles of eminent researchers: L. Auer (Austria), B. Baramidze (USSR), M. Baron (USSR), A. Borodulya (USSR), J. Cervós-Navarro (West Berlin), A. Chizhevsky (USSR), J. Fulton (USA), Y.-Ch. Fung (USA), P. Gaehtgens (West Germany), I. Gannushkina (USSR), M. Harper (United Kingdom), R.

Haynes (USA), D. Ingvar (Sweden), P. Johnson (USA), B. Klosovsky (USSR), A. Krogh (Denmark), B. Kuprianov (USSR), W. Kuschinsky (West Germany), N. Lassen (Denmark), E. Lightfoot (USA), H. Lipowsky (USA), V. Mamisashvili (USSR), Ch. Owman (Sweden), E. Pletchkova (USSR), M. Raichle (USA), M. Reivich (USA), H. Schmid-Schönbein (West Germany), B. Sjesjö (Sweden), Sh. Toidze (USSR), and B. Zweifach (USA). I wish to express my appreciation to the authors, as well as to the publishers, of these journals and books for permission to reproduce or modify the illustrations in this book.

I gratefully acknowledge the cooperation of Plenum Publishing Corporation in the production of the book.

For her moral support in the preparation of this book I thank my wife, Marina, who, as always, gave me confidence to carry on my favorite scientific work.

George Mchedlishvili

Contents

CHAPTER 1
CEREBRAL BLOOD FLOW: PERIPHERAL CIRCULATION

1.1. Functions of Cerebral Circulation   1
1.2. Central and Peripheral Circulation   3
1.3. Cerebral Vascular Bed: Integral Consideration of Its
     Structure and Function   9
1.4. Summary   15

CHAPTER 2
PRINCIPLES OF CEREBRAL BLOOD FLOW CONTROL.
A DEDUCTIVE APPROACH

2.1. Historical Sketch   17
2.2. Regulation of Cerebral Blood Flow from Viewpoint of
     Automatic Control   18
2.3. Types of Cerebral Blood Flow Control   22
2.4. Information about Disturbances Triggering Mechanisms
     of Cerebral Blood Flow Control   26
2.5. Coordination Systems of Cerebral Blood Flow Control   29
2.6. Vasomotor Mechanisms Controlling Cerebral Blood Flow . . .   31
2.7. Effectors of Cerebral Blood Flow Regulation   34
2.8. Efficiency Requirements of the Cerebral Blood Flow
     Control System   36
2.9. Physiological Mechanisms of Cerebral Blood Flow Control
     (from the present-day point of view).   39
2.10. Summary   41

CHAPTER 3
CEREBRAL ARTERIAL BEHAVIOR PROVIDING CONSTANT
CEREBRAL BLOOD FLOW, PRESSURE, AND VOLUME

3.1. Control of Constant Cerebral Blood Pressure and Flow . . .   43
3.2. Control of Constant Cerebral Blood Volume   57
3.3. Structural and Functional Features of the Vascular
     Effectors, the Major Brain Arteries   71
3.4. A Feedback Loop Responsible for the Active Maintenance
     of Constant Cerebral Blood Pressure and Flow   81

3.5. A Feedback Loop Responsible for the Control of Cerebral
      Blood Volume   92
3.6. Summary   94

CHAPTER 4

REGULATION PROVIDING AN ADEQUATE BLOOD SUPPLY
TO CEREBRAL TISSUE

4.1. Coupling between Blood Flow and Metabolic Rate in
      Cerebral Tissue   98
4.2. Regulation of Oxygen and Carbon Dioxide Levels in
      Cerebral Blood and Tissue 113
4.3. Organization of Pial Microvascular Effectors 122
4.4. Feedback Controlling Adequate Blood Supply to Cerebral
      Tissue and Constant Respiratory Gases in Blood   148
4.5. Summary 174

CHAPTER 5

PATHOLOGICAL ARTERIAL BEHAVIOR:
VASOSPASM AND VASOPARALYSIS

5.1. Vasospasm Relative to the Normal Behavior of Cerebral
      Arteries   178
5.2. Pathological Vasodilatation Relative to the Normal
      Behavior of Cerebral Arteries 184
5.3. The Objectives in Solving the Problem of Mechanisms of
      Pathological Behavior of Cerebral Arteries   188
5.4. The Essence of Pathological Arterial Behavior from the
      Standpoint of Vascular Smooth Muscle Physiology   189
5.5. Extrinsic Effects on Vascular Smooth Muscle That May Be
      Involved in the Development of Cerebral Vasospasm   195
5.6. Factors Inducing Pathological Vasodilatation in Cerebral
      Arteries   212
5.7. Disturbances in Smooth Muscle Cells That Provoke
      Arterial Pathological Responses 216
5.8. Compensatory Events Accompanying Pathological Arterial
      Responses 227
5.9. Summary 230

CHAPTER 6

TRANSPORT OF BLOOD AND OXYGEN TO BRAIN TISSUE

6.1. Fundamentals Determining the Rate of Microcirculation . . .   231
6.2. Flow Conditions in Minute Blood Vessels   242
6.3. Specific Phenomena Related to Blood Flow Rates in the
      Capillary Circulation 256
6.4. Red Cell:Plasma Ratio (Red Cell Concentration, Local
      Hematocrit) in Blood Flowing through Microvessels   274
6.5. Flow Conditions in Minute Blood Vessels following
      Vasomotor Disorders 291
6.6. Summary 293

AUTHOR'S NOTE   294
REFERENCES 297
INDEX   331

Chapter 1. Cerebral Blood Flow: Peripheral Circulation

This introductory chapter contains some general information on the circulatory system that is necessary for a more complete understanding of the next three chapters, which deal with the physiological behavior of the brain arteries that regulate cerebral blood flow. This chapter includes an outline of the structure and function of cerebral circulation portrayed as a typical representative of the peripheral circulation. It deals with the function of cerebral circulation and with general features of hemodynamics in the peripheral vascular bed; it will become evident why the classification of the circulatory system into the central and peripheral circulation is necessary. Finally, the functional organization of the peripheral vascular bed and circulation is outlined, with an emphasis on the cerebral circulatory system.

1.1. FUNCTIONS OF CEREBRAL CIRCULATION

Blood is continuously circulating in the brain. It is well known that the brain tissue needs a more constant, more highly regulated blood supply than any other part of the body. The following arguments may substantiate this assertion. The blood flow through the total human brain is about 750 ml per minute (Sokoloff, 1960). This means that 15% of the cardiac output, which at rest is 5000 ml per minute, passes through the brain, whose mass is only about 2% of the body weight. In one minute the brain utilizes on the average 49 ml of oxygen (Sokoloff, 1960). Assuming that the whole organism uses 250 ml of oxygen per minute, it follows that the cerebral tissue consumes about 20% of the total quantity of oxygen utilized by all tissues in the body.

It is well known that the main source of energy consumed by brain tissue is the oxidation of carbohydrates. The normal metabolism of the cerebral tissue is completely dependent upon a constant supply of blood-borne energy-producing materials, since the brain has negligible reserves of carbohydrates, and still less oxygen. Therefore, damage to the brain tissue has been regularly detected by neuroanatomists after only one or two minutes of complete cessation of cerebral blood flow at normothermy. This has never been observed in any other organ in the body. The high sensitivity of brain tissue to blood supply disturbances, on the one hand, and the comparatively high vulnerability of the cerebrovascular system, including its regulation, to different pathogenic factors, on the other hand, ex-

1

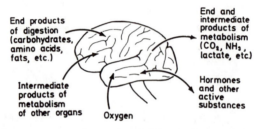

Fig. 1.1.   The purpose of cerebral blood flow, showing the sub-
            stances that are continuously transported to and
            from the brain tissue by the circulating blood.

plain why pathological changes of brain function are most frequently dependent on circulatory disorders. Different brain functions are certainly
not equally sensitive to circulatory deficiency: first speech and intel-
lectual activity become disturbed, then loss of consciousness appears and,
4–5 minutes after complete stoppage of blood flow in the brain, death of
the brain tissue occurs (Scheinberg and Joyne, 1952).

The main function of the brain circulation, similar to the peripheral
circulation in any part of the body, is the transport of various substances
to and from the tissue. Figure 1.1 presents the substances which are constantly transported by circulating blood to and from the brain. These substances are as follows: (1) Oxygen, which is transported from the lungs
to the brain and is utilized for oxidative metabolism. The constant oxygen supply to brain tissue is very important because the brain has a very
high metabolic rate. (2) Carbohydrates, amino acids, fats, and other end-
products of digestion, as well as intermediate metabolic products from
other organs, which represent the nutritive substances for brain tissue
metabolism. These products are utilized for the synthesis of high-energy
compounds, for maintaining the structure of the brain tissue elements, etc.
(3) Different intermediate and end-products of cerebral metabolism, primarily carbon dioxide, ammonia, etc., which are removed, since their presence in cerebral tissue would immediately cause disturbance of both cerebral blood flow and brain function. (4) Various physiologically active
substances, including hormones and vitamins, which are transported to and
from the brain. Among the active substances carried by the blood from the
brain, the hormones of the hypophysis should be mentioned first. Other
active substances, like insulin, thyroid hormone, serotonin, and many
others, as well as the vitamins, which are important for normal brain function, are transported from the sites of their peripheral penetration into
the blood, to the cerebral tissue.

The brain always has a priority over other organs in blood supply,
even though the other functions of the body may have to remain unfulfilled.
This priority in blood supply appeared in the evolution of living organisms and was probably determined not as much by the essence of the brain
as a body but for the benefit of the whole organism. Brain cells cannot
withstand a deficiency in blood supply, since they have less capacity for
anaerobic metabolism and, therefore, their metabolic reserves and survival
time after complete deprivation of blood supply are less in comparison
with other tissues of the body.

Although an uninterrupted blood flow everywhere in the cerebral vasculature is indispensable for the normal living brain, this does not mean
that the rate of cerebral blood flow is constant. The blood flow is period-

ically changed in particular regions of the brain both under normal and pathological conditions. First, the regional cerebral blood flow is coupled with the metabolic rate of brain tissue; this is necessary for normal functioning of cerebral tissue elements. This adjustment of cerebral blood flow to metabolism is a case of active control. Alternatively, the cerebral blood flow, pressure, and volume are maintained at constant levels despite circulatory changes outside the brain. Active control, leading either to expedient changes of cerebral blood flow or to its purposeful maintenance at a constant level, is particularly pronounced under pathological conditions when circulatory disturbances become harmful to brain function. Most forms of control of cerebral blood flow are achieved by the vasomotor behavior of the brain vessels and are always directed, on the one hand, to adjust the cerebral blood flow to brain functions and, on the other hand, to eliminate, as much as possible, pathological disorders in cerebral circulation.

1.2. CENTRAL AND PERIPHERAL CIRCULATION

In adult mammals blood circulation occurs in an integrated vascular system, where blood flows uninterruptedly in both oxygenated and deoxygenated circuits. However, from the functional standpoint, the system may be subdivided into the central and peripheral circulation.* Such a classification helps to better understand the purposes, hemodynamics, and control of the circulatory system.

The classification of the circulatory system into the central and peripheral circulation is based on the following factors: (a) anatomical differences, (b) functional characteristics, (c) the inherent circulatory parameters to be controlled, and (d) the different rheological properties of the blood flowing in large and small vessels.** However, no strict anatomical, functional, or hemodynamic boundary exists between the vessels of the central and peripheral circulation.

The central circulation involves, first, the distributing arterial subsystem starting from the left heart ventricle and including the aorta and all its branches, which feeds more than one organ. Furthermore, the central circulation includes a collecting venous subsystem composed of veins draining blood from the organs and carrying it through the venae cavae to the right atrium of the heart.

The central circulation functionally pertains to the whole organism and all its organs. It represents a kind of reservoir, from which all the organs, including the skin, adipose and other tissues throughout the body yield the necessary amount of blood, and another reservoir into which the blood is collected from the peripheral circulation itself. The description of the processes pertaining to the central circulation does not enter the scope of problems considered in this book, since they have been accurately presented in many special monographs devoted to circulation (see, e.g., Rushmer, 1961; Burton, 1972).

---

*Similar subdivisions may be probably also attributed to the pulmonary circulatory circuit. But this aspect has drawn less attention.
**The properties of blood flow in the larger vessels of central circulation and in the smaller vessels of peripheral circulation will be specially considered in Chapter 6 of this book.

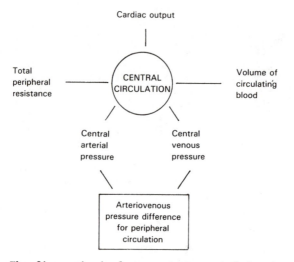

Fig. 1.2.   The five principal parameters pertaining to central
            circulation. Of these parameters, the central
            arterial and venous pressures, whose difference con-
            stitutes the perfusion pressure for particular per-
            ipheral beds, directly influence blood flow in in-
            dividual organs, especially the brain. See text for
            details.

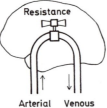

Fig. 1.3.   Principal factors that determine
            cerebral circulation according
            to the basic law of blood flow.

      In full accordance with the function performed by the central circula-
tion are the specific parameters characterizing this part of the circulatory system. There are several parameters of the central circulation which
must be maintained at certain levels in accordance with the circulatory
requirement of the whole organism. Probably, the most important parameter
of the central circulation is cardiac output per time unit. There are
also a number of other parameters, which are closely related with the
cardiac output, including the volume of circulating blood, the central
arterial pressure — in the aorta and its main branches, the overall peripheral vascular resistance — in the arterial system, the central venous
pressure — in the caval veins and their main branches (Fig. 1.2). However,
from the point of view of blood supply to an organ, the main physical
(hemodynamic) parameter characterizing the central circulation is the
arteriovenous pressure difference. Accordingly, the central circulation
has two parameters, namely the central arterial pressure and the central
venous pressure (often called the *systemic* arterial and venous pressures,
respectively), which must be maintained at constant levels in an organism
under normal conditions (Fig. 1.2). These pressures, to a great extent,

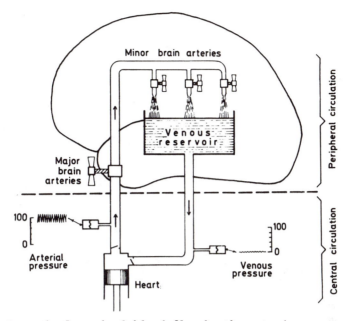

Fig. 1.4.   Control of cerebral blood flow by the arterio-venous pressure
            difference and the cerebral arterial resistance, which is, in
            turn, dependent upon active vasomotor responses of the major
            and minor cerebral arteries. See text for details.

determine the hemodynamics of the peripheral circulation, including the
hemodynamics of the brain itself (see Fig. 1.3).

     The peripheral, or regional, circulation (including the microcircula-
tion, i.e., the circulation in capillaries and adjacent small vessels) involves: (a) the arterial ramifications beginning from the largest branches,
which carry blood to the given region; (b) the capillaries and venules
where an interchange between the flowing blood and the tissue surrounding
the vessel walls occurs; and (c) the collecting veins which belong to the
given organ or region and carry blood out of its microcirculatory bed back
to the central circulation.

     The control of the peripheral circulation, including blood flow to the
brain, is basically accomplished by alterations in the peripheral vascular
resistance in an organ, which in turn induces the respective blood flow,
pressure, and volume changes in the peripheral vascular bed (Fig. 1.3).
The peripheral arteries, owing to their specific structure and function, act
as stopcocks to change the resistance, and thus, control peripheral blood
flow (see p. 10). All of these mechanisms control cerebral blood flow and are
shown schematically in Fig. 1.4. Under conditions when both the central
arterial and venous pressures are maintained at a constant level, the blood
flow in the peripheral circulation of any organ is adjusted by the width of
its arterial ramifications.

     Consequently, from the functional point of view, the main difference
between the central and peripheral circulation is that *blood pressure is
regulated in the central circulation, while blood flow is regulated in the
peripheral circulation of an organ*. This conception is schematically presented in Fig. 1.5.

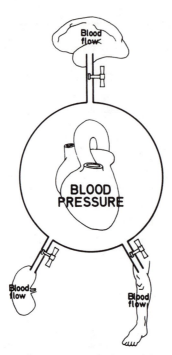

Fig. 1.5.   The main purpose and regulation of central
            and peripheral circulation. Blood pressure
            and blood flow, the most important param-
            eters of central and peripheral circulation,
            are steadily controlled under both physio-
            logical and pathological conditions. See
            text for details.

      Proceeding from this information, it should be obvious that the cen-
tral and peripheral circulations are closely interrelated. The relationship between the central and peripheral circulation is well defined in the
fundamental law of flow — the general principle of hemodynamics (Burton,
1972):

$$BF = \Delta P/R,$$

where BF stands for the blood flow in an organ, ΔP stands for the arterio-
venous pressure difference (pertaining to the central circulation; see
Fig. 1.2), and R stands for the resistance in the peripheral vascular bed.
Thus cerebral blood flow is directly proportional to the arterio-venous
pressure difference and inversely proportional to the cerebrovascular resistance. This relative effect of central and peripheral factors upon regional blood flow is presented schematically as a model in Fig. 1.6. The
left side of the figure shows the dependence of blood flow on the peripheral resistance when the arterio-venous pressure difference (or the perfusion pressure) is constant. The right side shows the dependence of blood
flow upon the arterio-venous pressure difference under conditions when the
peripheral resistance remains constant. Consequently, if the central
arterial and venous pressures are constant, the blood flow in a specific

A. CONSTANT ARTERIO - VENOUS
DIFFERENCE; CHANGES IN
VASCULAR RESISTANCE

B. CONSTANT VASCULAR RESISTANCE;
CHANGES IN ARTERIO - VENOUS
DIFFERENCE

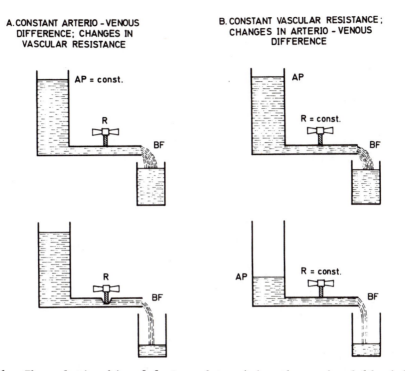

Fig. 1.6. The relationship of factors determining the regional blood flow
in a model. Shown schematically, these factors are: the peripheral resistance (R), determined by the peripheral vascular
width, and the arterio-venous pressure difference, dependent in
this case on the "arterial pressure" (AP) (in this model, the
"venous pressure" equals atmospheric pressure and remains constant). The effect of the peripheral resistance (when the
arterio-venous pressure difference is unchanged) is shown on
the left side of the figure. The effect of the arterio-venous
pressure difference (when the vascular width remains constant)
is shown on the right side of the figure.

organ depends solely on the resistance in its arteries; if the peripheral
resistance were constant, then the regional blood flow would be completely
dependent on the central arterial and venous pressures.

On the other hand, the central and peripheral circulations are also
comparatively independent of each other. There is much experimental evidence demonstrating the comparative independence of the central circulation
on changes in blood flow in individual organs under both physiological and
pathological conditions. Although the peripheral circulation regularly increases with rises in specific activity and metabolism of respective organs,
this does not usually cause changes in systemic arterial and venous pressures under physiological conditions. The considerable regional decrease
in blood supply to tissue due to pathological obstruction of peripheral
arteries in individual organs, resulting in ischemia, also may not cause
any regular changes in the systemic arterial pressure; this has been observed when ischemia affects even such important and highly sensitive parts
of the body as the cerebral cortex, for example following middle cerebral
artery occlusion (Klosovsky, 1951; Sundt and Waltz, 1971).

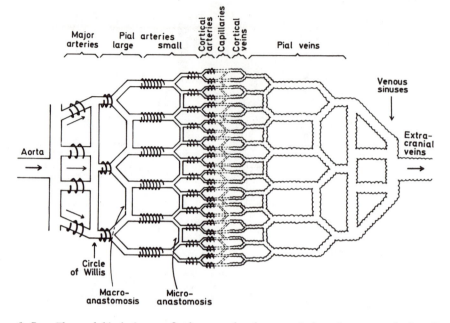

Fig. 1.7.   The subdivisions of the cerebral arterial and venous beds. Basic
            features which characterize the arterial branches are their abund-
            ant interconnections.   There are three main types of intercon-
            nections: (a) the largest anastomoses of the circle of Willis,
            (b) the pial macroanastomoses between the branches of the ante-
            rior, middle, and posterior cerebral arteries, and (c) the pial
            microanastomoses connecting the terminal branches on the cere-
            bral surface.   The arterial branches inside the brain substance
            are deprived of anastomoses, and only the capillaries form an
            uninterrupted microvascular network throughout the brain.   The
            venous branches and interconnections are similar to the arteri-
            al ones.

        Alternatively, peripheral circulation may also be, to a certain ex-
tent, independent of the central circulation because of active changes in
the peripheral resistance.   This phenomenon is especially well pronounced
in the organs, where the circulation is well regulated; in the brain blood
flow has been proved to be maintained at a constant level in spite of
changes of the systemic arterial pressure within limits of ~70-160 mm Hg
(see Chapter 3).   This constancy of peripheral circulation independent of
changes in the arterio-venous pressure difference is usually called "autoregulation" of the regional blood flow (see p. 81).

        Consideration of the peripheral circulation in general, in contrast
to the central circulation, signifies only that different peripheral vascular beds possess certain features common to the circulatory system.   But
this does not mean that the physiological and pathological events in the
peripheral circulation are similar in all organs.   Actually, considerable
differences in the control of peripheral blood flow have been found in different parts of the body, particularly in the brain, and this is why they
are usually considered separately (Johnson, 1978).   The present book deals
almost exclusively with the control and disturbances of the cerebral blood
flow.

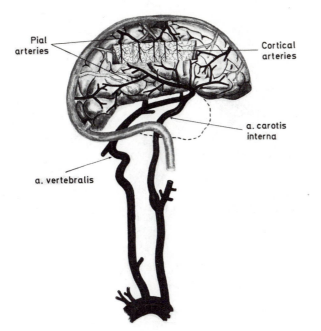

Fig. 1.8. Distribution of the main cerebral arteries and veins in the cere-
           bral vascular bed. See text for details. (Reproduced from Betz
           et al., 1974.)

1.3. CEREBRAL VASCULAR BED: INTEGRAL CONSIDERATION OF ITS
      STRUCTURE AND FUNCTION

     The peripheral (regional) vascular bed is composed of vasculature that
distributes blood from the arterial part of central circulation to the
capillary bed of a given organ or tissue, and then returns it to collecting
veins of central circulation. Consequently, the following types of blood
vessels compose the peripheral vascular beds: the medium- and small-sized
arteries, the capillaries, the small- and medium-sized veins, and, alternatively, the arterio-venous anastomoses, which are not present in the
vascular bed of the brain. All the aforementioned types of peripheral
blood vessels differ from each other both in wall structure and their function. However, we shall not consider the detailed anatomy of the peripheral blood vessels which has been described elsewhere in considerable detail
(Rhodin, 1962, 1980; Bader, 1963). The anatomical as well as physiological
characteristics of the cerebral vasculature are pointed out here only to
emphasize aspects which aid comprehension of the material included in the
subsequent chapters.

     General Anatomical Design of Cerebral Arterial Bed. The arterial sys-
tem of the brain, presented schematically in Fig. 1.7, starts with the
major arteries, the internal carotid and vertebrals, at the point where they
start carrying blood only, or mainly, to the brain. These arteries gradually ramify and anastomose with each other, inside the skull. They connect
at the base of the brain and form the so-called circle of Willis. From
this vascular circle three pairs of the anterior, middle, and posterior
cerebral arteries arise. The latter further ramify and anastomose on the
surface of the cerebral hemispheres and form the complex pial arterial bed
(Fig. 1.8). These surface vessels give off arterial branches, termed radi-

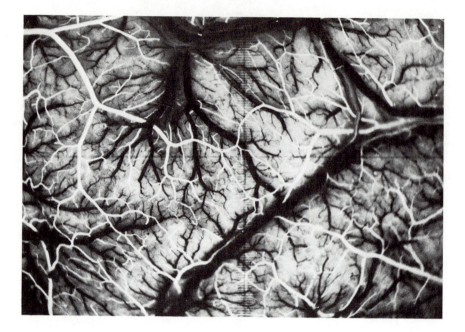

Fig. 1.9. This photomicrograph shows the pial arterial and venous networks
          on the brain surface. The pial arterial ramifications and macro-
          anastomoses shown are in the boundary zone of the anterior,
          middle, and posterior cerebral arteries in the temporal region
          of monkey *Cercopithecus sebaeus*. The arteries are shown in
          white, and the veins in black. (Reproduced with permission
          from Gannushkina et al., 1977b.)

al arteries, which dip into the brain substance, giving off further
branches, and finally produce the uninterrupted capillary network of the
cerebral tissue (Fig. 1.9). Comparatively larger arterial branches, arising from the arteries of the circle of Willis or its ramifications at the
base of the brain, supply the basal ganglia and the chorioid plexuses. The
branches of the vertebral and basilar arteries supply the brain stem and
the cerebellum.

    Arterial caliber in the cerebral circulation decreases at every
branching sequence, as in the rest of the body. The pial arterial system,
which is highly ramified and interconnected by anastomoses, has two types
of branchings: the bifurcations of the arterial trunks into branches
whose diameters do not differ greatly from each other and the offshoots of
smaller arterial branches from the trunks at approximately right angles
(see Chapter 4).

    The Arterial Walls. The main structural difference between the
arteries and other blood vessels — capillaries and veins — of the brain
(as in any organ) is a well-developed muscular coat in their walls (Rhodin,
1980). The muscular coat of the cerebral arteries consists of smooth
muscle layers that decrease with reduction of the arterial caliber. The
smallest arterioles which merge with capillaries consist of a single smooth
muscle layer in which the muscle cells gradually become separated from each
other.

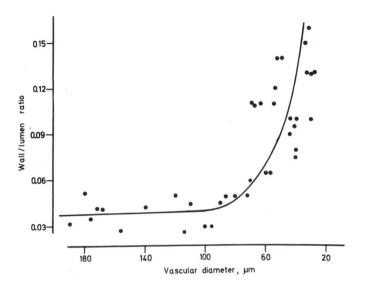

Fig. 1.10. The relative magnitude of the arterial smooth muscle layer, ex-
            pressed in terms of the ratio of wall thickness to pial arteri-
            al caliber in rabbits, is shown for pial arteries of different
            diameters. The significant increase in the relative size of
            the muscular coat in smaller pial arteries is related to their
            specific function (see pp. 104-106 in Chapter 4). (Reproduced
            from Mchedlishvili and Mamisashvili, 1974.)

     The muscular coat of the majority of cerebral arteries was found to
be somewhat thinner than that of the arterial vessels of the same caliber
in other organs (Lazorthes, 1961), but it is evident from known physiological data that the muscularis is sufficiently developed to change the
luminal size and vessel resistance. In contrast, the relative mass of the
muscular coat (relative to the total mass of vessel wall) in the walls of
the smaller pial arteries increases considerably. The arterial smooth
muscle layer, expressed in terms of a ratio of wall thickness to luminal
diameter, increases noticeably in the smaller pial arteries, smaller than
80-100 µm in diameter (Fig. 1.10).

     Cerebral arteries are richly innervated by both adrenergic and cholin-
ergic nerve fibers. The vascular nerve supply is more plentiful in large
cerebral arteries and decreases gradually with reduction of their caliber.
The innervation is considerably richer in those areas of the cerebral
arterial bed which show greater diameter changes. This was found, first,
in the cavernous portion of the internal carotid arteries (Borodulya and
Pletchkova, 1973), and, second, at the sites of sphincters of pial arterial offshoots and the precortical arteries (Baramidze et al., 1981, 1982).
The innervation of the major and pial arteries of the brain will be considered in more detail in Chapters 3 and 4.

     Structure and Function of Capillaries. The cerebral capillaries are
a direct continuation of the smallest arterioles that represent terminal
branches of the radial arteries. The latter penetrate the brain substance
either over a small area within the cortex or for a longer distance, to the
white substance and deeper brain structures. During ontogeny the cerebral
capillary bed originates from the radial arterial branches penetrating the

embryonic brain substance. The density of the capillary network varies significantly throughout the adult brain (Scharrer, 1962; Lierse, 1963) and is certainly coupled with the metabolic rate of the surrounding tissue. Therefore, the capillary network is very dense in the ground substance, containing mostly cellular elements, and comparatively sparse in the white substance formed from myelinated nerve fibers. The cerebral cortex incorporates two networks: a superficial one, where the majority of vessels are arranged parallel to the cerebral surface, and a deeper one surrounding the pyramidal cells. The design of capillary beds is also exceedingly variable in different brain structures and is related to the arrangement of the varying brain regions. The detailed investigation of the specific capillary networks in different parts of the brain provide the basis of description of angioarchitectonic areas of the brain (Pfeifer, 1940), based on the anatomy of every specific part of the brain and on their cytoarchitecture.

The structure of capillary walls (Rhodin, 1980) is well adjusted to the performance of their main function, i.e., efficient transport of different substances across their walls from the blood stream to the surrounding tissue and back. Accordingly, no muscle or other specific contractile cells are found in the walls of the true capillaries and, therefore, they cannot be involved in an active control of blood flow inside them by primary changes of their lumina, as is the case with the arterial vessels of the peripheral circulation. The walls of the capillaries consist of one layer of flat endothelial cells. Their outer surface rests on a basement membrane formed by a continuous layer of ground substance which separates the endothelium and the surrounding astroglial processes.

The capillaries have a minimal possible diameter of approximately 5 μm to allow the transport of the deformed red cells along their lumina. Therefore, the capillaries occupy a minimal space in the tissue and provide a relatively great surface of their wall area for transport of oxygen and other materials through the vascular wall. The capillaries form a continuous plexus inside the whole brain substance. However, because of a low intracapillary blood pressure and small lumina, this does not permit a collateral blood inflow from the neighboring capillary network in cases when the feeding arterioles become occluded (Gannushkina, 1958). Thus the capillary system of the brain, though uninterrupted in the brain substance (Klosovsky, 1951), cannot provide a normal microcirculation in capillaries deprived of a normal blood supply from the respective arterioles.

Structure and Function of Cerebral Veins. The cerebral veins, which are thin-walled similar to other peripheral veins, drain blood from the cerebral capillaries back to the central circulation (see Fig. 1.7). The blood flows through two groups of cerebral veins: the superficial veins, comparable to the pial arterial bed, and the deep veins that correspond to the arteries supplying the basal ganglia; the latter collect blood into the great cerebral vein of Galen. The blood from the cerebral veins is drained into the cerebral sinuses and then into the extracranial veins, mainly the jugular veins of the neck.

The pressure in the cerebral veins is very low, almost equal to the pressure in the cerebrospinal fluid. The pressure gradient between the cerebral capillaries and the central venous trunks is small, and blood flows along the intracranial veins with a relatively low (but greater than capillary) velocity. This is explained by the fact that the lumen of the individual veins, and therefore the cross-sectional area of all the veins draining blood from the brain, is relatively large in comparison with the arterial system.

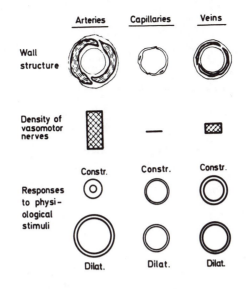

Fig. 1.11.   Scheme of the behavior of different blood vessels
             related to wall structure. The comparatively thick
             muscular layer and high density of vasomotor nerves
             account for considerable constriction and dilata-
             tion ability of peripheral arteries. These re-
             sponses are less pronounced in the veins (especial-
             ly in the cerebral veins, which are devoid of a
             continuous muscle layer), and absent in the capil-
             laries. Therefore, only the regional arteries are
             anatomically and functionally adjusted to control
             peripheral resistance. See text for details.

The walls of the smallest cerebral veins resemble those of the large
capillaries. The larger vein walls are composed of many collagenous and
few elastic fibers. The smooth muscle layer inside their walls is incomplete, except for the largest pial veins — especially at the sites where
they merge with the venous sinuses (Alexandrovskaya, 1955). The responses of intracranial veins to different vasoactive substances have been
found to be insignificant in comparison with extracranial veins of the
same caliber (Orlov et al., 1977). But detectable venoconstriction was discovered following topical microapplication of noradrenaline in $vivo$ in concentrations of $10^{-6}-10^{-3}$ M to the walls of cat pial veins (Ulrich et al.,
1981). Similar effects have been observed under in $vitro$ conditions
(Edvinsson et al., 1983). It is quite probable that the capacitance function of the cerebral veins is decreased compared to other veins of the
body; it seems unlikely that large volumes of blood could be stored inside
the rigid skull. Thus, the main function of the cerebral veins is blood
drainage from the cerebral capillaries to the extracranial veins.

However, the larger veins of the head outside the skull, which drain
into central veins, have shown active physiological responses to various
humoral and neural effects (Orlov and Priklonskaya 1980; Pearce and Bevan,
1981). In all probability, these active areas of venous outflow adjacent
to the brain control blood drainage from the brain. This means of control
explains, to a certain extent, the experimental results of the effects of
sympathetic stimulation and of catecholamines following intraarterial ad-

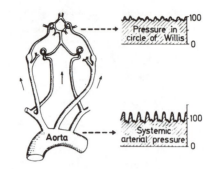

Fig. 1.12.   Damping of systemic arterial
             pressure pulsatile fluctua-
             tions along the major arter-
             ies of the brain. (From
             Mchedlishvili et al., 1977.)

ministration — the capacitance of intracranial vessels was unrelated to
the resistance in cerebral arteries (Tkachenko, 1979).

   Cerebrovascular resistance is determined by functional behavior of
specific brain vessels. The well-defined muscular layer in cerebral
arterial walls actively constricts or dilates upon exposure to various
humoral and neural control stimuli, thus regulating the blood circulation
in the whole brain and in specific regions. As in other peripheral blood
vessels of the body, the functional behavior of cerebral arteries is closely related to wall structure (Fig. 1.11).

   For many years the main regulators of regional circulation were
thought to be the smallest precapillary arterioles, where the resistance,
according to Poiseulle's law, should be the greatest. In accordance with
this concept, the major arteries of the brain were thought not to participate actively in the control of cerebral blood flow. However, beginning in
the late 1950s, evidence started to show that even the largest cerebral
arteries are actively involved in the control of brain circulation due to
the pronounced ability of their walls to actively change their widths within a large range (Mchedlishvili, 1959a, 1960b, 1972; Heistad et al., 1978).
Furthermore, these arteries have been found to play an important role in
damping the pulsatile fluctuations of the arterial pressure of blood flowing into the skull. The arterial pressure recorded at the beginning and
end of the major cerebral arteries shows that the pulsatile fluctuations
of arterial pressure decrease considerably inside the skull at the circle
of Willis (Fig. 1.12). In contrast to the major brain arteries, however,
pial arterial walls had always been believed to actively change their lumina during regulation and pathological changes of the cerebral circulation.

   With respect to the functional behavior of cerebral arteries, it is
important to note that the anatomical surroundings of both the major and
pial arteries are readily displaced fluids (blood in the venous sinuses,
or cerebrospinal fluid in the subarachnoidal channels), and, consequently,
the vessels can easily change their diameter within wide limits. In contrast to this, the intracerebral arteries and arterioles, like the majority
of other arteries of the body, are closely surrounded by tissue structural
elements, which creates the extravascular pressure (see also p. 108 in Chapter 4). The actual vasomotor reactivity of the intracerebral blood vessels
remains much less investigated than that of the major and pial vessels be-

cause of their inaccessibility for direct *in vivo* observations. Existing experimental data, concerned with the responses of these arteries, are still few in number and sometimes contradictory (see pp.108-111 and 119-120 in Chapter 4).

   Redistribution of Blood. Another important function of the cerebral arterial system is to redistribute blood among various brain regions. This capability is related, in particular, to the presence of numerous inter-arterial anastomoses along the cerebral arterial bed, starting from the major arteries of the brain and terminating at the smallest pial arterial branches (see Fig. 1.7). Interarterial anastomoses are much more numerous in the brain than in any other part of the body.

   Although all four major arteries of the brain are interconnected in the circle of Willis, blood is not mixed in it under normal conditions. Blood from each major artery is distributed strictly to the respective blood vessels of the ipsilateral side of the brain: from the internal carotid arteries to the cerebral hemispheres and from the vertebral arter-ies to the posterior fossa, i.e., to the cerebellum and brain stem. This has been convincingly demonstrated in experiments where radio-opaque materials and dyes were injected into the individual major arteries (Schmidt, 1950; Holmes et al., 1958; Himwich et al., 1965). This ipsi-lateral distribution can be explained by an absence of blood flow in the anastomoses of the circle of Willis under normal conditions, since no pressure gradient exists at the terminal segments of the major arteries of the brain. Blood flow appears in the anastomoses only if a major artery becomes occluded, resulting in a collateral blood supply to the area previously fed by the occluded artery. It is interesting to note that even blood from the vertebral arteries is distributed only to the ipsi-lateral parts of the brain due to laminar flow in the basilar artery (Holmes et al., 1958; McDonald and Potter, 1951).

   There are numerous interarterial anastomoses in the pial arterial sys-tem (Klosovsky, 1951; Duvernoy et al., 1981). The pial anastomoses may be classified into two types: those belonging to the larger pial arteries, and those located at the branches of the smallest pial arterial. The larger anastomoses connect regions supplied by branches of the anterior, middle, and posterior cerebral arteries in both hemispheres of the brain. These anastomoses are located in specific areas of the cerebral surface (see Fig. 1.13) called pial arterial boundary zones. They provide a col-lateral blood supply to the respective brain regions when either the an-terior, middle, or posterior cerebral arteries, or their branches, become oc-cluded.

   Many other types of interarterial anastomoses are distributed over the entire surface of both cerebral hemispheres at the different branches of the pial arterial bed (Fig. 1.7). These microanastomoses connect either two precortical arteries or a precortical artery with an adjacent small pial arterial branch. The role of the pial microanastomoses in the control of adequate blood supply to the smallest areas of the cerebral cortex seems to be very important and will be specially considered in Chapter 4. No interarterial anastomoses connecting the smallest arterial branches have been found *inside* the cerebral cortex (Klosovsky, 1951; Duvernoy et al., 1981).

1.4. SUMMARY

   The function of the cerebral blood circulation is to transport to and from the brain various substances that are necessary for its normal me-

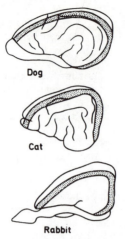

Fig. 1.13. Schematic distribution of pial
            arterial boundary zones on the
            brain surface of dogs, cats,
            and rabbits, where the majority
            of anastomoses connect the
            branches of the anterior, mid-
            dle, and posterior cerebral
            arteries. (Reproduced with
            permission from Klosovsky,
            1951.)

tabolism and function. The cerebral circulation is constantly regulated to
provide the brain with an adequate blood supply and to eliminate all possible disturbances, which repeatedly appear in the course of life. The
cerebral blood flow is a typical representative of the peripheral circulation (versus the central circulation), which is regulated in living organisms mainly by the behavior of cerebral arteries.

Chapter 2. Principles of Cerebral Blood Flow Control
A Deductive Approach

This chapter deals with the physiological systems controlling cerebral blood flow. Regulation occurs via active physiological processes, which change the cerebral blood flow in a specific direction: either by stabilizing some parameters, or by adjusting the others to the related functions. When the physiological mechanisms regulating cerebral blood flow are operating normally, the control is completely achieved in the healthy organism. However, when disturbances of cerebral blood flow become excessive during disease, the regulation is achieved only partially, and the compensation for such disturbances varies under different circumstances.

This chapter contains an attempt at deductive analysis of the functions of the physiological systems regulating the cerebral blood flow, proceeding from the viewpoint of automatic control. Therefore, the reader will find less concrete experimental data and more general speculation. A "systemic" consideration of the problem of cerebral blood flow control seems to be important at present, when so much confusing experimental material has been accumulated in the world's scientific literature. This chapter should help to provide an insight into the problem as a whole and a better understanding of what is actually known about the physiology and pathology of cerebral blood flow control. A suggested style of thinking for future experimentation will be presented.

2.1. HISTORICAL SKETCH

Several conceptual trends in physiological thought concerning the mechanisms regulating cerebral blood flow existed during the 19th and 20th centuries. The earliest was the Monro-Kellie doctrine (cited by Hill, 1896) which postulated that there are three incompressible constituents inside the skull: cerebral tissue, cerebrospinal fluid, and blood. Therefore, the amount of the blood and, hence the cerebral blood flow, should remain constant under any physiological and pathological condition. The doctrine rejected the possibility of active control of cerebral blood flow.

By the end of the 19th century, evidence had accumulated to show that cerebral blood flow may, nevertheless, change (Hill, 1896). Although the diameter of the cerebral blood vessels was still believed to be unchanged, cerebral blood flow was thought to be controlled by changes in systemic arterial and/or venous pressures. Hence, cerebral perfusion pressure was considered as the main regulator of brain blood supply.

   The role of the central arterial pressure as an effector of cerebral
blood flow control would have been certainly proved if there were some
evidence that the cerebral circulation could actually be corrected by its
changes. Since the last century, many researchers have been interested in
whether or not the central arterial pressure rises in response to a deficiency in blood supply to brain tissue. Increases in the central arterial pressure were observed after occlusion of carotid arteries (this phenomenon had been described by Magendie as far back as 1838); however, this
response was later proved to be the result of the carotid sinus reflex
(Hering, 1937; Heymans and Niel, 1958). It was later proven in experiments
where the cerebral arteries were occluded (Mchedlishvili and Ormotsadze,
1963; Waltz et al., 1966) that even an identified deficiency of blood
supply to cerebral tissue does *not* cause an elevation of the central arterial pressure. The absence of the hypertensive response during an identified
ischemia in cerebral tissue is also well known in neurological and neurosurgical practices. The only exceptions are cases of elevation of the
arterial pressure during deficient blood supply to those cerebral areas related to arterial pressure regulation, particularly the brain stem (Klosovsky, 1951; de la Torre et al., 1962; Dickinson, 1965). Therefore, despite
the fact that the systemic arterial pressure can affect cerebral blood flow
to a certain degree, it cannot be considered as an effector of cerebral
blood flow control even under conditions of decreased blood supply to the
brain.

   The next concept concerning the control of cerebral blood flow was developed in the 1930s when studies by Forbes and associates (Forbes et al.,
1937; Forbes and Cobb, 1938; Fog, 1937, 1939) showed that the pial arteries
can actively constrict and dilate. Thus, the cerebrovascular resistance
became a topic of interest in the study of cerebral blood flow control and
research carried out in the 1940s and 1950s clarified its role (Schmidt,
1950; Klosovsky, 1951; Kety, 1960). At that time the control of dilatation and constriction of cerebral blood vessels was thought to be due only
to the direct effect of humoral agents, like carbon dioxide and oxygen.

   In the 1960s and 1970s researchers attempted to analyze the circulatory phenomena responsible for cerebral blood flow control by studying the
specific activity of particular portions of cerebral arteries and neurohumoral influences on cerebral blood vessels (Mchedlishvili, 1964, 1972;
Lübbers, 1972; Betz, 1972; Purves, 1972; von Essen, 1973; Olesen, 1974;
Edvinsson and MacKenzie, 1977; Kuschinsky and Wahl, 1978). Further read-
ings on the main trends of this period can be found in the Proceedings of
the International Symposia on Cerebral Blood Flow held in different coun-
tries (Ingvar and Lassen, 1965; Ingvar et al., 1968; Mchedlishvili, 1969a;
Ross Russel, 1971; Langfitt et al., 1975; Harper et al., 1975; Mchedlishvili, Kovách, et al., 1977; Owman and Edvinsson, 1977; Ingvar and Lassen,
1977a; Mchedlishvili, Purves, et al., 1979; Gotoh et al., 1979; Raichle et
al., 1981).

   Concepts concerning the physiological mechanisms controlling cerebral
blood flow, which replaced each other during the 19th and 20th centuries,
are schematically summarized in Fig. 2.1.

2.2. REGULATION OF CEREBRAL BLOOD FLOW FROM VIEWPOINT
      OF AUTOMATIC CONTROL

   The control of cerebral blood flow is one of many homeostatic mechanisms which are steadily operating in living organisms and control various
functions. All control systems are governed by certain general principles
although they control quite different functions.

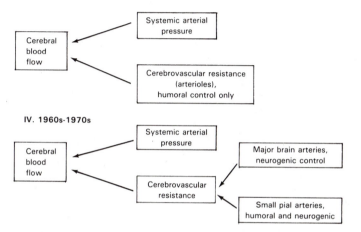

I. 19th CENTURY

Cerebral blood flow = constant

II. PRIOR TO 1930s

Cerebral blood flow ← Systemic arterial pressure

III. 1940s-1950s

Cerebral blood flow ← Systemic arterial pressure
← Cerebrovascular resistance (arterioles), humoral control only

IV. 1960s-1970s

Cerebral blood flow ← Systemic arterial pressure
← Cerebrovascular resistance ← Major brain arteries, neurogenic control
← Small pial arteries, humoral and neurogenic

Fig. 2.1. Hypothetical mechanisms for the active control of cerebral blood flow in different periods of scientific thought during the last two centuries. See text for details. (Reproduced from Mchedlishvili, 1980a.)

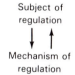

Subject of regulation

Mechanism of regulation

Fig. 2.2. Bilateral interaction of the subject and the mechanism of regulation ensuring physiological regulation. (Reproduced from Mchedlishvili, 1981b.)

The control system of any physiological function comprises two parts: (a) the subject of regulation, i.e., the system to be controlled, including a collection of interacting subsystems which are in need of coordination, and (b) the regulatory mechanism of the subject, which provides for the necessary degree of coordination between parts of the system being regulated. The interaction of these two principal parts of the control system ensures smooth operation of the entire system; any changes or disturbances in the subject being regulated results in activation of the con-

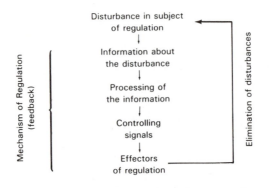

Fig. 2.3.   Interconnections between the
            links of a regulatory system.
            See text for details.

trol mechanism which, in turn, affects the subject being regulated, thus
attaining control (Fig. 2.2).

In the case of control of cerebral blood flow, as with any other function in the body, physiological control mechanisms are triggered by disturbances such as primary decrease in blood supply or excessive increase
in cerebral blood volume. In response to such disturbances, a control
mechanism becomes active by adjusting cerebral blood flow to the new conditions, with the aim of eliminating the disturbance within the limits of
the system. The mechanisms of control usually consist of several interconnected links: (1) afferent information indicating the type of disturbance
in the subject being regulated, (2) processing of this information, usually by specific nervous centers, (3) the transmission of regulatory signals
originating either from the nervous centers or operating outside them (e.g.,
in the vascular smooth muscle or in the surrounding tissue), and (4) the
vascular effectors of regulation within the circulatory system. Together
these links provide the cerebral blood flow system with a feedback mechanism of control. An outline of a physiological mechanism controlling cerebral blood flow is shown schematically in Fig. 2.3.

The type of afferent information in the cerebral blood flow control
system can vary. It can arise from the degree of stretch of vascular smooth
muscle caused by changes in the intravascular pressure, from diffusion of
vasoactive metabolic substances accumulated in the tissue, or from specific
nervous receptors located either in the vessel walls or in the surrounding
tissue. The information from these receptors is transmitted to the nervous
centers by specific afferent pathways.

Regulatory signals appear in response to the afferent information.
They can be seen in response to stretch of the arterial smooth muscle
(myogenic mechanism), or in the direct effect of metabolites or other
active substances on the vessel walls (humoral mechanism), or in the efferent vasomotor effects on specific blood vessels (neurogenic mechanism). In
the latter case, regulatory signals are commonly generated in specific
neuron association centers, which also coordinate changes pertaining to
the control of other related physiological processes, e.g., the hemodynamics of the systemic circulation.

The effectors of regulation are the specific blood vessels in the circulatory bed, which respond primarily to the aforementioned regulatory signals and effect the appropriate hemodynamic responses occurring in the vascular bed by adjusting the cerebral blood flow to new conditions.

A. Simple regulating loop   **B. Complex regulating loop**

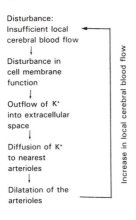

Disturbance:
Insufficient local
cerebral blood flow

↓

Disturbance in
cell membrane
function

↓

Outflow of K⁺
into extracellular
space

↓

Diffusion of K⁺
to nearest
arterioles

↓

Dilatation of the
arterioles

Increase in local cerebral blood flow

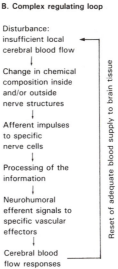

Disturbance:
insufficient local
cerebral blood flow

↓

Change in chemical
composition inside
and/or outside
nerve structures

↓

Afferent impulses
to specific
nerve cells

↓

Processing of the
information

↓

Neurohumoral
efferent signals to
specific vascular
effectors

↓

Cerebral blood
flow responses

Reset of adequate blood supply to brain tissue

Fig. 2.4. Simple and complex control loops, which maintain an adequate
           blood supply to cerebral tissue in response to insufficient
           blood flow. See text for details.

     The parts of the regulatory mechanism form control loops, which start
from the subject to be regulated, i.e., from the vascular system of the
brain or the surrounding tissue, and terminate on cerebral blood vessels.
It follows from the aforementioned information that there are two types of
control loops of cerebral blood flow regulation: (a) simple control loops
which operate exclusively locally, for instance, the direct myogenic response of the vascular smooth muscle to stretch or the direct effect of
a humoral agent from tissue on the vascular walls, and (b) complex control
loops, such as the neurogenic control of the cerebral blood flow, which in-
corporate elements of the humoral and myogenic mechanisms. Complex control loops can operate both locally and distantly. These two types of
regulatory mechanisms are presented schematically in Fig. 2.4, and will be
discussed thoroughly below and in the following chapters.

     The efficiency of the cerebral blood flow control system has gradual-
ly developed during phylogeny and ontogeny. Due to these processes, the
control mechanisms of cerebral blood flow evolved in the most efficient
way to reach the aim of regulation. The presently known criteria of efficiency of cerebral blood flow control will be considered in this chapter.

     One way to increase understanding of cerebral blood flow regulation is
to use a problem-solving approach.

     The solution of the problem of cerebral blood flow control will not
be achieved unless its constituting problems (subproblems) are solved. To
this end, the problem is to be considered as a whole and its structure is
to be defined. The aim of outlining the structure of the problem includes,
first, the estimation of its dimensions, i.e., the recognition of all the
constituent subproblems which should be solved to achieve solution of
the whole problem.
     The constituents of the problem of control of the cerebral blood flow
(Mchedlishvili, 1981b) are as follows: (a) the subjects, and hence the
aims, of the control; (b) the information about disturbances in the subject

PHYSIOLOGICAL MECHANISM
OF CEREBRAL BLOOD FLOW REGULATION

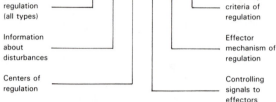

Fig. 2.5. The subproblems that need to be solved to achieve
           solution of the whole problem of physiological regu-
           lation of cerebral blood flow. (Reproduced from
           Mchedlishvili, 1981b.)

to be regulated by the cerebral blood flow system; (c) the coordination
centers that process afferent information; (d) the regulatory signals to the
vascular effectors of cerebral blood flow control; (e) the effector mechanisms of regulation of cerebral blood flow, including the identification
of the vascular effectors and the subsequent hemodynamic events in the
vascular system; and (f) the criteria needed for efficient control of cerebral blood flow. All the enumerated problems are to be approached with respect to solving the whole problem. Figure 2.5 shows schematically the
structure of the problem of cerebral blood flow control.

It appears obvious that a system analysis of a biomedical problem may
be valid only at the current level of knowledge and therefore can be outlined only for the time being. As soon as a significant body of new knowledge is accumulated, the graphs must be revised to specify not only the
new objectives, but also reformulate the whole problem.

2.3. TYPES OF CEREBRAL BLOOD FLOW CONTROL

To apply the deductive method for the analysis of physiological control of cerebral blood flow, first, one must identify the various mechanisms of such control. All types of controls must be specified in this
case. In fact, the statement that "cerebral blood flow is regulated" is
actually devoid of concrete meaning. Therefore, it is necessary to define
what is actually to be controlled in the case of cerebral blood flow.

In order to specify the different types of cerebral blood flow control, we should first establish the criteria of their adequate classification. Probably the first criterion that needs to be defined is the specific subject of the control, i.e., what is actually to be regulated. Next,
criteria for the kind of regulating system involved in reaching the particular aim of cerebral blood flow control should be specified. Two types
of physiological controls may be identified. In the first group we single
out the control aimed at stabilization of certain parameters which must be
held constant despite changes in others. These parameters include the
cerebral blood pressure and flow, which need to be stabilized against
changes in the perfusion pressure (chiefly the changes of systemic arterial
pressure), and the cerebral blood volume against changes in the blood inflow to the brain and outflow from the cranial case. In the second group, the
parameter to be primarily controlled is the rate of blood flow, which must

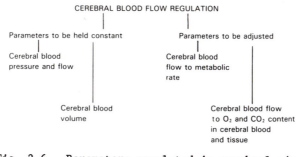

Fig. 2.6.   Parameters regulated in cerebral cir-
            culation.

be coupled with the metabolic rate (the latter being, in turn, related to
the level of activity) of cerebral tissue. Furthermore, the cerebral blood
flow must be adjusted to the oxygen and carbon dioxide content in the cerebral blood and tissue (Fig. 2.6).

     In addition to the specific aims and character of cerebral blood flow
control, there are several criteria which are related to the physiological
mechanisms of the control system: (a) The source of information which
turns on the control mechanism. The information conveys the specific disturbances that are to be eliminated (for instance, increased blood pressure
in the cerebral arteries, excessive accumulation of blood in cerebral veins
resulting in distension of their walls, deficient blood supply to cerebral
tissue where the actual blood flow does not meet the metabolic needs, etc.).
(b) The specific control loop, including localization of coordinating centers, where the information is processed, the whole regulatory system is
controlled and, in particular, the controlling signals that specifically
alter cerebral blood flow are initiated. The centers can be localized in
several parts of the brain (e.g., in the brain stem and hypothalamus) or
can be diffusely arranged in particular areas of the brain where local
blood flow is regulated. The type of regulatory signals to the blood vessels may vary (e.g., diffusion of specific metabolic substances or efferent vasomotor nerve outflow by specific pathways).   (c) The specific vascular effectors that determine circulatory phenomena in the brain during
cerebral blood flow control. These effectors are primarily the arteries
of specific localization (e.g., the major arteries, the pial arterial ramifications, and the intracerebral arteries and arterioles).

     The criteria for identification of the types of cerebral blood flow
control are schematically shown in Fig. 2.7.

     Advances in physiological knowledge of cerebral blood flow have gradu-
ally elucidated the specific types of its control. The different types of
cerebral blood flow control have long been known. Clarification of their
identities, however, occurred only recently, when thorough analysis of the
physiological processes of cerebral blood flow control became particularly
essential. The classification of the types of cerebral blood flow control
presented below may seem at first to be somewhat artificial, since the
specific types are closely related and their control loops may operate
simultaneously under natural conditions. Nevertheless, the classification
is very important for a better understanding of the complex control mechanisms. Four types of cerebral blood flow control were first definitively
identified at the Fourth Tbilisi Symposium on Cerebral Circulation in 1978

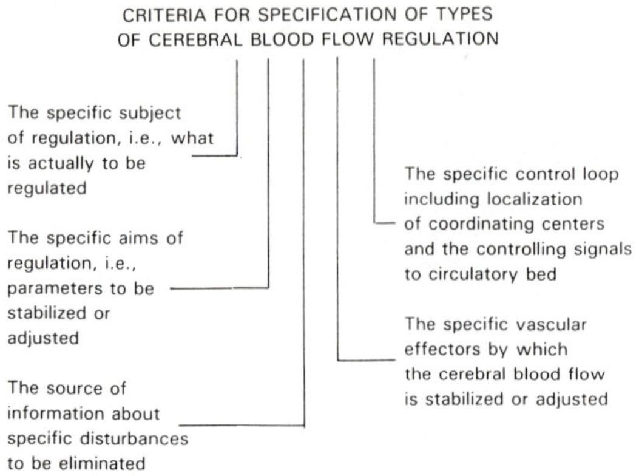

CRITERIA FOR SPECIFICATION OF TYPES
OF CEREBRAL BLOOD FLOW REGULATION

The specific subject
of regulation, i.e., what
is actually to be
regulated

The specific aims of
regulation, i.e.,
parameters to be
stabilized or
adjusted

The source of
information about
specific disturbances
to be eliminated

The specific control loop
including localization
of coordinating centers
and the controlling signals
to circulatory bed

The specific vascular
effectors by which
the cerebral blood flow
is stabilized or adjusted

Fig. 2.7. Criteria by which the particular types of cerebral
blood flow regulation can be identified. Some of
the criteria (e.g., the subjects and the aims of
regulation) are specific for each particular type,
while the others (e.g., the sources of information,
the control loops, and the vascular effectors) can
participate in several types of regulation. See
text for details.

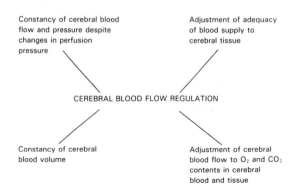

Constancy of cerebral blood
flow and pressure despite
changes in perfusion
pressure

Adjustment of adequacy
of blood supply to
cerebral tissue

CEREBRAL BLOOD FLOW REGULATION

Constancy of cerebral
blood volume

Adjustment of cerebral
blood flow to O_2 and CO_2
contents in cerebral
blood and tissue

Fig. 2.8. Schematic drawing of the four types of cerebral
blood flow regulation, which have been identified
at the Fourth Tbilisi Symposium on Cerebral Circulation (Mchedlishvili et al., 1979) according
to the criteria presented schematically in Fig.
2.7. See text for details.

(Mchedlishvili, Purves, et al., 1979; Mchedlishvili, 1980b). They are presented schematically in Fig. 2.8 and are described below:

1. An adequate blood supply to cerebral tissue is needed to ensure
that the cerebral blood flow rate meets the metabolic needs of the tissue.
This type of cerebral blood flow control was identified at the end of the
19th century (Roy and Sherrington, 1890), despite the prevailing Monro-
Kellie doctrine of that period (see p. 17). This control means that the
rate of cerebral microcirculation is coupled to the rate of metabolism of

the surrounding tissue. When the adequacy of blood supply is disturbed (because of primary changes either in cerebral blood flow or in metabolism) the specific responses of the cerebral blood vessels lead to recovery of sufficient microcirculation. For instance, if the blood flow becomes insufficient either because of an increase in neuronal activity and a corresponding rise in the tissue metabolic rate, or because of occlusion of a feeding arterial branch, the appropriate cerebral blood vessels undergo dilatation, resulting in a decrease in vascular resistance, and hence a restorative increase in blood flow.

2. The adjustment of cerebral blood flow to the oxygen and carbon dioxide content in the cerebral blood and tissue is directed toward maintenance of blood gas tensions at necessary levels. This type of cerebral blood flow control was actually identified as far back as the 19th century, when a distinctive cerebral vasodilatation was observed during asphyxia (Donders, 1851). Others studied this thoroughly in the 1930s (Lennox and Gibbs, 1932). It became obvious from many studies that hypoxemia, and hence oxygen deficiency in the brain, as well as hypercapnia, immediately cause cerebral vasodilatation and an increase in cerebral blood flow. On the other hand, hyperoxia and hypocapnia result in cerebral vasoconstriction with an ensuing decrease in cerebral blood flow rate. Constant levels of oxygen and carbon dioxide are thus restored in brain tissue.

3. Constant cerebral blood pressure and flow are maintained despite changes in perfusion pressure; this occurs by a form of control which was identified in the 1930s when cerebral arterial constriction was observed during rises in systemic arterial pressure, and vice versa (Fog, 1937, 1939). In the early 1950s it was proved that cerebral blood flow can remain constant, and therefore partly independent, of the systemic arterial pressure changes (Carlyle and Grayson, 1956). According to Poiseuille's law, CBF = CPP/CVR, where CBF is the cerebral blood flow, CPP is the cerebral perfusion pressure, and CVR is the cerebrovascular resistance. Thus, cerebral blood flow may be maintained at constant levels when cerebrovascular resistance is actively changed in an opposite direction to changing pressures, i.e., if it becomes increased (due to cerebral vasoconstriction) during rises in systemic arterial pressure, or decreased (due to cerebral vasodilatation) during drops in systemic arterial pressure.

4. Constancy of cerebral blood volume is an important condition for homeostasis of the brain in the rigid skull. This volumetric type of cerebral blood flow regulation was identified at the end of the 1950s (Mchedlishvili, 1959a). Blood volume increases in the cerebral vasculature either because of an enhanced blood inflow from the central arterial system due to cerebral vasodilatation, or as a result of reduced outflow of blood from the brain into the central veins. Excessive accumulation of blood occurs mainly in the cerebral venous bed, partly in the brain capillaries and possibly in smaller arteries. The only way to decrease excessive cerebral blood volume by the circulatory system is through restriction of blood inflow into the cerebral vessels by constriction of larger cerebral arteries. Thus, a new balance between amounts of inflowing and outflowing blood is established, leading to normalization of cerebral blood volume.

Circulatory disturbances, as well as the physiological mechanisms operating for their elimination, are closely related to each other under normal conditions. In an organism a single disturbance may appear (a necessary condition for physiological experiments that analyze the events involved in cerebral blood flow control), or, more often, probably disturbances appear in various combinations with each other. For instance, a

significant rise in the systemic arterial pressure causing an increase of
cerebral perfusion pressure should cause an increased blood inflow to the
brain; this results in excessive cerebral blood flow, pressure, and volume,
as well as in inadequate blood and oxygen supply to brain tissue. Therefore, all these disturbances come to be eliminated by cerebral vasoconstriction. However, the nature of these disturbances is different, and
therefore there are specific differences in the mechanisms of their elimination by physiological means. The mechanisms are affected by afferent information about the disturbances, efferent effects controlling the cerebral
blood vessels and, in some instances, also by specific vascular effectors
(e.g., the larger and smaller arteries) involved in respective hemodynamic
changes occurring in the cerebral vasculature. These physiological events
will be discussed in detail both in the present and subsequent chapters.

Under normal conditions different types of cerebral blood flow control
mechanisms operate not in isolation but in various combinations. There is
evidence not only for synergism, but for antagonism, of these mechanisms,
which may decrease the efficiency of the control of the blood supply to the
brain.

An example of *synergism* between two types of control is the maintenance of a constant cerebral blood flow and pressure despite changes in systemic arterial pressure, while control of an adequate blood supply to cerebral tissue is also maintained. If changes in the perfusion pressure become too great, control by the major arteries might become insufficient to
maintain a constant cerebral blood flow and pressure, and disturbances in
adequate blood supply to the brain tissue would inevitably appear. In
this situation the small arteries respond by performing a second stage of
the cerebral blood flow control, which tends to maintain an adequate blood
supply to cerebral tissue (Mchedlishvili, Mitagvaria, et al., 1973). For
details see Chapters 3 and 4.

An *antagonistic* relationship of cerebral blood flow control can occur
during a postischemic state, asphyxia, or a considerable increase in neuronal activity throughout the cerebral hemispheres. In this case, two
types of control mechanisms having opposing effects start to operate simultaneously. The rise in the metabolic demand causes dilatation of the
small arteries, which results in an increase in blood supply to the brain
and in cerebral blood volume. Then the excessive cerebral blood volume
must be reduced by another control mechanism, i.e., by constriction of the
major arteries of the brain (Mchedlishvili, 1960b, 1960c, 1960d). These
oppositely directed vascular responses, i.e., constriction of the major and
dilatation of the minor arteries, seem to be an inherent mechanism for cop-
ing with the aforementioned disturbances (see Chapters 3 and 4 for details).
Under these conditions, the overall cerebrovascular resistance, and hence
the cerebral blood flow, is equal to the algebraic sum of the mentioned
segmental resistances. The total resistance can in this case either be increased, resulting in reduction of cerebral blood flow, or, on the contrary,
it can be decreased, causing an increased cerebral blood flow.

2.4.   INFORMATION ABOUT DISTURBANCES TRIGGERING MECHANISMS
OF CEREBRAL BLOOD FLOW CONTROL

Physiological mechanisms of cerebral blood flow control are triggered
by information about disturbances appearing in the cerebral circulation
(Fig. 2.3). The four main types of disturbances have been described
in the previous section concerning the types of cerebral blood flow control: (a) alterations in perfusion pressure causing changes in cerebral

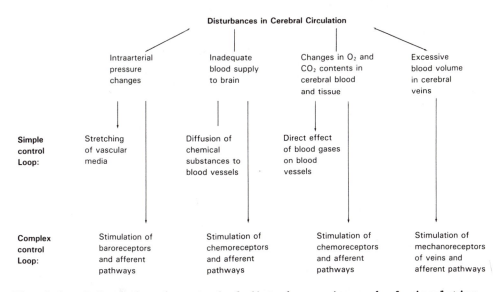

Fig. 2.9. Information about typical disturbances in cerebral circulation
           can be transmitted through simple control loops or through com-
           plex control loops. See text for details.

blood pressure and random alterations of blood flow rate in the brain; (b)
excessive increase in the cerebral blood volume causing distension of the
walls of cerebral veins and possibly other vessels; (c) excessive increases or decreases in oxygen and/or carbon dioxide levels in cerebral
arterial blood and/or cerebral tissue causing metabolic disturbances; and
(d) an inadequate blood supply, which does not meet the metabolic needs of cerebral tissue and also results in disturbances in tissue metabolism. Information about all these disturbances should activate the control mechanisms of the cerebral blood flow.

     According to present-day physiological knowledge, the peripheral cir-
culatory system of mammals possesses the following three devices to provide
information to the control system about disturbances in cerebral circulation and/or related processes: (1) different degrees of stretch of vascular smooth muscles; (2) diffusion of vasoactive substances in tissue from
the place of their origin to the site of their effect; and, (3) afferent
neural impulses from specific receptors and afferent pathways. The information could enter either of two paths (see p. 21 and Fig. 2.4): a
simple control loop, i.e., representing direct effects on the vessel wall
(its stretch or the effect of the vasoactive substances that diffuse
through the vessel wall), or a complex control loop with a specific center of
regulation involving afferent neural pathways (Fig. 2.9).

     If we now consider every type of cerebral blood flow control, we can
mention all the possible forms of information about the specific disturbances in the cerebral circulation and in the related processes.

     Alterations in systemic arterial pressure cause changes in the trans-
mural pressure of cerebral arteries, thus supplying the brain with blood.
This also occurs at the periphery of arterial occlusions. These pressure
changes cause deviations in the stretch of arterial walls from the inside
and may result in a direct reaction on vascular smooth muscle known as the
Baylyss effect: increases in stretch result in contraction and increases

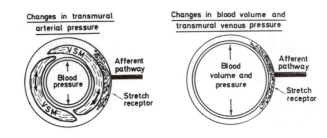

Fig. 2.10.   Information about changes in the intraarterial pressure (left)
              can initiate regulation by stretch of the vessel walls, as well
              as activation of baroreceptors in the vessel walls. Informa-
              tion about changes in intravascular volume and pressure in
              cerebral veins (right) can be transmitted only by activation
              of specific neural pathways, since these vessels contain a
              sparse muscle layer in their walls.

in the tone of smooth muscle cells, and vice versa. In addition, information about changes in intravascular pressure may be transmitted by specific
baroreceptors located in the arterial walls to appropriate afferent pathways. It is well known that the carotid sinus, which monitors arterial
blood carried to the brain, contains an accumulation of mechanoreceptors
(baroreceptors, or pressoreceptors) that specifically react to stretch of
the arterial walls. Numerous receptors, including baroreceptors, have
also been found along the larger and smaller cerebral arteries (Kuprianov
and Zhitsa, 1975); their functions have not been sufficiently elucidated.
All baroreceptors in cerebral arterial walls can inform the regulatory system about changes in transmural pressure once the systemic arterial pressure has been altered. Possible modes of information about changes in intravascular pressure are shown schematically in Fig. 2.10 (left).

Changes in cerebral blood volume occur primarily in the cerebral
veins, partly in capillaries, and little, if any, in smaller arteries. Information about the degree of stretch of the walls of these blood vessels
triggers responses in the major cerebral arteries (see Chapter 3), which
are located far from the blood vessels where the information has originated. Therefore neither stretch of vessel walls with increased blood volume nor diffusion of vasoactive substances can be involved in transmission of information about the changes. The information is, in all probability, conducted by neural pathways from numerous receptors that have been
identified in the walls of cerebral veins and minor cerebral arteries (Kuprianov and Zhitsa, 1975), although their physiological role has not yet
been investigated in detail. The source of the afferent information during
disturbances in cerebral blood volume is shown schematically in Fig. 2.10
(right).

Information about changes in oxygen and carbon dioxide levels in cerebral arterial blood and cerebral tissue can originate from several sources.
Changes in O_2 and CO_2 levels can directly cause specific responses in vascular walls. Changes in the metabolism of cerebral tissue may also occur,
resulting in the production of diffusible vasoactive substances, which
cause specific responses of the arterial walls. Finally, changes in the
oxygen and carbon dioxide content in blood or tissue can affect specific
chemoreceptors. Such receptors were found long ago in the carotid sinuses.
A similar kind of chemoreceptor may be present along cerebral vessel walls.
Many receptors were morphologically identified in cerebral vessels, but

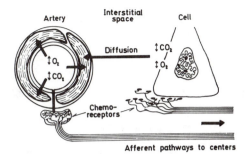

Fig. 2.11.   Hypothetical routes of information about
             changes in oxygen and carbon dioxide con-
             tent in cerebral blood and tissue. The
             information can be transferred in two
             ways: by direct effects on vascular
             smooth muscle from blood and tissue, and
             by activation of the chemoreceptors in
             the vessel walls and tissue that respond
             to changes in oxygen and carbon dioxide
             levels.

their physiological function has not yet been sufficiently studied. It is
quite probable that they play a chemoreceptive role by detecting oxygen and
carbon dioxide tension changes and by transmitting information about disturbances in the chemical composition in cerebral arterial blood and/or in
brain tissue. The information from these receptors is conveyed via corresponding afferent pathways and initiates regulation of cerebral blood flow.
Different routes of information about oxygen and carbon dioxide levels in
arterial blood and cerebral tissue are presented schematically in Fig. 2.11.

Primary alterations in blood supply to the brain result in specific
disturbances in cerebral tissue metabolism. Information about these disturbances may spread in two main ways. First, the metabolic changes may
result in an accumulation in the interstitial space of vasoactive metabolites, e.g., H^+, K^+, adenosine, etc., which can diffuse through the walls
of adjacent arteries and cause responses that help re-establish an adequate
blood supply to the tissue. The second way of transmitting information
may be neurogenic: metabolic changes in cerebral tissue affect sensitive
neural structures, i.e., specific chemoreceptors or other similar structures. Information from these receptors may spread by afferent pathways
to the site of regulatory areas that trigger specific vascular responses
which, in turn, lead to the restoration of an adequate blood supply to
cerebral tissue.

Information about the disturbances in cerebral circulation and related processes should provide both qualitative and quantitative data to
the organism about the disturbances. Thus, changes in cerebral blood
flow will tend to accurately eliminate disturbances which trigger the control responses of cerebral blood vessels and flow.

2.5.   COORDINATION SYSTEMS OF CEREBRAL BLOOD FLOW CONTROL

We know that every physiological function is closely related to, and
balanced with, many others in the body. The same is true for local blood

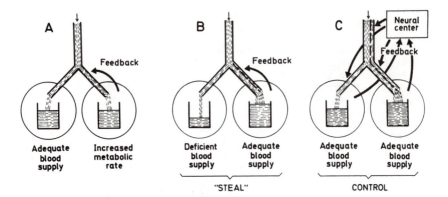

Fig. 2.12.   Schematic diagram of the coordination of cerebral blood flow
              control. An increased metabolic rate in tissue triggers a
              physiological feedback to the feeding artery directed toward
              increasing the blood supply to tissue (A). The subsequent
              vasodilatation results in an adequate blood supply to the re-
              gion, but inevitably causes a deficient blood supply to adja-
              cent regions, called the "steal phenomenon" (B). However, if
              the vascular responses are coordinated by a neural center,
              then feedback to the respective arteries should provide ade-
              quate blood supply to all areas of the organ (C).

flow in any single area of the central nervous system. Therefore, when
blood flow is actively changed by regulation in a given tissue region, this
could cause circulatory disturbances in adjacent tissue areas. An example
of this is the so-called "steal phenomenon" (Symon, 1969) which occurs when
the vascular activity is increased in a brain region. This area receives
an increased blood flow, but can cause a deficient blood supply in an adjacent region, or regions. To prevent a "steal," the process of blood flow
control spreads to "higher levels" of the feeding vessels, i.e., to the
larger arteries, which should provide a sufficient amount of blood to both
regions (Fig. 2.12). Therefore, the regulatory system performs properly
only when the control of adjacent vascular regions is coordinated and
hence the appearance of new disturbances is prevented.

     It seems, however, that not all control systems of cerebral blood
flow could provide such coordination. Indeed, how could the direct myogenic responses in cerebral arteries to stretch or to vasoactive metabolites from brain tissue provide for the coordination of the local vascular
responses with those of the adjacent vascular areas? Proceeding from our
present-day physiological knowledge it seems obvious that it is primarily
the neurogenic control loop that coordinates cerebral blood flow control
in adjacent areas. Therefore we may conclude that only neural mechanisms
properly control cerebral blood flow (in the sense of eliminating the
primary disturbances) and prevent simultaneous occurrence of new circulatory disturbances in adjacent regions.

     Information about disturbances in cerebral blood flow should reach
specific neural centers, i.e., neuron association areas which are able not
only to regulate regional cerebral blood flow, but also to coordinate
changes in adjacent vascular regions. Functions of these centers generally include: (a) receiving information about both primary disturbances and
related functions, and (b) processing the information and initiating con-

trolling signals that cause specific vascular responses leading to elimination of the disturbances. These events are coordinated in related brain
areas.

     Since there are different types of cerebral blood flow control that
are triggered by specific disturbances and eliminated by distinct means,
it is hard to imagine that all types of control could originate in the same
neural center. It seems probable that there are at least two types of centers regulating cerebral blood flow. There may be one common center, or
centers, for those types of cerebral blood flow control that regulate the
blood supply to the whole brain via the major arteries. This center may be
active, for instance, when cerebral blood flow and pressure remain constant
despite changes in the systemic arterial pressure or when cerebral blood
volume is regulated. Activation may also occur during regulation of the
oxygen and carbon dioxide levels in cerebral arterial blood.

     Another type of control center may regulate changes in regional cere-
bral blood flow triggered by changes in the metabolic demands of brain
tissue. It seems improbable that a common center could couple regional
blood flow regulation with regulation of local metabolism or with oxygen
and carbon dioxide level changes. Regulation of the latter occurs at the
smallest branches of pial or intracerebral arteries (see Chapter 4). This
form of control should be performed by neurons located somewhere nearby,
or even inside, the area where the regulation of blood flow is being carried out. Spreading of the area involved in the circulatory changes would
then involve other groups of neurons in the control. Only when circulatory
changes become widespread in the brain may some general center become involved in the events of cerebral blood flow control.

     Consequently, the function of the neural centers of cerebral blood
flow control is, on the one hand, to eliminate specific disturbances that
trigger the cerebral blood flow control mechanism and, on the other hand,
to regulate processes in adjacent areas so their normal function is not
disturbed (Fig. 2.13). When the limits of the control system are restricted, the centers are, in all probability, responsible for "choosing the
lesser of two evils" — providing maximum control and minimizing resultant
disturbances.

2.6. VASOMOTOR MECHANISMS CONTROLLING CEREBRAL BLOOD FLOW

     Vasomotor regulation of vascular effectors is an important link in
the control loop of cerebral blood flow regulation (see Fig. 2.3). The
types of regulatory signals causing specific responses in the cerebral
blood vessels involved in this control may vary (see Fig. 2.14): (a) signals, which arise inside the vascular walls, particularly in smooth muscle
cells, in response to the degree of stretch (myogenic effects), and (b) efferent signals that spread by vasoactive substances that diffuse to vascular smooth muscle and cause specific arterial responses (humoral effects).
The latter signals require the availability of specific vasoactive substances that either circulate in the blood or originate inside the vascular walls or near specific brain vessels. (c) The efferent signals can
also be vasomotor nerve impulses that reach blood vessel walls from efferent nerves and affect vascular smooth muscle by means of specific neurotransmitters (neurogenic effects). These efferent neurogenic effects are
transmitted by vasomotor nerve fibers originating in neurons pertaining to
cerebral blood flow regulation; the fibers terminate on the specific blood
vessels to be regulated and cause specific reactivity of their smooth

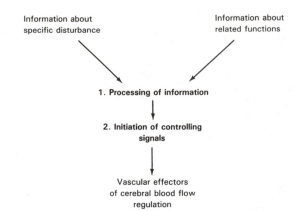

Fig. 2.13. Two types of functions performed by centers
            regulating cerebral blood flow. Informa-
            tion on physiological events to be regulat-
            ed affect the vascular effectors involved
            in the regulation. See text for details.

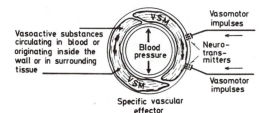

Fig. 2.14. Presently assumed types of vasomotor con-
            trol of cerebral arteries involved in regu-
            lation of cerebral circulation. See text
            for details.

muscles. In the normal organism, all these regulatory effects on vascular
smooth muscle can operate simultaneously or in various combinations. However, from a physiological standpoint the specific role of each particular
type of signal in cerebral blood flow control must be analyzed.

From what we presently know about vascular physiology, we can assume
that the vasomotor mechanisms controlling cerebral blood vessels may be
either similar or different in various types of cerebral blood flow control. To maintain constancy of cerebral blood flow despite changes in
systemic arterial pressure, two kinds of vasomotor mechanisms may occur:
(1) direct responses of vascular smooth muscles to various degrees of
stretch, and (2) neurogenic vasomotor signals.

The regulatory mechanisms of blood volume, triggered in response to
excessive blood accumulation in cerebral veins, cause constriction of brain
arteries and restriction of blood inflow into the cerebral vasculature.
Neurogenic signals are assumed to be involved in this regulation. Direct
myogenic responses of arteries probably do not occur since blood accumulation and increase in transmural pressure take place chiefly in the veins,
while direct vascular responses actually appear in quite different blood

vessels, namely in the larger arteries. The involvement of a purely humoral affect on the cerebral arteries in this type of cerebral blood flow
control should also be excluded, because it would be hard to imagine some
specific vasoconstrictor substance which could be accumulated in the vicinity of arterial walls under these specific conditions. Therefore, only
neurogenic effects on the arterial walls are thought to occur during this
type of cerebral blood flow control.

When oxygen and carbon dioxide levels in cerebral arterial blood and
brain tissue change, direct myogenic responses to stretch are probably not
involved, because primary stretching changes of arterial walls do not occur. Thus,
two kinds of efferent signals on the cerebral arteries may be transmitted
during this type of cerebral blood flow control. First, the humoral mechanism may operate, i.e., the direct effect of oxygen and/or carbon dioxide
on vascular smooth muscle from inside arteries when levels of arterial
blood gases undergo primary changes. Another humoral mechanism cannot be
excluded in this example: primary changes in oxygen and/or carbon dioxide
levels in tissue and secondary effects of other vasoactive substances
originating from tissue elements (e.g., hydrogen ions) may influence cerebral arterial activity from the outside (see Chapter 4). Secondly, the
neurogenic mechanism also cannot be excluded from this type of cerebral
blood flow control. Specific receptors sensitive to oxygen and carbon dioxide changes in blood, located either in the carotid sinus region, somewhere close to cerebral arterial walls, in brain tissue, or the meninges,
can trigger efferent vasomotor impulses spread by vasomotor nerves to
specific cerebral blood vessels pertaining to this type of cerebral blood
flow control.

An adequate blood supply to cerebral tissue can also be provided by
two kinds of efferent signals to respective cerebral arteries. Humoral
effects on arterial walls occur by signals of those vasoactive substances
(e.g., hydrogen and potassium ions, adenosine, etc.), which originate in
the tissue as soon as its blood supply becomes inadequate. Such substances
might diffuse to appropriate arterial walls and cause their vasomotor responses, thus correcting the blood flow rate and changing it to a level
adequately coupled with the metabolic needs of the tissue. However, it
must be taken into consideration that not all vasoactive substances can
readily reach the proper blood vessels by diffusion. The pial arteries on
the brain surface are easy to investigate but are comparatively far from
the source of substances that originate in the deeper layers of cerebral
cortex. As for intracerebral arteries and arterioles, they are in an immediate position to possible sources of vasoactive metabolic substances
but are almost inaccessible for direct investigation. On the other hand,
there may also be neurogenic effects on vascular walls. Efferent regulatory signals, originating in specific neurons related to this type of cerebral blood flow control, can travel to arteries that regulate cerebral
circulation by appropriate efferent neural pathways.

The different efferent signals mentioned above can reach the vascular
walls both at different times and simultaneously. It is difficult, however, to properly analyze the vasomotor mechanisms which operate to some
extent, or do not participate at all, in cerebral blood flow control under
natural conditions.

The neurogenic mechanism was rejected by the majority of leading
authorities in the field, as a mechanism of cerebral blood flow control,
until 1960 (Kety, 1960). The main reason was that the dissection or stimulation of respective vascular nerves did not give rise to pronounced
cerebral effects compared to those observed in other vascular regions of

the body. Proceeding from consideration of data published in that period, this author came to the conclusion (Mchedlishvili, 1972, p. 99): "If neural effects were always as weak as this, regulation of cerebral circulation would be impossible. On the other hand, the absence of lucid results in these experimental investigations provided sufficient grounds for the conclusion that nervous control over the cerebral circulation is in fact absent or nearly so. However, it could also indicate that the methods used for detection were unsuitable for the purpose. For example, it could be claimed that artificial stimulation or transection of vascular nerves, techniques often used to investigate these problems, like the direct application of neurohumoral agents to the vessels (externally or internally), could disturb normal circulation in the brain. Quite logically it was suggested that under these conditions the mechanisms of regulation that have evolved in circulation in the brain are more refined than those in other parts of the body, and they quickly correct experimentally induced disturbances of normal circulation. For this reason, experimental results have so far been unclear or even negative." And indeed, from the late 1960s throughout the 1970s, researchers accumulated a large body of evidence that neurogenic effects play an important role in the cerebral blood flow control. Nevertheless, many problems remain unsolved, namely the identification of neural receptors in cerebral blood vessels and brain tissue, the afferent and efferent neural pathways, the localization and function of the neural centers pertaining to the cerebral blood flow control, etc. These problems are in need of further thoughtful experimentation.

2.7. EFFECTORS OF CEREBRAL BLOOD FLOW REGULATION

In the majority of studies related to cerebral blood flow control (where the cerebrovascular resistance was considered as its major determinant), the specific effectors in the cerebral arterial system have neither been investigated nor properly considered. Since only the cerebral blood flow was usually recorded, the results could not possibly show how different brain vessels participate in both the control and the disturbances of cerebral circulation. Therefore it was customarily assumed that either regulation of cerebral blood flow is affected by the "cerebral vessels" (without specifying which vessels) or, alternatively, the leading role was ascribed to the "arterioles." Although originally the term "arterioles" had the concrete meaning of the smallest precapillary arteries, the walls of which contain a single layer of smooth muscle cells, later on it was applied to all small arteries (even up to 300-500 µm in caliber) capable of changing their lumen within wide ranges. In all probability the concept of the leading regulatory role played by the arterioles was originally based on Poiseuille's law, according to which the resistance was assumed to be highest in the smallest blood vessels, i.e., the arterioles. Actually, however, the control of regional blood flow primarily implies an ability of the blood vessels to *change* the flow appropriately. Thus, it is the regional segments of arteries which should be considered as the important vessels in the control of cerebral blood flow; they actually affect the *changes* in cerebrovascular resistance under natural conditions.

The specific effectors of regulation of cerebral blood flow can be identified under conditions when the functional behavior of various parts of the cerebral arterial system is investigated during different types of regulation. To this end, it was essential that the research methods used should yield not indirect data but concrete and quantitative information concerning the functional behavior of specific parts of the cerebral arterial system. As a result of investigations carried out starting in the early 1960s, different patterns of functional behavior (with respect to control of cerebral blood flow) have been found in at least three different parts of the arterial system of the brain: (a) the major arteries, including the internal carotid and vertebrals, as well as the adjacent larger arteries at the base of the brain; (b) the pial arteries whose branches and anastomoses are distributed over the cerebral hemispheres; and (c) the smallest intra-cerebral (parenchymal) arteries and arterioles, which are converted to capillaries. These parts of the cerebral arterial system differ in their anatomical location, the structural peculiarities and innervation of their walls, and, finally, distinctive physiological properties. It has been shown that these parts of the arterial system of the brain may behave differently with respect to the characteristic direction of their responses (constriction or dilatation) during every type of control of cerebral blood flow. Under specific conditions the responses of the above-mentioned arterial segments can be either in concert or else relatively independent.

The role of the major arteries of the brain in regulating cerebral circulation, as well as in the development of vasospasm, has been demonstrated in the majority of vertebrates, including man. This function is apparently also present in animals in which the internal carotid arteries have become obliterated and the carotid system supplies blood to the circle of Willis via branches of the external carotid artery and the *rete mirabile* located inside bone (e.g., in cats) (Mchedlishvili, 1964, 1972).

Although the muscle layer in the walls of pial arteries is comparatively thin (Lazorthes, 1961), it can actively change their lumen within wide ranges. The responses of pial arteries have been observed in numerous studies, probably since these arteries are the most easily approachable part of the cerebral vascular bed (Forbes et al., 1937; Forbes and Cobb, 1938; Fog, 1937, 1939; Klosovsky, 1951; Mchedlishvili, 1968, 1972; Kuschinsky and Wahl, 1978; MacKenzie et al., 1979; Wei et al., 1980; Auer, 1981). Unlike the pial arteries, the functional behavior of parenchymal arteries and arterioles located inside the brain substance, between pial arteries and cerebral capillaries, remained the least investigated part of the cerebral arterial bed. Only a few experimental studies concerned with the functional behavior of these arteries have been published in the world's scientific literature. Results have been obtained with morphometrical investigation of the arteries following brain tissue *in situ* fixation under specific experimental conditions (Mchedlishvili, Baramidze, et al., 1967, 1974-1975; Sadoshima et al., 1980). These results are still scarce and do not provide conclusive data on the characteristic functional behavior of intracerebral arteries under specific conditions.

The blood supply to cerebral tissue is regulated by small pial arteries while the larger pial arteries, and especially the major arteries of the brain, do not participate in this control. This appears to be logical from an anatomical viewpoint: deficiencies, as well as excesses, of blood supply are generally local, especially under physiological conditions and, therefore, should be primarily regulated by local means. The functional behavior of the pial arterial effectors pertaining to this type of cerebral blood flow control will be considered in more detail in Chapter 4.

The best way to clarify the role of the effectors of cerebral blood flow control is to investigate their behavior during specific types of control of cerebral circulation. In so doing the specific purpose of the type of control studied should be taken into consideration, and proceeding from the available results it must be decided if the reaction of the arteries studied fulfills this purpose.

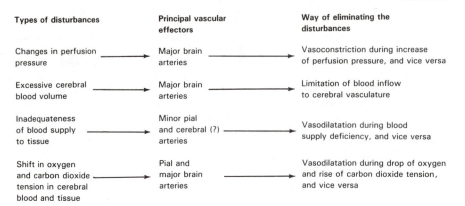

Types of disturbances	Principal vascular effectors	Way of eliminating the disturbances
Changes in perfusion pressure ⟶	Major brain arteries ⟶	Vasoconstriction during increase of perfusion pressure, and vice versa
Excessive cerebral blood volume ⟶	Major brain arteries ⟶	Limitation of blood inflow to cerebral vasculature
Inadequateness of blood supply to tissue ⟶	Minor pial and cerebral (?) arteries ⟶	Vasodilatation during blood supply deficiency, and vice versa
Shift in oxygen and carbon dioxide tension in cerebral blood and tissue ⟶	Pial and major brain arteries ⟶	Vasodilatation during drop of oxygen and rise of carbon dioxide tension, and vice versa

Fig. 2.15. Presently known functional behavior of vascular effectors regulating cerebral blood flow. See text for details.

The systematic investigation of the functional behavior of different parts of the cerebral arterial bed under experimental conditions carried out in the last two decades led the present author to the following conclusion about the nature of the specific vascular effectors (Mchedlishvili, 1972, 1980a). The major arteries of the brain have been shown to be responsible for the control of the constancy of blood supply to the brain despite changes in systemic arterial pressure; they also restrict excessive blood from filling the cerebral vascular system. However, the major arteries of the brain never dilate in response to a deficiency of blood supply to cerebral tissue and, hence, their functional behavior does not determine the maintenance of sufficient brain blood supply. This function has been proved to be performed by the minor cerebral arteries, especially the smaller pial arterial blood vessels which represent the specific effectors of regulation of the levels of tissue oxygen and carbon dioxide. Present data about the functional behavior of the vascular effectors regulating cerebral blood flow are summarized in Fig. 2.15.

The two previously mentioned concepts regarding vascular effectors of cerebral blood flow control which originated from Poiseuille's law and from evidence published in the 1960s and 1970s are demonstrated schematically in Fig. 2.16.

2.8. EFFICIENCY REQUIREMENTS OF THE CEREBRAL BLOOD FLOW CONTROL SYSTEM

The physiological system regulating cerebral blood flow (Mchedlishvili, 1981b), similar to other body functions, had gradually developed in the course of evolution. The degree of efficiency of work in the system has been determined in the evolutionary process by the requirements of the function to be performed. In the case of cerebral blood flow, the requirements were particularly high, since the blood supply to the brain must be steadily regulated (i.e., stabilized and adjusted — see pp. 24-25) not only in the entire brain but also independently in small areas. In addition, brain tissue is extremely sensitive to any circulatory disturbance. This is considerably more pronounced for neurons than for any other cellular elements in the body. Therefore, the controlling system of blood flow in the brain has become even more efficient than that in any other organ. Accordingly, all types of cerebral blood flow control should be executed with maximum efficiency, although the requirements for such efficiency have not yet been sufficiently understood.

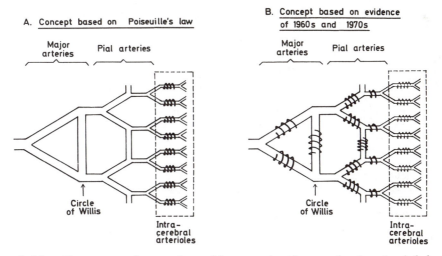

Fig. 2.16. The types of vascular effectors in the cerebral arterial bed
            thought to regulate cerebral blood flow, according to
            Poiseuille's law (A) and from the evidence accumulated in the
            1960s and 1970s (B).

    The efficiency needs for the system of cerebral blood flow control are
related to both the anatomical and physiological properties of the cerebrovascular bed. We are in a position to consider only those criteria which
are known by the present author (Mchedlishvili, 1980a). But other criteria
in need of further research may also exist.

    One requirement for efficiency of the system regulating cerebral blood
flow is *the optimal selection of the possible vascular effectors of control.*
An increase or decrease in cerebral blood flow can be achieved in different
ways, i.e., by a change in the perfusion pressure or in the resistance in
some specific part (or parts) of the cerebral arterial bed, such as the
major, pial, or intracerebral (parenchymal) arteries. It is now obvious
that control of cerebral blood flow is usually achieved in the most ratio-
nal way. For instance, during a local increase in the metabolic needs of
cerebral tissue in the cortex, an increase in its blood supply does not result from a rise in systemic arterial pressure, since this would entail an
increase of the perfusion pressure for the whole brain and for all other
organs of the body as well. Nor does it occur due to a decrease in resistance in the major brain arteries, as blood flow would become inadequate in
all other parts of the brain. Further, enhanced local blood flow in response to increased metabolic demands of the tissue does not result from
dilatation of the parenchymal arterioles either, as this would entail compression of the tissue adjacent to the blood vessel walls. What does occur in this case is dilatation of the respective small pial arteries,
which allow for an increase in blood flow only in those regions of the
cortex where the metabolic needs are increased (Mchedlishvili, 1972, 1980a).

    Another example of this efficiency requirement is the maintenance of a
constant blood flow and pressure in the cerebral vasculature despite
changes in systemic arterial pressure. This control is achieved primarily
by changes in resistance in the major, i.e., internal carotid, vertebral
and larger pial arteries (Mchedlishvili, 1980a). Use of the small pial
arteries as effectors of the regulation would interfere with the simultaneous control of the adequate blood supply to cerebral microvascular
beds.

     Another efficiency requirement of the cerebral blood flow control sys-
tem is *the maximum economical use of the vascular bed for regulation.* This
is related both to the anatomy and function of the cerebral vascular system. The anatomy of the arterial branches provides for a minimum energy
cost during blood flow in the larger pial arteries that is thought to be
related to the size of angles and radii in branching arteries that provide
minimum resistance (according to Rosen, 1967). Investigation of the geometry of pial arterial branches in rabbits has shown that branch angles and
radii with a diameter greater than 100 μm provide minimum resistance
(Mamisashvili et al., 1977). In the smaller pial arteries (less than 100
μm) in rabbits, the actual relation of angles and diameters in branches
probably causes considerable resistance under normal conditions. However,
when vasodilatation occurs during deficiency of blood supply to the cerebral cortex (during significant arterial hypotension, functional and postischemic hyperemias), this results in changes that minimize resistance to
blood transport through vessels (see Chapter 4, pp.124-129) and hence allows the maximum blood flow through the microvascular bed (Mamisashvili et
al., 1977).

     The third requirement for efficiency is *the maximum speed of opera-
tion of the control system* of cerebral blood flow. This feature is related
to the anatomy of the system. The richness of anastomoses between cerebral
arteries provides for a fast redistribution of blood among the individual
parts of the vascular bed. A sufficiently large amount of anastomoses connect the major arteries in the circle of Willis; the large branches of the
pial arteries (the branches of the anterior, middle, and posterior cerebral
arteries) are also interconnected on the cerebral surface (see Chapter 1,
pp. 9-10); finally, arterial microanastomoses in the terminal network of the
minor pial arteries are abundant. The small arterial circles thus formed
in this region, along with the specific behavior of these vessels (see
Chapter 4, pp. 129-135), provide for a fast redistribution of blood into
the microvascular regions of the cerebral tissue as soon as their metabolic
needs are increased, while the adjacent regions do not exhibit blood supply
deficiencies. The maximum speed of operation of the control system of
cerebral blood flow is also related to behavior unique to cerebral blood
vessels. The system permits a very rapid change in resistance and hence a
rapid redistribution of blood to various parts of the brain. The rapidity
of the system is provided for by the following presently known peculiarities of the cerebral vascular bed. There is considerable bending along
the course of major arteries of the brain (both in the internal carotids
and vertebrals) where turbulence readily appears in blood flow (Stehbens,
1961). This should result in a tangible change in resistance when luminal
changes occur even though they may be relatively insignificant (Mchedlishvili, 1968). In addition, active vascular regions have been discovered in
the branches of small pial arteries, i.e., the sphincters at offshoots of
smaller branches from larger trunks, as well as the precortical arteries
at the entry of pial terminal branches into the cerebral cortex. These microvascular effectors provide for a fast and effective redistribution of
blood among the smallest areas of cerebral cortex when the microcirculation is regulated (see Chapter 4, pp. 135-137).

     There is no doubt that in addition to these requirements for the ef-
ficiency of the control system of cerebral blood flow there are some others
related to the accuracy of functioning of the system, related to the optimal selection of the control loops of regulation, etc. But present knowledge of physiological events in the control system of cerebral blood flow
seems to be insufficient for consideration of these criteria, and further
investigations in this field are needed.

2.9. PHYSIOLOGICAL MECHANISMS OF CEREBRAL BLOOD FLOW CONTROL (FROM THE PRESENT-DAY POINT OF VIEW)

Proceeding from the foregoing information, there are several important objectives which must be met in order to elucidate the physiological mechanisms involved in every type of control of cerebral blood flow. The objectives were formulated for discussion purposes at the Fourth Tbilisi Symposium on Cerebral Circulation held in 1978 (Mchedlishvili, 1977b; Mchedlishvili, Purves, et al., 1979). These objectives (slightly changed for the present edition) are enumerated below in order to assist the reader with a better understanding of the content of Chapters 3 and 4 in this book. In this way the reader can more easily learn the extent to which the mechanisms of the particular types of cerebral blood flow control have been solved. The objectives are as follows:

The maintenance of constant cerebral blood flow and pressure despite changes in perfusion pressure (1.0).

1.1. To identify the regulation effectors, i.e., the cerebral arteries, which provide control of constant cerebral blood pressure and flow despite changes of systemic arterial pressure;

1.2. To identify the characteristics of smooth muscle responses to stretch in different parts of the cerebral arterial bed, taking into account their structure and actual functional state (constriction and dilatation);

1.3. To find out whether or not the pure myogenic responses, typical in smooth muscle cells in certain cerebral arteries, provide for the control of constant blood flow and pressure in the brain under conditions of changes in systemic arterial pressure;

1.4. To discover the anatomy and function of receptors, as well as afferent and efferent neural pathways, by which the physiological mechanism of neurogenic control operates;

1.5. To localize and determine the function of the central nervous structures ("centers"), which maintain the constancy of cerebral blood pressure and flow despite changes in cerebral perfusion pressure;

1.6. To ascertain the possible types of neurotransmitters responsible for appropriate arterial behavior during changes in systemic arterial pressure.

The maintenance of constancy of blood volume in cerebral vasculature (2.0).

2.1. To identify the effectors that are responsible for elimination of excessive blood volume in cerebral vasculature and restriction of brain volume during edema;

2.2. To discover the anatomy and function of neural receptors, as well as afferent and efferent pathways, by which the neurogenic mechanism of elimination of excessive cerebral blood volume operates;

2.3. To localize and determine the function of central nervous structures which maintain control of constant blood volume in cerebral vasculature;

2.4.   To ascertain the possible types of neurotransmitters involved in cerebral vascular behavior maintaining constant blood volume in brain vasculature.

The mechanism adjusting the cerebral blood flow to changes in oxygen and carbon dioxide tension in cerebral blood and tissue (3.0).

3.1.   To identify the effectors in the control of cerebral blood flow during changes in oxygen and carbon dioxide tension in cerebral blood and tissue;

3.2.   To ascertain the smooth muscle responses of appropriate cerebral blood vessels as effectors to the *direct action* of oxygen and carbon dioxide, or related substances, on the vascular walls acting from within or without;

3.3.   To determine the relationship (in quantity and in time) between oxygen and carbon dioxide tension and the responses of the specific vascular effectors of this type of cerebral blood flow control;

3.4.   To ascertain the anatomy and function of nervous receptors, and of afferent and efferent pathways that adjust cerebral blood flow to changes in oxygen and carbon dioxide tension in blood and tissue;

3.5.   To localize and determine the function of central nervous structures which provide for the adjustment of cerebral blood flow to changes in oxygen and carbon dioxide levels in cerebral blood and tissue;

3.6.   To ascertain the neurotransmitters responsible for the peripheral and central neurogenic processes controlling cerebral blood flow.

Control of adequate blood supply to cerebral tissue (coupling of blood flow and metabolic rate) (4.0).

4.1.   To identify the vascular effectors in the brain that provide for this type of control of regional cerebral blood flow;

4.2.   To investigate the direct responses to humoral factors of specific cerebral vessels that act as effectors of the regulation of adequate blood supply to cerebral tissue.   These may be the messengers for the coupling of tissue metabolism and regional blood flow;

4.3.   To identify the vasoactive humoral factors that might be responsible for the coupling of tissue metabolism and flow rate in respective regions of cerebral tissue;

4.4.   To ascertain the relationship (both in quantity and in time) between the action of humoral factors involved in the vasomotor effects and the responses of the specific arteries that are the effectors of this control of local blood flow;

4.5.   To investigate the anatomy and function of nervous receptors, as well as afferent and efferent pathways, providing for neurogenic control of regional cerebral blood flow;

4.6.   To localize and determine the function of the neuronal "centers" controlling adequate blood supply to smaller areas of cerebral tissue;

4.7. To ascertain the possible neurotransmitters taking part in the neurogenic mechanism providing for the coupling of regional cerebral blood flow and metabolic rate in appropriate areas of brain tissue.

2.10. SUMMARY

Using the deductive approach, the author considers all the possible links of the control system of cerebral blood flow. This will contribute to evaluation of the specific results of experimental studies of all types of cerebral blood flow control considered subsequently in Chapters 3 and 4 of this book. The deductive approach is an efficient mode of defining the main points and emphasizes the need for further research in the field of cerebral blood flow control.

Chapter 3. Cerebral Arterial Behavior Providing Constant
Cerebral Blood Flow, Pressure, and Volume

Cerebral blood flow, pressure, and volume are the three physiological parameters that must be maintained at a certain level to provide adequate blood supply to the brain. These parameters are to a great extent dependent on circulatory processes occurring outside the skull, i.e., in the central circulation (see Chapter 1). The control systems that maintain these circulatory parameters at physiological levels are triggered by disturbances related to changes in central arterial and venous pressures, on the one hand, and to disturbances of blood inflow or outflow from the brain on the other. These cerebral blood flow disturbances usually occur in the whole cerebral vascular system; this is also true for operation of the physiological mechanisms of their elimination.

As we mentioned in Chapter 2 (p. 34), the prevailing physiological theory for many years was that peripheral blood flow throughout the body is regulated exclusively by the smallest arterioles, where the resistance to flow is greatest under conditions of rest. The larger cerebral arteries, especially the internal carotid and vertebral arteries, were considered to be arteries of an elastic type, like the other largest arteries in the body, and thus were not believed to be involved in the regulation of peripheral blood flow. However, from the hemodynamic point of view, the determining factor of peripheral blood flow regulation is not the value of resting vascular resistance but the actual level of vessel resistance changes under regulatory conditions.

The analysis of functional behavior of the cerebral vascular bed by conventional physiological methods (e.g., stimulation of vascular nerves, application of vasoactive substances, etc., to estimate blood flow changes) cannot be assumed to be conclusive. These methods cannot evaluate the natural behavior of the various vessels involved in blood flow regulation. In order to ascertain the actual involvement of specific cerebral vessels in control of blood flow, as well as their normal functional behavior, another experimental approach appears to be more appropriate. This involves experiments under conditions in which the physiological mechanisms

controlling cerebral blood flow are functioning normally, i.e., maintaining
some circulatory parameters at constant level, adapting cerebral blood flow
to changes in the metabolic demands of brain tissue, or compensating for
disturbances in cerebral circulation. To this end, various circulatory
changes within the brain can be produced experimentally, and the behavior
of specific portions of the cerebrovascular system can be studied under
these conditions. Investigations under pathological conditions are highly
informative because they can provide a particularly wide range of experimental conditions under which mechanisms controlling cerebral blood flow
can be detected (Mchedlishvili, 1968, 1972). However, it must be stressed
that just the acute pathological changes are preferred in this case because an actual pathological process, complicating the proper analysis of
events, has not yet developed. When, however, the general behavior of specific cerebral vessels had been discovered in such investigations, conventional
physiological methods (i.e., stimulation and division of vascular nerves,
the direction of action of physiologically active substances on the vessels,
and so on) can be used in their analysis. This broad outline has been the
general plan followed in current investigations of the functional behavior
of particular parts of the cerebral arterial system.

3.1.   CONTROL OF CONSTANT CEREBRAL BLOOD PRESSURE AND FLOW

Blood perfusion pressure in the brain, as for any other organ of the
body, is the arterio-venous pressure differences. This is the difference
between the arterial pressure at the portals of the brain (i.e., the aorta
and carotid arteries) and the venous pressure close to the venous sinuses
of the skull (i.e., the jugular and the upper, or cranial caval veins).*
Under normal conditions both the central arterial and venous pressures are
actively kept constant by special control systems: the mean arterial pressure is equalized to approximately 100 mm Hg and the venous pressure is
close to zero. Thus, the blood perfusion pressure for the brain of young,
healthy humans and the majority of other mammals is about 100 mm Hg.

Since both the central arterial and venous pressures contribute to the
level of cerebral perfusion pressure, it is necessary to consider the influence of each of these pressures under varying conditions. The central
arterial pressure can rise and drop because of changes in either the cardiac output or the total peripheral resistance, but these variations are
usually minor both in size and duration under physiological conditions.
However, under the influence of pathological factors changes in arterial
pressure can be very significant: it can increase up to 300 mm Hg or drop
to zero (see Fig. 3.1). The central venous pressure constitutes a small
fraction of the arterial pressure, and its level is usually close to zero,
i.e., atmospheric pressure. Under physiological conditions central venous
pressure changes very slightly; it can only rise (but certainly not drop)
under pathological conditions, mostly due to cardiac insufficiency or exposure to high, cranially directed centrifugal force, up to about 20 mm Hg
(see Fig. 3.1). It follows from these considerations that the central, or
systemic, arterial pressure makes a much greater contribution to the cerebral perfusion pressure, i.e., to the arterio-venous pressure difference

---

*Sometimes the blood perfusion pressure of the brain is defined as the dif-
ference between the central arterial and the intracranial pressures. This
definition is in principle incorrect, although the cerebral perfusion
pressure may be estimated as the difference between the systemic arterial
and the intracranial pressures, since the latter is *approximately* equal
to the systemic venous pressure.

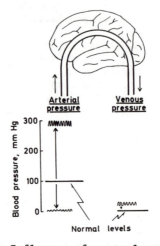

Fig. 3.1.   Influence of central arterial and
            venous pressures on cerebral per-
            fusion pressure. Owing to the
            essentially greater physiological
            ranges of central, or systemic,
            changes in arterial pressure (as
            well as to the frequency of occur-
            rence), cerebral perfusion pres-
            sure changes are more significant-
            ly affected by changes in central
            arterial pressure than in central
            venous pressure.

for the brain. The arterial contribution may be approximately 15 times
greater than that of the central venous pressure. In addition, changes in
central arterial pressure occur much more frequently than changes in venous
pressure under physiological and pathological conditions. This is probably
why, when considering cerebral blood flow regulation related to changes in
the cerebral perfusion pressure, we should stress that this regulation has
developed in evolutionary processes related to changes in the central
arterial pressure and not to those in the venous pressure (Ekström-Jodal
et al., 1969); thus, we will stress only alterations in arterial pressure,
which are certainly more important with regard to changes in cerebral perfusion pressure.

   Maintenance of Constant Cerebral Blood Flow Despite Changes in Perfusion Pressure. As already mentioned in Chapter 1 (p. 6), in accordance
with the general principles of hemodynamics: CBF = CPP/CVR, where CBF is
the cerebral blood flow, CPP is the cerebral perfusion pressure, and CVR
is the cerebrovascular resistance. Therefore, the cerebral blood flow is
directly proportional to the cerebral perfusion pressure. This means that,
all other conditions being equal, a rise in perfusion pressure must result
in an equivalent increase in the cerebral blood flow, and vice versa. This
relationship, shown in Fig. 3.2 (left side) was thought during the first
few decades of the present century to determine cerebral blood flow. This
was when biomedical thought was still under the influence of the Monro-
Kellie doctrine which stated that the diameter of cerebral blood vessels
must remain unchanged under all conditions (see p 17-18). However, due to

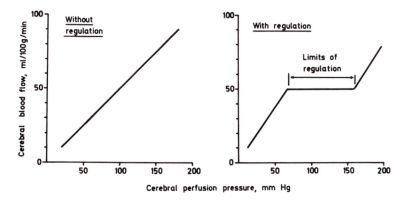

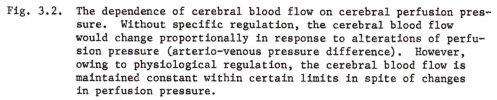

Fig. 3.2.   The dependence of cerebral blood flow on cerebral perfusion pressure. Without specific regulation, the cerebral blood flow
would change proportionally in response to alterations of perfusion pressure (arterio-venous pressure difference). However,
owing to physiological regulation, the cerebral blood flow is
maintained constant within certain limits in spite of changes
in perfusion pressure.

progress in techniques of cerebral blood flow investigation in animals and
humans, the researchers proved quite convincingly in the 1950s that under
normal conditions cerebral blood flow is kept constant when the mean arterial pressure increases or decreases. For instance, during a drop in arterial pressure in dogs, the blood flow in the brain decreases comparatively
less than in other organs (Kovách et al., 1959). The critical level of reduced arterial pressure, under which cerebral blood flow begins to decrease,
was found to be 50-60 mm Hg in experiments with monkeys (Meyer and Denny-
Brown, 1955) and 30 mm Hg in cats (Carlyle and Grayson, 1956). Many similar investigations were carried out in unanesthetized humans with quantitative measurements of cerebral blood flow using the Kety-Schmidt technique.
These studies convincingly proved that despite an increase or decrease in
systemic arterial pressure within certain limits, cerebral blood flow remains constant — near its normal values of 50 ml per 100 g brain tissue per
minute (Lassen, 1959; Kety, 1960).

This stability of cerebral blood flow within certain limits of perfusion pressure change convincingly proves that an active control mechanism exists.
The manifestation of this control is shown schematically in Fig. 3.2 (right
side). The upper and lower limits of cerebral perfusion pressure, within
which stability of cerebral blood flow is actively maintained, are the de-
signated limits of this type of regulation.

The limits of cerebral blood flow control are far from uniform (see
Fig. 3.3). Diverse limits may be observed not only in different species
but also in different representatives of the same species. For instance,
when the lower limits of control were investigated in healthy young persons, they were found to be quite different in different individuals: in
some the limits were comparatively high (e.g., 89 mm Hg), but very low in
others (29 mm Hg) (Finnerty et al., 1954). Even in the same subject, depending upon its state, these limits may vary considerably. This regulation of cerebral blood flow is readily disturbed, similar to other physiological control systems in humans, especially under pathological conditions.
A special test involving an artificial gradual decrease in systemic arteri-

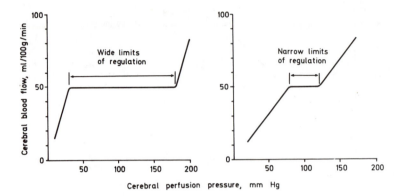

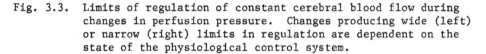

Fig. 3.3.   Limits of regulation of constant cerebral blood flow during
            changes in perfusion pressure. Changes producing wide (left)
            or narrow (right) limits in regulation are dependent on the
            state of the physiological control system.

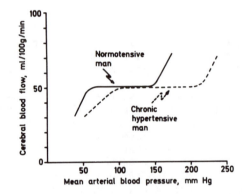

Fig. 3.4.   Shift in the curve of the cerebral blood
            pressure—blood flow relationship toward
            higher levels of systemic arterial pres-
            sure in patients with chronic hyperten-
            sive disease. See text for details.
            (Modified by permission from Lassen,
            1978.)

al pressure with simultaneous estimation of cerebral blood flow was performed on patients for determination of the limits of this regulation. This
test may result in correct decisions regarding the necessity of neurosurgical operations (Arutiunov et al., 1972). In healthy, well-adapted
organisms, the limits of this type of cerebral blood flow regulation may
be greatly expanded. This is seen during pathological states when cerebral
blood flow regulation has adapted to new conditions, e.g., to high arterial
pressure in humans and animals, when cerebral blood flow may not increase
despite high arterial pressure (Kety, 1960; Dickinson, 1965; Jones et al.,
1976). This phenomenon is shown schematically in Fig. 3.4.

     The principal physiological mechanism of this type of cerebral blood
flow regulation can be understood in relation to the hemodynamic principle

of flow that has been repeatedly mentioned in this book. Indeed, from the
relationship CBF = CPP/CVR it is clear that to keep the cerebral blood flow
(CBF) constant when the cerebral perfusion pressure (CPP) has changed in
either direction, the cerebrovascular resistance (CVR) must also change proportionally in the same direction. For instance, if the systemic arterial
pressure has increased, then a respective increase in the cerebrovascular
resistance is required to maintain constant cerebral blood flow. The cerebral blood flow would likewise remain stable during a decrease in systemic
arterial pressure if cerebrovascular resistance also decreases. Hence, the
considered cerebral blood flow regulation must necessarily involve active
changes in the resistance to flow in the cerebral vasculature. This, in
turn, is regulated in the organism by active vasomotor responses of cerebral arteries.

     Disturbances in cerebral blood flow related to changes in cerebral
perfusion pressure appear when the aforementioned type of regulation of
cerebral blood flow becomes insufficient. This insufficiency means that
the cerebrovascular resistance is not changed by appropriate feedback in
the respective direction or in proportion to systemic arterial pressure
changes. Therefore, alterations appear in both blood flow and pressure in
the brain vasculature, which increase with a rise in systemic arterial
pressure and decrease with its drop. This can occur in two cases: when
the control system of the cerebral blood flow does not function properly,
or when the actual changes in systemic arterial pressure are beyond the
limits of regulation (see Figs. 3.2-3.4).

     Disturbances in the normal functioning of the control system of cere-
bral blood flow can result from different causes — mostly from the effects
of various pathological factors. Considerable restrictions on the limits,
and sometimes even complete disappearance, of this type of cerebral blood
flow regulation have been demonstrated under different pathological conditions, i.e., after brain trauma (Sagawa and Guyton, 1961; Reivich et al.,
1969), considerable hypercapnia (Lassen, 1964; Häggendal and Johansson,
1965; Harper, 1965), hypoxia (Häggendal, 1968; Freeman, 1968), and cerebral ischemia (Symon et al., 1976). Disturbances of this type of cerebral
blood flow regulation can also be caused by pathological changes in the
arterial walls themselves, including principally functional changes (vasospasm, pathological dilatation; see Chapter 5 of this book), or those accompanied by gross structural changes in the vascular walls (e.g., sclerosis of any kind).

     The extent of pathological disorders in cerebral circulation caused
by changes in perfusion pressure is dependent on the degree of change.
Because a directly proportional relationship exists between cerebral perfusion pressure and cerebral blood flow, disorders of the latter increase
with increased change in the perfusion pressure. Furthermore, the initial
functional state of a given artery, manifested in its specific luminal
diameter, should play an important role in its myogenic, as well as neurogenic, responses to changes of intravascular pressure. Arteries have been
observed to follow the relationship (law of Laplace): $T \approx Pr/d$, where T
is the tangential tension of the vascular wall, P is intravascular pressure, r is the radius of the vascular lumen, and d is the thickness of the
vascular wall (Damask, 1978). If r is decreased, vasoconstriction should
occur in response to a smaller increase in smooth muscle tension.

     The pathological effects of a systemic arterial pressure drop on the
brain are shown schematically in Fig. 3.5. The extent of these pathological changes in brains exposed to a deficient blood supply is also dependent on the responsiveness of specific brain structures to ischemia.

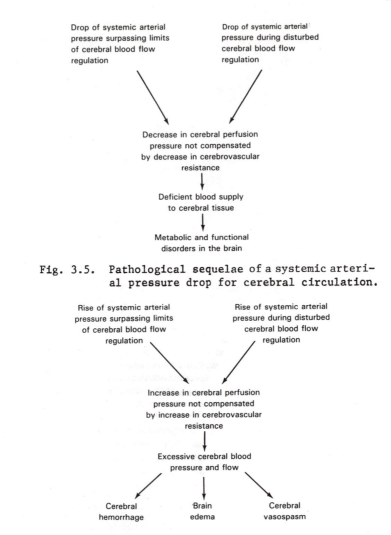

Fig. 3.5. Pathological sequelae of a systemic arterial pressure drop for cerebral circulation.

Fig. 3.6. Pathological sequelae of a systemic arterial pressure rise for cerebral circulation.

This is in turn related to their inherent sensitivity to lack of oxygen,
as well as to their ability to adapt to a deficient supply. Thus, neurons
are much more vulnerable in this respect than glial cells. A deficient
blood supply to brain tissue, which has not surpassed certain limits, may
be compensated for by a respective reduction in the oxygen consumption and
metabolic rate of the brain tissue (Meyer, 1968). But if the cerebral
blood flow drops below approximately 15%, then typical ischemic disturbances in brain tissue metabolism and function occur. The lack of oxygen
and nutrient supply causes an immediate decrease in the amount of glucose
and glycogen, as well as high-energy compounds, adenosine triphosphate and
phosphocreatine, with a concomitant increase in the concentration of lactic
acid and inorganic phosphate in brain tissue (Sjesjö, 1978).

On the other hand, excessive cerebral blood pressure and flow, caused
by rises in systemic arterial pressure and breakthrough of regulation, also
results in various disturbances, which are mainly related to considerable

rises in intravascular pressure in the cerebral vasculature (Fig. 3.6).
Among these disturbances are the following: (a) Disruption of the cerebral arterial walls, especially if they have been pathologically changed,
e.g., in sites of arterial aneurysm that result in hemorrhage into cerebral tissue, brain ventricles, or the subarachnoid space. (b) Damage to the
blood—brain barrier and excessive fluid filtration from the blood stream
into cerebral tissue, especially if the latter had already been changed and
predisposed to edema formation. (c) Vasopasm which can develop during rises in
intravascular pressure if the cerebral arterial walls are predisposed to
its development (see Chapter 5); in these cases the vasospasm appears as a
pathological manifestation of cerebral blood flow regulation. The flow
regulation causes vasoconstriction, which is necessary in this case but
excessive in size and duration, and can result, in turn, in a deficient
blood supply to respective areas of the brain.

Identification of the vascular effectors providing constant cerebral
blood pressure and flow, despite changes in central arterial pressure, is
an important step in the elucidation of physiological mechanisms of this
type of cerebral blood flow regulation (see Chapter 2, pp. 34-36). The
vascular effectors providing any type of cerebral blood flow regulation
can be identified only if the functional behavior is compared in different
parts of the cerebral arterial bed under the specific conditions of operation
of the control mechanisms, e.g., when the systemic arterial pressure has
been primarily changed and the cerebral blood flow is still maintained at
a constant level. Early experimental studies related to this problem were
concerned with the pial arteries, which were the easiest to approach. In
the well-known experiments with cats, carried out in the 1930s by Forbes
and his associates, it was observed that following a decrease in arterial
pressure to about 70 mm Hg (caused by bleeding, or by stimulation of the
vagus or other nerves) dilatation of pial arteries occurs — the lower the
pressure, the greater the arterial dilatation (Fog, 1937; Forbes et al.,
1937). Opposite vascular responses have been detected during elevation of
systemic arterial pressure (caused by stimulation of splanchnic nerves or
occlusion of the abdominal aorta); vasoconstriction occurs only when the
arterial pressure rises by more than 20% of its initial level and is particularly pronounced when the initial pressure is low (Fog, 1939). These
pial arterial responses have been further substantiated by other researchers and were thought to maintain constant cerebral blood flow despite
changes in systemic arterial pressure.

However, an attentive consideration of these experimental results
casts doubt on the authors' conclusion that the pial arteries are responsible for the regulation of cerebral blood flow under these conditions.
Why do the pial arterial responses appear only when the degree of arterial
pressure change is so great? Actually, even the smallest fluctuations in
systemic arterial pressure (the pulsatile fluctuations, in particular)
have been found to be primarily eliminated on the way from the aorta to
cerebral blood vessels (Söderberg and Weckman, 1959; Tkachenko, 1964;
Ayala and Himwich, 1965).

One argument against a primary role of the pial arteries in this type
of cerebral blood flow regulation is that the specific latent period of the
vascular response, which was not mentioned in the experiments by Fog and
Forbes, was found to be rather long and surprisingly variable in different
pial arteries, even those located adjacently on the cerebral hemispheres
(Fig. 3.7). The latent period lasts 20-240 seconds for vasodilatation
which occurs following arterial hypotension, and 15-205 seconds for vasoconstriction related to hypertension (Mchedlishvili, Nikolaishvili, et al.,
1976). A rather long latency of the pial arterial responses, about one

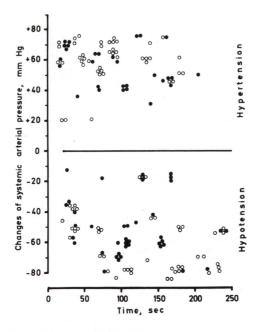

Fig. 3.7.   Latent period of pial arterial responses
to changes in systemic arterial pressure.
The onset of the pial arterial responses
in rabbits related to changes in the systemic arterial pressure during arterial
hypertension (stepwise increases in systemic arterial pressure by ≈70 mm Hg
caused by intravenous infusion of noradrenaline) and hypotension (stepwise decreases in systemic arterial pressure by
≈60 mm Hg caused by bleeding) is shown.
Every point demonstrates the onset of a
vascular response, either constriction
(during hypertension) or dilatation (during hypotension), as a function of the
time interval following the initiation
of changes of the arterial pressure (ab-
scissa). White circles denote pial
arteries having an initial diameter over
100 μm and black circles denote those
under 100 μm. (Reproduced from Mchedlishvili, Nikolaishvili, et al., 1976.)

minute in duration, has also been reported in other experiments (Wahl and
Kuschinsky, 1979). It seems improbable that the pial arteries would directly respond to simultaneously occurring changes in intravascular pressure
after such a long and rather variable latent period.

The magnitude of the responses of pial vessels of different diameter
further substantiates the reasoning above: the responses (especially
dilatation) are considerably greater in minute blood vessels (those having
an initial diameter under 100 μm in the rabbit) than in larger vessels
(Fig. 3.8). These results cannot be due to direct responses of arterial

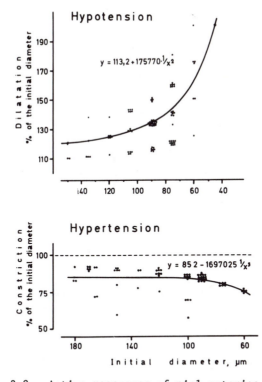

Fig. 3.8. Active responses of pial arteries to
           changes in systemic arterial pressure.
           The active constrictor responses and
           especially the dilator responses of
           the smaller pial arteries to changes
           in systemic arterial pressure in rab-
           bits are considerably more pronounced
           than those of the larger vessels, al-
           though the degree of intravascular
           pressure changes are positively cor-
           related with vessel size (i.e.,
           greater in the larger than in smaller
           vessels). Arterial hypertension
           (stepwise increase in the arterial
           pressure by ≈70 mm Hg) was produced by
           intravenous infusions of noradrenaline,
           and arterial hypotension (stepwise de-
           creases in the arterial pressure by
           ≈60 mm Hg) was produced by bleeding.
           (Reproduced from Mchedlishvili, Niko-
           laishvili, et al., 1976.)

walls to changes in intravascular pressure, since the pressure changes
should be considerably greater in the larger than in the smaller vessels
under experimental conditions (Mchedlishvili, Nikolaishvili, et al., 1976).

    Thus, there are strong points in favor of the conclusion that active
diameter changes in the pial arteries are actually not direct responses to
changes in the blood pressure, but rather responses to the altered blood
supply to respective areas of cerebral tissues (see Chapter 4). The great

variability of the latent periods of individual pial arterial responses may be explained by respective variability in the actual blood supply to adjacent small areas of the cerebral cortex. This variability is evident regardless of the direction of circulatory disturbances, i.e., whether the blood flow is deficient due to a drop in systemic arterial pressure, or excessive because of its elevation.

While investigating pial arterial behavior under conditions of systemic arterial pressure changes, it has been concluded that it is only the larger pial arteries — from the circle of Willis to vessels 200 μm in diameter — that may be involved in the regulation of cerebral blood flow. The smallest pial and intracerebral arterioles appear to be relatively unresponsive to acute changes in the blood pressure within limits from 100 to 150 mm Hg, i.e., when the blood supply to the cortex has probably not been disturbed because it was already controlled (Kontos et al., 1978). The involvement of the minute pial arteries in the regulation of adequate blood supply to cerebral tissue will be considered in Chapter 4 of this book.

The role of the major arteries of the brain (internal carotid and vertebral arteries) as the probable vascular effectors of this type of cerebral blood flow control drew attention at the end of the 1950s. Initial evidence was obtained in experiments with rabbits, and is presented in Fig. 3.9. In spite of repeated experimentally induced increases in central arterial pressure to the same level (in response to intravenous adrenaline injection), the pressure in the circle of Willis, which was initially raised, later remained unaltered. Thus, the recorded increase in the pressure gradient along the major arteries was direct evidence for a respective rise in the resistance of these blood vessels, indicating their constriction (Mchedlishvili, 1960a). Since the direct effect of catecholamines (and adrenaline, in particular) on the major cerebral arteries is rather small (see below, Fig. 3.36), their constrictor response during rises in arterial pressure is, in all probability, a manifestation of the control mechanism that maintains constant blood pressure, and hence flow, in the brain despite changes in perfusion pressure.

The role of major arteries of the brain in the maintenance of constant cerebral blood pressure and flow despite changes in central arterial pressure has been further substantiated by estimations of the arterial resistance. An example of these experimental results is presented in Fig. 3.10. A stepwise increase in the inlet pressure of the internal carotid artery over a total range of about 120 mm Hg results in a respective rise in the computed vessel resistance and leads to slight changes in the outlet pressure recorded in the circle of Willis (Mchedlishvili, Mitagvaria, et al., 1973). These results provide further evidence that the regulation of cerebral blood pressure and flow is primarily performed by the major arteries. Independent responses of these arteries during changes in cerebral perfusion pressure have been observed recently in investigations in which the resistance in the major cerebral arteries in dogs has been estimated from the arterial pressure gradient along their course and the cerebral blood flow. These experiments have demonstrated that the resistance decreased significantly in the major arteries during reductions in systemic arterial pressure caused by hemorrhage (Heistad et al., 1978). The involvement of the major brain arteries in the maintenance of constant cerebral blood flow despite drops in systemic arterial pressure has also been substantiated by the finding that the regulation by the carotid arteries was found to be more pronounced than regulation by the vertebral arteries in rhesus monkeys; this correlates with the respective nerve supply of the vessels (Tomita et al., 1982).

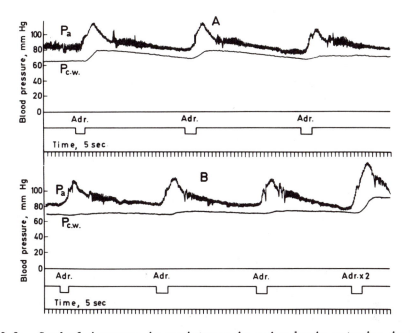

Fig. 3.9. Gradual increase in resistance in major brain arteries in the
           course of repeated elevation of systemic arterial pressure. A
           simultaneous record of arterial blood pressure in aorta (P_a)
           and in circle of Willis ($P_{c.w.}$) was made, the difference of
           which reflects the resistance in the major cerebral arteries in
           an experiment with rabbits (trace B is a direct continuation of
           trace A). In the course of repeated rises in the aortic pres-
           sure by intravenous administration of equal doses of adrenaline
           (5.4 μM), the $P_{c.w.}$, which initially rose, stopped increasing
           during subsequent rises in aortic pressure (at the seventh in-
           jection, the dose of adrenaline was doubled). The increase in
           resistance in major brain arteries estimated in this fashion
           proves that the vessels become constricted in response to ele-
           vations of the aortic pressure, thereby providing for constant
           cerebral blood pressure and flow despite increases in cerebral
           perfusion pressure. (Reproduced from Mchedlishvili, 1960a.)

    These results are actually comparable to those obtained in other
studies where the attenuation of arterial pulse fluctuations along the
major arteries of the brain has been demonstrated. The simultaneous recording of blood pressure fluctuations in the aorta (or its branches) and
the circle of Willis indicate that pulsatile fluctuations are considerably
decreased toward the skull. This has been detected not only with mercury
manometers in earlier studies (Bouckaert and Heymans, 1933; Opdyke, 1946),
but also by means of electromanometers which have less inertia (Söderberg
and Weckman, 1959; Ayala and Himwich, 1965; Tkachenko, 1964) and piezo-
manometers (Moskalenko and Filanovskaya, 1967). These authors, however,
did not consider this as an active contribution of the major brain arteries;
they believed other factors were involved, in particular the curvature
along the course of these vessels (Klosovsky, 1951). The relatively slower fluctuations of systemic arterial pressure (such as respiratory waves
and third-order waves of Traube-Hering) are also significantly decreased,
or even completely eliminated, along the course of the major arteries to-

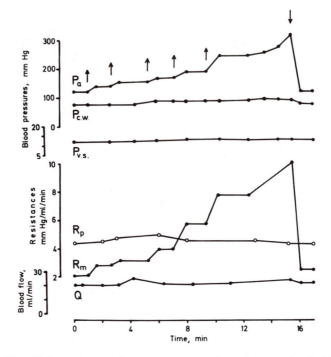

Fig. 3.10.   Maintenance of constant pressure in cerebral blood
vessels despite increases in the inlet pressure of
the major arteries. The results of an experiment
using dogs, in which the inlet pressure of major
brain arteries (an analog of the central arterial
pressure, P_a) has been increased stepwise (arrows
directed to top), showed that the outlet pressure
of the arteries, i.e., the pressure in the circle
of Willis ($P_{c.w.}$), remained unchanged. This phenomenon is related to the calculated rise in resistance in the major brain arteries (R_m), while the
resistance in the smaller brain vessels peripheral
to the circle of Willis (R_p) remained unchanged.
When the steadily rising arterial pressure (P_a)
reached a certain limit (approximately 250 mm Hg),
a spontaneous increase in resistance in the major
arteries (seen as a rise in P_a and R_m, but $P_{c.w.}$
remained constant) took place. This was probably
due to significant decreases in their luminal
radii (r), according to the Laplace relationship
$T \approx P \times r$ (Damask, 1978). When T (the vascular
wall tension) overcomes the P (intravascular pressure), further decreases in the vascular lumen are
seen. (Reproduced from Mchedlishvili, Mitagvaria,
et al., 1971.)

ward the base of the brain. The rise in tone in arterial walls at every
mount in arterial pressure has been proven by an increase in the velocity
of pulse waves that spread from the aorta to the circle of Willis (Nadareishvili, 1962). The significance of anatomical peculiarities and of the
active responses of the major arteries of the brain in attenuation of the

amplitude of pulsatile fluctuations of arterial pressure have been studied
more recently (Mchedlishvili, Ormotsadze, et al., 1977; Toidze et al.,
1983).

Thus, substantial experimental evidence has been obtained for the
active involvement of the brain major arteries (primarily the internal and
vertebral arteries) in the maintenance of a constant cerebral blood pressure and flow despite changes in the brain perfusion pressure (Fig. 3.11).
The smaller blood vessels, located in the periphery of the circle of Willis,
particularly the minute pial arteries, may respond when the central arterial pressure has changed, but this is, in all probability, a secondary
(backup) system. This mechanism operates only in cases when the primary
vascular mechanism, i.e., the major arteries of the brain, proves to be insufficient to provide a constant blood pressure and flow in the cerebral
vasculature.

The vascular effectors providing this type of cerebral blood flow regulation have been selected in the evolutionary process by the same principle
that applies to other kinds of regulation of circulatory processes, i.e.,
the most efficient way. The major arteries of the brain efficiently maintain normal cerebral blood pressure and flow in the whole brain at essential

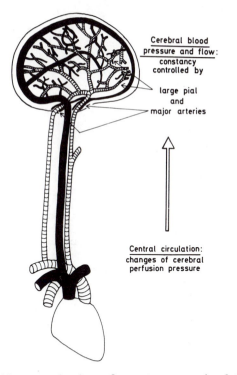

Fig. 3.11.   Regulation of constant cerebral blood
              pressure and flow by vascular effectors
              despite changes in systemic arterial
              pressure. Regulation occurs through
              responses of the major brain arteries
              (internal carotid and vertebral arter-
              ies), as well as the larger pial
              arteries, which are induced by changes
              in the systemic arterial pressure.

levels despite changes in central arterial pressure. It would be less efficient to use small pial arteries as the effectors in this case, since
this would interfere with the function of the regulatory mechanism that
controls adequate blood supply to minute areas of cerebral tissue, i.e.,
the coupling of microcirculation and metabolic needs in cerebral tissue.

3.2. CONTROL OF CONSTANT CEREBRAL BLOOD VOLUME

Although the blood volume in each part of the vascular bed is changeable, the mean blood volume can be estimated with a certain degree of accuracy. It is known (Mellander and Johansson, 1968; Tkachenko, 1979) that
the blood volume is distributed among the body's arteries, capillaries,
and veins in such a way that almost three-fourths of the blood is stored in
the peripheral venous bed (Fig. 3.12). We can assume that the blood volume is comparably distributed in the brain vessels.

Volumetric Equilibrium within the Skull. The brain in the vertebrate's
body, unlike other organs, sits inside a rigid bony skull. The skull cavity
contains basically three noncompressible components, namely the cerebral
tissue (which is composed of approximately 80% water and can be considered
incompressible), and two fluids: the blood inside the cerebral vasculature
and the cerebrospinal fluid in the brain ventricles and subarachnoid spaces
(Fig. 3.13). From the physical point of view, neither of these intracranial
components can be changed in mass without an oppositely directed, and quantitatively similar, change in other components. This relationship between the
intracranial components had been understood as early as the end of the 18th
and beginning of the 19th centuries when the Monro-Kellie doctrine was formulated. According to this doctrine, the cerebral blood volume, and hence the
cerebral blood flow, are kept constant due to the hermeticity of the skull.
Though the postulate of the doctrine is in principle correct, the conclusion
concerning constancy of cerebral blood flow is wrong (see Chapter 2, p. 18).
Events related to that postulate were erroneously supposed to be absolute,
not relative, in living bodies. Evidence soon came forward to counter the
absolutes of the Monro-Kellie doctrine: first, the relative compliance of
the non-bony components of the cerebral and especially of the spinal cavity
walls; second, the possibility of displacement of the cerebrospinal fluid
inside the cavity; third, relatively insignificant alterations in arterial
vessel diameter, and thus their volume, which are still sufficient to change
the cerebrovascular resistance and regional cerebral blood flow within broad
limits; fourth, the dissipation of the volume changes of pial arteries
(i.e., the vessels, which experience pronounced diameter changes under
natural conditions) over the whole intracranial cavity, since their walls
are actually surrounded by easily displaced cerebrospinal fluid.

However, the initial postulate of the Monro-Kellie doctrine is in principle correct, and excessive accumulations of blood in the skull must cause
displacement of other components in its interior. For instance, an excessive accumulation of blood in cerebral vasculature should inevitably cause
an increase in intracranial pressure, a decrease in cerebrospinal fluid
volume, or compression of cerebral tissue. Therefore, it should not be
surprising that a special control mechanism eliminating this disturbance
in the cerebral circulation has appeared in the evolutionary process of
the vertebrates.

Balance of Blood Inflow to, and Outflow from, the Brain. As is schematically shown in Fig. 3.13, the constancy of cerebral blood volume is
maintained by a balanced blood inflow to, and outflow from, the skull.
Considering possible disturbances in cerebral blood volume, it should be

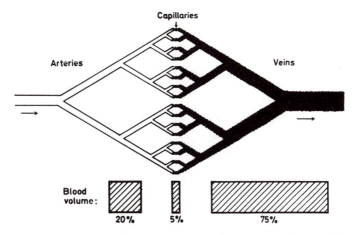

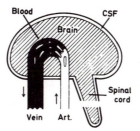

Fig. 3.12.   Relative blood volumes in the arterial, capillary,
             and venous ramifications of a peripheral circula-
             tory bed. The blood volume is greatest in the veins,
             due to the comparatively wide lumina of these ves-
             sels, and is smallest in the capillaries, although
             the total cross-sectional area of the capillary bed
             is significantly greater than the veins and the
             arteries, since the mean length of the capillaries
             is comparatively small.

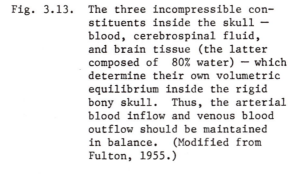

Fig. 3.13.   The three incompressible con-
             stituents inside the skull —
             blood, cerebrospinal fluid,
             and brain tissue (the latter
             composed of 80% water) — which
             determine their own volumetric
             equilibrium inside the rigid
             bony skull. Thus, the arterial
             blood inflow and venous blood
             outflow should be maintained
             in balance. (Modified from
             Fulton, 1955.)

emphasized that decreases represent an insignificant problem for steady
state of the brain, compared to an increased blood volume. An excessive
volume of blood in the cerebral vasculature may appear in the two following cases. First, surplus inflow of blood into the cerebral vessels from
the central arterial system may occur while the outflow through the veins
is insufficient to keep the normal intracranial blood volume constant;
this leads to excessive blood accumulation in the cerebral vasculature

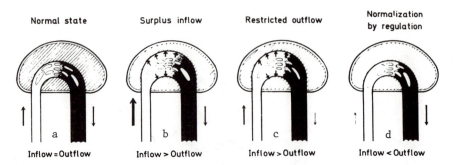

Fig. 3.14. Cerebral blood volume changes and their regulation. The main
causes of excessive accumulation of blood in cerebral vasculature (the size of the arrows specify the blood flow intensity
in both feeding arteries and draining veins) are: (b) surplus
inflow of arterial blood to the brain and (c) restricted venous blood outflow from it. The physiological control system
to eliminate this disturbance operates to reduce the blood inflow by the constriction of the major feeding arteries (d).

(Fig. 3.14). The second cause of accumulation of excessive cerebral blood
volume may be by restriction of blood outflow into the extracranial veins
from inside the skull, resulting in an accumulation of blood in the cerebral vessels (Fig. 3.14).

Surplus blood volume in the skull primarily accumulates in the distended cerebral veins, and only partly in the capillaries, and the smallest amount, if any, in the arteries. The elimination of these changes in
the cerebral blood volume might be fulfilled in principle by two hemodynamic events: by an increased blood outflow from the brain to the extracranial venous bed, or by a restricted inflow of blood to the brain from the
extracranial arteries. The active tools in the cranial venous beds to increase the outflow of blood from inside the skull can be efficient, although
the walls of the intracranial veins, in contrast to the venous vessels of
the same caliber in other parts of the body, are deprived of a continuous
muscular layer (see Chapter 1). Cranial veins have been shown to respond
to sympathetic stimulation and vasoconstricting agents (Auer et al., 1982).
However, the cerebral venous pressure was found to be linearly related to
the extracranial venous pressure (Mchedlishvili, Sikharulidze, et al.,
1980), thus indicating the absence of an active "autoregulatory" control,
which was just described for the cerebral arterial system. This linear
relationship between cerebral blood volume and systemic venous pressure
changes (Fig. 3.15) is thus evidence in favor of a relatively negligible
role of cerebral veins in the control of cerebral circulation.

Unlike the physiological peculiarities of the cerebral venous bed,
the brain arteries are both structurally and functionally adjusted to control the blood inflow to the brain. Therefore it appears natural that only
the arterial vascular mechanisms are responsible for eliminating excessive
cerebral blood volumes and maintaining it in a normal range. All possible
causes of disturbances of cerebral blood volume, as well as the basic mechanism of their elimination, are schematically presented in Fig. 3.14.

Thus the regulation of constant cerebral blood volume can be achieved
in all probability only by the regulation of the blood inflow from central

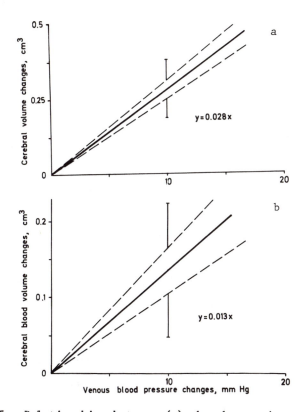

Fig. 3.15. Relationships between (a) the changes in venous pres-
            sure and cerebral volume and (b) the changes in ven-
            ous pressure and cerebral blood volume. The mean
            slope of the linear pressure-volume relationships
            (the regression coefficient) were obtained in experi-
            ments with open skulls in rabbits. The dotted line
            circumscribes the area of mean errors in the regres-
            sion coefficients and the vertical lines show its
            standard deviations. See text for details. (Repro-
            duced from Mchedlishvili, Sikharulidze, et al.,
            1982.)

arteries to brain vasculature. This control can be expressed as the functional relationship between blood inflow-outflow balance and cerebral blood
volume, as is schematically shown in Fig. 3.16. If the balance becomes
positive, entailing accumulation of excessive blood inside the skull (due
to excessive blood inflow to or deficient blood outflow from the skull), a
regulatory mechanism, maintaining constant (naturally within certain limits)
cerebral blood volume in cerebral vasculature, starts to operate. This
regulation of cerebral blood volume is described below. However, if the
balance is shifted to the negative side because of a deficient blood inflow to the brain, the cerebral blood volume should also be maintained
within certain limits. Physical factors (including the rigidity of the
skull, the cerebrospinal fluid pressure, the mechanical properties of the
brain, etc.) play, in all probability, an important role in the maintenance of constant cerebral blood volume, especially when the balance of
blood inflow and outflow is shifted to the negative side. Relationships

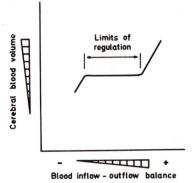

Fig. 3.16. Diagrammatic representation of cerebral
            blood volume regulation. The active
            control system of cerebral circulation
            maintains a constant cerebral blood vol-
            ume within certain limits in spite of
            changes in cerebral blood inflow—outflow
            balance. See text for details.

between the biophysical factors maintaining intracranial fluid mechanics
are considered in detail in the monograph by Moskalenko et al. (1980).

Evidence for the existence of an active control mechanism maintaining
constant cerebral blood volume was first obtained in the late 1950s, which
is later than the other presently known types of cerebral blood regulation
(see Chapter 2, pp. 24-25). The other types of cerebral blood flow regulation (i.e., of an adequate blood supply to cerebral tissue, of a constant
blood-gas content in cerebral blood and tissue, as well as a constant
cerebral blood flow and pressure despite changes in systemic arterial pressure) were discussed even when the appropriate regulatory mechanisms, in
particular the specific vascular effectors, were still unknown. The mechanism of regulation of cerebral blood volume, however, was discovered
simultaneously with the corresponding vascular effectors which maintain
constant blood volume in the brain vasculature. Actually, the endeavor of
investigating the vascular effectors regulating the cerebral blood flow
under various conditions led to the discovery of this particular type of
control, i.e., of the constant cerebral blood volume.*

In experiments with rabbits the simultaneous occlusion of all jugular
veins at the neck surprisingly did not produce venous blood stagnation in
the brain (with all the known characteristic features of this disturbance
in peripheral circulation), but rather a deficient blood inflow to the
brain. However, this phenomenon could not be explained by the constriction
of either the pial or intracerebral vessels. At that time, no appropriate
physiological techniques for ascertaining the behavior of the major brain
arteries (i.e., the internal carotid and vertebral arteries) were available. Techniques were developed (see below) and evidence was later obtained, proving that the major arteries of the brain are responsible, as
vascular effectors, for this cerebral blood flow regulation under these

_____

*The majority of articles containing the experimental evidence cited in
 the following paragraph were published in Russian and have been further
 summarized elsewhere in English (Mchedlishvili, 1964, 1972).

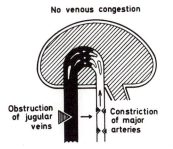

Fig. 3.17. An experimentally produced obstruction
of venous blood outflow from the brain
through the jugular veins results in
constriction of the major brain arteries, thus eliminating excess blood volume in the cerebral vasculature.

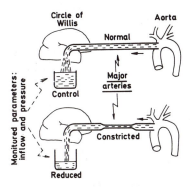

Fig. 3.18. An estimation of the functional state
of major brain arteries, i.e., the internal carotid and vertebral arteries,
can be made by monitoring arterial
blood inflow to, or blood pressure in,
the circle of Willis (with controlled
arterial pressure in the aorta), as
shown.

circumstances (Mchedlishvili, 1959a). The crucial experiment demonstrating
this regulatory mechanism, which eliminates excessive blood accumulation in
the brain and hence provides a constant cerebral blood volume, is schematically demonstrated in Fig. 3.17.

    Physiological Techniques Applied for Estimating the Behavior of Major
Brain Arteries. These arteries, unlike pial vessels, are not easily accessible for direct examination *in vivo*. Their surgical exposure, even very
carefully accomplished, for direct observation, results in disappearance
of the natural vascular responses of these arteries. Therefore, indirect
methods have had to be applied. Such physiological methods for discovery
of the arteries' behavior were gradually developed and applied in animal
experiments in the course of the 1960s. The principles of the techniques
are as follows.

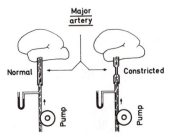

Fig. 3.19.   Resistography of the isolated internal
             carotid artery of dog *in situ*. Estima-
             tions of the resistance, and hence the
             vessel tone, reflect circulatory changes
             in the isolated internal carotid artery
             (with ligated connections to extra-
             cranial arteries) in dogs. The artery
             is continuously perfused with a constant
             output pump of autogenic blood or arti-
             ficial perfusion fluid. The perfusion
             pressure of the artery is recorded. See
             Fig. 3.20 and text for details.

Initially the blood inflow to, or blood pressure in, the terminal of
the major arteries, i.e., in the circle of Willis, is recorded. If the
pressure in the aorta is known (and if necessary can be kept constant),
then a decrease in blood flow in the major arteries or drop in pressure in
the circle of Willis indicates that the major arteries have constricted,
and vice versa. Schematically this principle for investigation of arterial
behavior is presented in Fig. 3.18. Application of these techniques has
made it possible from the very beginning to record the active responses of
the major brain arteries in rabbits (Mchedlishvili, 1960b, 1960c, 1960d).
Likewise, an indicator of constriction of these arteries is the reduction
of blood flow which can be recorded if the flow is estimated simultaneously
with the pressure gradient in the vessels (Mchedlishvili, Akhobadze, et al.,
1962; Mchedlishvili and Gabashvili, 1965).

A method for computation of the resistance along both the major arteries and the smaller vessels located distal to the circle of Willis has been
developed based on a mathematical model, where the values of the pressure
drop along the cerebral vascular bed have been used for calculations
(Mchedlishvili, Mitagvaria, et al., 1971, 1973). The resistance in the
major brain arteries has correspondingly been computed from the pressure
gradient along these vessels and the values of the cerebral blood flow
(Heistad et al., 1978).

Another method which gives direct data on the functional behavior of
the major brain arteries are measurements of resistance in the isolated internal carotid arteries in dogs when either the blood from the animals'
aortas, or Ringer-Krebs bicarbonate solution from a reservoir, is pumped
(using a constant-output pump) into the artery (the surgical procedure and
the application of the method have been described elsewhere; see Mchedlishvili, Ormotsadze, et al., 1967a; Mchedlishvili and Ormotsadze, 1970, 1979).
The schematic design of the method is given in Figs. 3.19 and 3.20. When
the artery becomes constricted the continuously recorded perfusion pressure
rises in proportion to the vasoconstriction. Another modification of the
technique (Mamisashvili et al., 1983) involves estimates of vascular responses in terms of flow changes in the artery (Fig. 3.21).

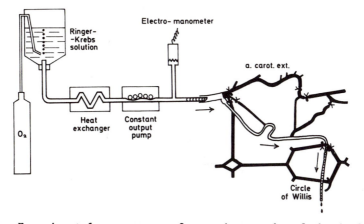

Fig. 3.20.   Experimental arrangement for resistography of the isolated in-
             ternal carotid artery (i.e., with all vascular connections to
             extracerebral vessels ligated) of dogs *in situ*. The pump pro-
             vides a constant output of perfusion fluid into the artery.
             The fluid then flows out of the artery through a catheter in-
             troduced in its peripheral portion in a retrograde direction.
             Increases in the resistance of the artery under investigation
             result in rises in the perfusion pressure, and vice versa.
             (Modified from Mchedlishvili, 1972.)

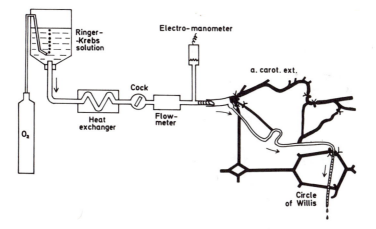

Fig. 3.21.   Experimental arrangement for flowmetry of isolated internal
             carotid artery of dogs *in situ*. The perfusion pressure re-
             mains constant at any given level. The perfusion fluid flows
             out of the artery through a catheter introduced in its periph-
             eral portion in a retrograde direction. Changes in the vascu-
             lar resistance bring about proportional changes of flow in the
             isolated artery. (Reproduced from Mamisashvili et al., 1983.)

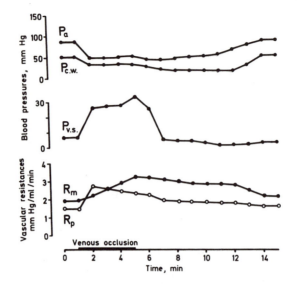

Fig. 3.22.   Increase in resistance in major brain arteries in re-
             sponse to rises in cerebral venous blood pressure and
             volume. During a four-minute occlusion of the crani-
             al vena cava in the dog, the pressure in the venous
             sinuses of the brain ($P_{v.s.}$) rises considerably,
             while the arterial pressures in the aorta (P_a) and
             the circle of Willis ($P_{c.w.}$) drop due to reduced ven-
             ous return to heart. The computed vascular resis-
             tance in the major brain arteries (R_m) shows its gradu-
             al increase in this period, while the resistance at
             the periphery of the circle of Willis (R_p) rises ini-
             tially, then starts to decrease. See text for the
             details of these oppositely directed vascular re-
             sponses of the major and the pial arteries. (Repro-
             duced from Mchedlishvili, Mitagvaria, et al., 1971.)

     Further evidence for an active contribution of the major cerebral
arteries in response to excessive blood accumulation in the brain was obtained in a variety of experimental conditions in which the blood volume
was increased primarily in cerebral vasculature by different means: either
by hindrance of blood outflow (e.g., occlusion of the cranial caval vein or
transverse centrifugation of the animals) or by excessive blood inflow to
the brain (asphyxic, postischemic, or even functional hyperemia in the
whole brain).

     The identification of vascular effectors of this particular type of
cerebral blood flow regulation requires determination of the specific
cerebrovascular portion (or portions), which becomes regularly constricted,
and hence tends to reduce the blood inflow to the brain, in response to increased cerebral blood volume. For this purpose the behavior of major and
pial arteries had to be studied under conditions of excessive blood accumulation in the cerebral vasculature. The widely opened skull is a very
suitable experimental preparation for this purpose, since purely physical
factors, which make considerable contributions to the maintenance of volumetric equilibrium within the skull under normal circumstances, are completely excluded when the skull has been opened. Thus, the involvement of the

vascular phenomena in the maintenance of a constant cerebral blood volume
can be most clearly elucidated.

During occlusion of the cranial caval vein with ensuing venous blood
stagnation inside the skull of dogs, it was impossible to adequately record
the behavior of major brain arteries (by the methods available in the
1960s). As soon as the blood flow in the vena cava was recovered, the pres-
,sure difference between the aorta and the circle of Willis was found to be
increased by about 36% of its initial value, which provided evidence that
the resistance increased in the major brain arteries (Mchedlishvili, Akhobadze, et al., 1963). The computation of resistance in these arteries during the venous occlusion (Fig. 3.22) further clarified a progressive increase in resistance after caval venous occlusion, while the vascular resistance at the periphery of the circle of Willis (presumably in pial
arteries) increased initially, then began to decrease progressively (Mchedlishvili, Mitagvaria, et al., 1971). Direct investigation of the pial
arterial diameter has shown that they regularly respond with dilatation,
especially the minute vessels: smaller pial arteries (30–45 μm in diameter) dilate by 85–175%, while larger arteries (80–120 μm in diameter) dilate only by 20–60%. The largest pial arteries (over 225 μm in diameter)
have the opposite tendency: they constrict at the first occlusion of the
caval vein but begin to show exclusively the dilatatory response with repeated occlusions (Mchedlishvili, Akhobadze, et al., 1963). Thus it may
be concluded that it is only the major cerebral arteries that regularly constrict under these conditions, and this vascular response is, in all probability, directed to elimination of the excessive blood accumulation in
cerebral vasculature. As for the simultaneous dilatation of pial arteries,
it is a typical characteristic of these vessels to improve the blood supply
to cerebral tissue, which suffers from hypoxia and hypocapnia during venous
occlusion (see Chapter 4 for details).

Evidence for existence of this specific type of cerebral blood volume
regulation has also been obtained in the studies by Moskalenko and his associates: in humans with implanted gold electrodes for diagnostic electroplethysmography, an active normalization of increased blood volume has been
observed during an orthostatic maneuver (Moskalenko et al., 1964). In
animal experiments with transverse acceleration, the intracranial blood
volume and pressure have been found to stop rising despite continuing centrifugation; direct examination indicated tangible constriction of the
arteries of the circle of Willis (Weinstein, 1970). Clinical evidence of
a similar nature has been further reported by Kaasik (1979a): the angio-
grams often reveal constriction of the intracranial portions of internal
carotid arteries in patients with increased cerebral blood volume, whereas
the extracranial parts of these vessels remain normal. Consequently, an
increase in cerebral blood volume, caused by obstruction of venous blood
outflow from the skull, is regularly associated with constriction of major
brain arteries resulting in an increase in resistance to blood flow along
the path to the circle of Willis.

An analogous constrictor effect of the major brain arteries has been
discovered under conditions of increased cerebral blood volume due to excessive blood inflow to the brain. This has been described to occur when
a widespread and pronounced dilatation of small cerebral arteries occurs
during (a) systemic asphyxia, (b) postischemic states involving the whole
brain, and (c) extensive functional hyperemia of the cerebral hemispheres.

Widespread pial arterial dilatation following obstruction of tracheotomy tubes has been detected repeatedly (see pp. 118–119). The coincident

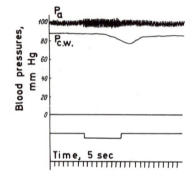

Fig. 3.23.   Constriction of major brain arteries
seen in response to asphyxia. Following tracheotomy tube occlusion, the
pressure in the circle of Willis ($P_{c.w.}$)
decreases while the pressure in the
aorta (P_a) remains constant. The pressure gradient increases by a mean of
22% under these conditions, indicating
an increase in resistance in the major
brain arteries. Record from an experiment carried out with "chest-head
preparation" in a rabbit. (Reproduced
from Mchedlishvili, 1962.)

constriction of the major arteries has been shown under these conditions with
a variety of experimental techniques: measurements of the pressure gradient along the major arteries (independent of whether the blood pressure
rises considerably or is maintained constant in the aorta) (Fig. 3.23),
recordings of blood flow in the major brain arteries, and computation of
the resistances in large and small cerebral arteries (Fig. 3.24), as well
as resistography of the isolated internal carotid artery in dogs (Mchedlishvili, 1960b, 1962; Mchedlishvili and Gabashvili, 1965; Mchedlishvili,
Mitagvaria, et al., 1971). Thus, constriction of the major brain arteries
has been consistently shown by different experimental techniques during
the asphyxic increase in cerebral blood volume (due to a considerable dilatation of pial arteries). This vasoconstriction has been interpreted as
an active regulation of cerebral circulation, directed at withdrawing excess blood from cerebral vasculature. But this vasoconstriction appears
to be caused not by the direct effect of hypercapnia, which has been shown
to further dilate these arteries (Heistad et al., 1978), but rather by an
excessively increased blood volume inside the brain.

A similar phenomenon has also been observed following cerebral
ischemia. The postischemic, or reactive, hyperemia, related to dilatation
of the pial arteries, is certainly a manifestation of adequate blood flow
regulation directed at eliminating the sequences of a deficient blood supply to brain tissue (see Chapter 4). In experiments with rabbits, following temporary stoppage of cerebral blood flow (due to exsanguination and
subsequent reinfusion of blood), the pressure gradient along the major
brain arteries increased considerably (on the average, by 177%) (Fig.
3.25), thus indicating an increase in their resistance (Mchedlishvili,
1960d). Similar results have been obtained in the postischemic states of
dogs by using both estimates of pressure gradients in the major arteries
of the brain and of resistography of circulatory isolated internal carotid
arteries (Mchedlishvili, Akhobadze, et al., 1962a; Mchedlishvili, Baramidze,

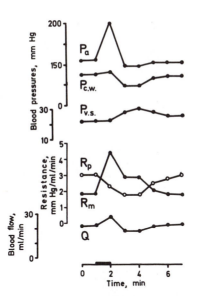

Fig. 3.24.   Resistance changes in major and minor
             brain arteries during asphyxia. Fol-
             lowing tracheotomy tube occlusion in
             dogs, the pressure in the aorta (P_a)
             rises while in the circle of Willis
             ($P_{c.w.}$) it drops with a simultaneous
             increase in pressure in venous sinuses
             ($P_{v.s.}$). The computed vascular re-
             sistance increases considerably in the
             major cerebral arteries (R_m), indicat-
             ing constriction, but decreases in
             vessels peripheral to the circle of
             Willis (R_p), probably due to pial
             arterial dilatation (see pp. 118–119
             in Chapter 4). (Reproduced from Mched-
             lishvili, Mitagvaria, et al., 1971.)

et al., 1968; Mchedlishvili, 1972). A pronounced increase in cerebral
blood volume in the postischemic state has thus been found to be regularly
accompanied by constriction of major brain arteries.

     Another experimental model resulting in widespread dilatation of minor
cerebral arteries (presumably the pial arteries) with an ensuing increase
in cerebral blood volume has been produced by increasing neuronal activity
throughout the cerebral hemispheres following intracarotid injection of a
convulsive drug, strychnine. Figure 3.26 shows that spike activity appears
periodically in the electrocorticogram with an ensuing decrease in oxygen
tension and enhancement of cerebral blood flow. The computed resistance
in blood vessels located distal to the circle of Willis decreased with
every attack of convulsive activity. This is evidence of dilatation of the
smaller brain arteries. The major brain arteries have an opposite tendency.
The latter vascular response is actually comparable to the vasoconstriction
detected during the asphyxic and postischemic hyperemias in the cerebral
cortex. The vasoconstriction of the major cerebral arteries is also probably directed toward normalizing excess blood volume in the cerebral vasculature under these specific experimental conditions.

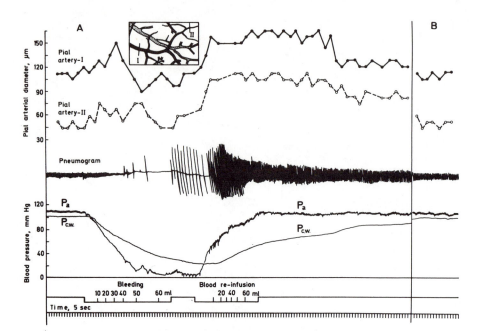

Fig. 3.25. Cerebrovascular responses following transitory stoppage of ce-
            rebral blood flow. Following a drop in systemic arterial pres-
            sure (P_a) to zero and its subsequent recovery (with recovery
            of cerebral blood flow), the pressure in the circle of Willis
            ($P_{c.w.}$) decreases, signifying an increase in the resistance in
            major brain arteries. Simultaneously, the pial arteries, espe-
            cially the smaller vessels (see the schematic drawing at the
            top), undergo marked dilatation. (Reproduced from Mchedlish-
            vili, 1960d.)

Thus, a great deal of evidence has accumulated for the existence of an
active control of constant blood volume, as a specific type of cerebral
blood flow regulation. This regulatory mechanism starts to operate as soon
as an excessive amount of blood accumulates inside the skull, regardless of
the cause of the disturbance, i.e., restriction of blood outflow from the
skull or excessive blood inflow from the central arteries to the brain.
These experimental data have further shown that the effectors of this type
of cerebral blood flow regulation are the major brain arteries, i.e., mainly the internal carotid and vertebral arteries, which constrict as soon as
the cerebral blood volume becomes increased due to any cause. The reduction of arterial blood inflow to the brain facilitates the recovery of
normal blood volume because of reestablishment of normal balance between
the inflow and outflow of blood to and from the skull. The feedback loop
of this regulation is shown in Fig. 3.27.

Unlike the constriction of the major brain arteries being regularly
observed under the conditions of increased cerebral blood volume, the pial
arteries respond, as a rule, with dilatation, which is probably due to
primarily deficient blood supply to the cerebral cortex under the conditions reported (asphyxia, postischemic state, increased neuronal activity,
venous blood stagnation). Only one conclusion may be drawn from these considerations: it is the major brain arteries that are the vascular effectors that regularly constrict under these circumstances and lead to elimina-

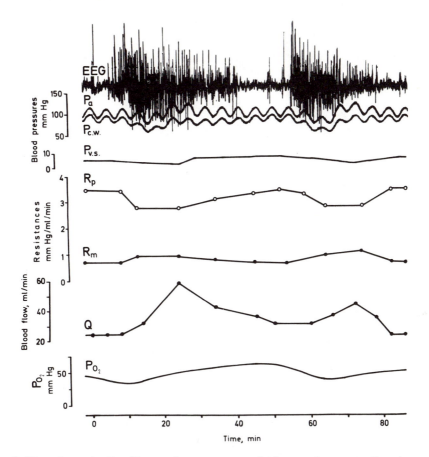

Fig. 3.26. Oppositely directed responses of the resistance of major and
            pial arteries during widespread functional hyperemia. Func-
            tional hyperemia in the cerebral hemispheres of dogs occurring
            simultaneously with periods of convulsive activity (seen in the
            EEG) in the cerebral cortex (caused by intracarotid administra-
            tion of 10 mg strychnine) results in enhanced cerebral blood
            flow (Q), increased pressure in venous sinuses ($P_{v.s.}$), and in-
            creased cortical P_{O_2}. During hyperemia, resistance in the
            small cerebral arteries peripheral to the circle of Willis (R_p)
            decreases, but the resistance in the major brain artery (R_m)
            has a tendency to simultaneously increase. P_a is the pressure
            in the aorta; $P_{c.w.}$ is the pressure in the circle of Willis.
            See text for details. (Reproduced from Mchedlishvili, Ormo-
            tsadze, et al., 1973).

tion of excessive blood volume from the cerebral vasculature. Because of
the oppositely directed responses of the larger and smaller cerebral arteries (constriction of major and dilatation of pial arteries), the cerebral
blood flow rate changes reflect the actual net cerebrovascular resistance
in every individual case.

     Disturbances Related to Increased Cerebral Blood Volume. Cerebral
blood volume *can* be increased in spite of the presence of several physical

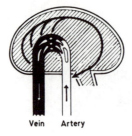

Vein   Artery

Fig. 3.27.   Diagram of the presumable feedback
            which operates in response to increas-
            ed cerebral blood volume and results
            in constriction of the major brain
            arteries, thus re-establishing the
            normal blood inflow-outflow balance.
            See text for details.

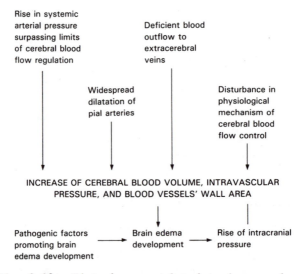

Fig. 3.28.   Disturbances related to increased ce-
            rebral blood volume.

factors (rigid skull box, incompressible cerebrospinal fluid, and almost
incompressible brain tissue), assisting in the maintenance of constant
blood volume inside the skull, as well as the aforementioned physiological
mechanism, which eliminates the excess accumulations of blood inside the
brain. Volume increases occur in two circumstances: either the disturbing hemodynamic factor (the excessive blood inflow or deficient blood outflow) are excessively great or the regulatory mechanism of the constant
cerebral blood volume is insufficient and does not properly provide control. The excessive blood volume accumulation in cerebral vasculature can
be harmful for the brain due to the following reasons. Increased blood
volume in brain vessels is always related to rises in the cerebral intravascular pressure, as well as to expansions in the cerebral blood vessel
wall area. These two changes represent important factors which promote
excessive water filtration from the blood stream into the brain tissue.

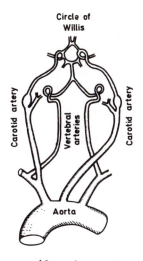

Fig. 3.29.   Diagram (from human X rays) of the four
             major brain arteries — two carotid and
             two vertebral — originating from the
             aortic arch and interconnected by large
             anastomoses at the base of the cerebrum
             where they form the circle of Willis.
             (Reproduced from Mchedlishvili, 1968.)

Therefore, if the brain tissue has been previously exposed to some pathogenic factors (trauma, hypoxia, etc.), then an increase in cerebral blood
volume considerably augments brain edema development (Mossakowski et al.,
1980; Mchedlishvili, Mossakowski et al., 1984). In addition, an increase
in cerebral blood volume immediately causes changes in the cerebrospinal
fluid pressure with ensuing symptoms such as headache.

     Figure 3.28 presents schematically the disturbances related, as
causes or effects, to cerebral blood volume increases.

3.3. STRUCTURAL AND FUNCTIONAL FEATURES OF THE VASCULAR
      EFFECTORS, THE MAJOR BRAIN ARTERIES

     Anatomic and Physiological Considerations. The major arteries of the
brain include primarily the internal carotid (to the periphery of the foramen
caroticum) and the vertebral (approximately to the periphery of the first
cervical vertebra) arteries. From the viewpoint of hemodynamics, these
four arteries cannot be considered separately in mammals, since they are
interconnected by large arterial trunks both at their origin (aortic arch)
and inside the skull, where they form the circle of Willis (Fig. 3.29).
Therefore, the major arteries of the brain operate as a unique vascular set.
Similar arterial sets include, in all probability, those of the large
arterial ramifications at the base of the brain, including the circle of
Willis, as well as the anterior, middle, and posterior cerebral arteries,
although their functional behavior has not been sufficiently investigated.

     The major arteries of the brain developed in the evolutionary process
of vertebrates from the anterior part of the dorsal aortic system (Romer,

1956). First there was only one pair of major arteries, the internal carotid arteries, that supplied the brain with blood (in fishes, amphibians,
and birds), but in the majority of mammals a second pair of arteries, the
vertebral arteries, was added. However, we encounter considerable anatomical variety in the set of major arteries in different mammal species
(Klosovsky, 1951). In some (ox, goat, marsupials) the main sources of
blood supply to the brain are the carotid arteries, while the vertebral
arteries are comparatively small. In other mammals (bats, guinea pigs,
lemurs, etc.) the vertebral arteries play a more important role in blood
supply to the circle of Willis, and the carotid arteries are insignificant.
Human beings and most laboratory animals occupy an intermediary position:
both carotid and vertebral sets are important for the blood supply to the
brain. In addition, there are considerable species-variations in blood
supply from the carotid arteries. For instance, in the cat family the internal carotid arteries are rudimentary and may even be obliterated; the
circle of Willis is supplied primarily via the developed branches of external carotid arteries, namely internal maxillary arteries, that create
multiple, complex anastomoses, the so-called *rete mirabile*, which are, in
turn, connected to the circle of Willis.

This great variability of anatomical arrangements of major arteries
of the brain is astonishing in different species of mammals. As a result,
neither phylogeny nor ontogeny give any basis for determining the priority
of any of the mentioned modes of blood supply to the brain (Klosovsky,
1951).

As we have already mentioned, until the end of the 1950s it was not
even considered that the internal carotid and vertebral arteries might exhibit any active physiological responses and be involved in the regulation
of cerebral blood flow. Some earlier experimental results, which can now
be interpreted as a manifestation of this arterial operation, remained un-
appreciated before by researchers. For instance, the simultaneous recording of blood pressure in aortic branches and in the circle of Willis actually revealed variations in vascular resistance along the major arteries of
the brain (Hürthle, 1889; Biedl and Reiner, 1900), but this was then interpreted in quite a different way, since the authors completely ignored the
possible involvement of these large arteries in the regulation of blood
supply to the brain. More recently an active spasm-like constriction of
internal carotid arteries has been observed by neurosurgeons in patients,
following mechanical stimulation of their vessel walls (Pool, 1957), as
well as after administration of X-ray contrast media into their lumina
(Brain, 1957; Raynor and Ross, 1960). This evidence brought forward the
possibility of active constriction of the major arteries of the brain, but
did not provide a proof of their active involvement in the regulation of
cerebral circulation.

The unexpected discovery in 1957 of the involvement of cerebral major
arteries in the active physiological regulation of blood supply to the
brain has already been described (Mchedlishvili, 1972, pp. 2-3; see also
p. 60): in experiments with rabbits the *in vivo* excision of part of the
parietal cortex (for microscopical investigation) immediately after occlusion of the jugular veins resulted in unexpectedly slight bleeding. Subsequent investigations showed that this resulted from constriction of all
the major arteries in the brain. This vascular response was interpreted
as a compensatory response, i.e., as a manifestation of cerebral circulatory regulation, since venous stagnation had not been found in the brain
under these circumstances. In later years an active role of the major
arteries in the regulation of blood supply to the whole brain was demonstrated in numerous studies under different experimental conditions (see

pp. 64-71). A long time was required, however, to establish the truth of
this finding.

Morphological Basis for a Neurohumoral Control of Major Brain Arteries.
Unlike other large arteries, which are generally elastic, the internal carotid and vertebral arteries are muscular; they have numerous layers of
smooth-muscle cells and relatively less elastic and collagen structures inside their walls. Only the initial (cervical) portion of these arteries
is predominantly an elastic type, like the other large arteries of the
body. The prominent muscular layer of the internal carotid arteries inside
the bony canals and venous sinuses contains smooth-muscle cells arranged
circularly or obliquely to the direction of the artery (Ter-Grigorian,
1962; Mchedlishvili, Kaufman, et al., 1971).

The active portions of the internal carotid and vertebral arteries
are difficult to approach surgically during life. Furthermore, they stop
responding to vasoactive substances, such as serotonin, as soon as their
bony surrounding has been surgically opened (the author's observations).
Once their regulatory function was discovered, one of the first problems
was to identify the arterial segments where the "closing mechanism" is
located, i.e., where the most pronounced active diameter changes in these
arteries might occur. To examine this problem their walls were fixed *in
vivo* by intra-arterial infusion of 20% formalin in ethanol under conditions
of experimental vasospasm produced by prolonged perfusion with isotonic
saline with a high potassium concentration (see Chapter 5) in anesthetized
rabbits and dogs. The arteries were subsequently studied in serial microscopic sections as well as in corrosion preparations made by filling their
lumina with self-hardening plastics and subsequent dissolving of the surrounding tissues in concentrated hydrochloric acid. The study revealed
that maximal constriction of the arteries occurred in the bends along their
course — within the cavernous sinuses for the carotid arteries and at the
distal part of the vertebral arteries near the skull.

During contraction of the muscular layer, the inner elastic membrane
of the internal carotid arteries becomes highly folded, and in some places
doubles, while pulvinate swellings project from the vessel walls into its
lumen. Thus the constriction of these arteries is frequently not concen-
tric, so that in places the lumen becomes stellate or even flattened in
shape (Mchedlishvili, 1959b; Mchedlishvili, Kaufman, et al., 1971). This
must be of considerable physiological consequence, because these changes
in vascular lumen shape (local invaginations, twistings, and so on) are
bound to give rise to turbulence in the flow of blood and thus cause a
sharp increase in intravascular resistance.

The walls of the major arteries in the brain appear to be particularly
rich in their supply of nerve fibers originating from the autonomic (sympathetic, vagus, etc.) and somatic (especially cranial) nerves (Klosovsky,
1951; Lazorthes, 1961; Fang, 1961; Kuprianov and Zhitsa, 1975). The internal carotid plexus consists of bundles of medullated and nonmedullated
nerve fibers, and contains nerve cells, both singly and in groups. In
addition to branches arising from superior cervical sympathetic ganglia, this
plexus also receives branches from the optic, occulomotor, trochlear, tri-
geminal, and abducent nerves. Branches from the glossopharyngeal, vagus,
and superior laryngeal nerves have also been described. The nervous plexus of the vertebral arteries receives, in addition to sympathetic branches
(from the inferior and middle cervical ganglia), branches from the vagus
nerves and from the first to eighth cervical spinal nerves.

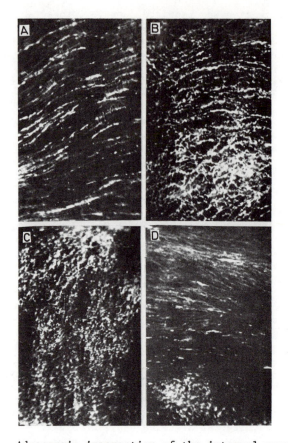

Fig. 3.30.   Adrenergic innervation of the internal carotid ar-
             tery. These photomicrographs show the localization
             of the catecholamines in nerves stained by the
             Falck-Hillarp histochemical technique in various
             portions of the internal carotid artery of the dog.
             (A) Cervical portion of the artery: brightly lumi-
             nescent, parallel nerve bundles in superficial layers
             of the adventitia; (B) cranial portion of the ar-
             tery: dense plexus of adrenergic fibers in the ad-
             ventitia (many of them show a granular character);
             (C) curvature of the artery: dense nerve plexus of
             thin varicose adrenergic fibers at the border of
             the muscular coat; (D) curvature of the artery:
             terminals of adrenergic nerve fibers in superficial
             strands of muscular tissue in the middle sheath.
             Magnification, 114×. See text for details. (Re-
             produced with permission from Borodulya and Pletch-
             kova, 1973.)

    The innervation of the human and animal internal carotid arteries has
been investigated histologically by silver impregnation techniques from
the carotid sinus to the circle of Willis (Borodulya, 1965; Kuprianov and
Zhitsa, 1975; Motavkin and Chertok, 1980). Receptors are richly represented in the region of the carotid sinus. Different receptors have also been
found in the cranial part of the vessel, especially in the region of the

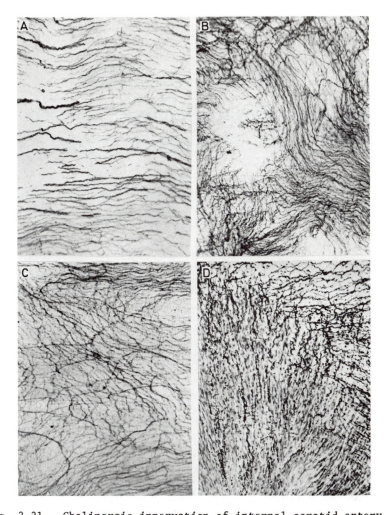

Fig. 3.31. Cholinergic innervation of internal carotid artery.
These photomicrographs show acetylcholinesterase
stained by the Koelle-Gomori histochemical technique
as an index of the cholinergic nature of the nerves,
in various parts of the internal carotid artery of
the dog. (A) Cervical region of the vessel: plexus
of cholinesterase nerve fibers running parallel in
superficial adventitial layers; (B) cranial segment
of the artery: dense plexus of cholinergic fibers
in the deep adventitial layers of the curvature of
the internal carotid artery; (C) cranial portion of
the artery: plexus of acetylcholinesterase nerve
fibers at the border of muscular coat in the region
of the curvature; (D) cranial segment of the artery:
the cholinergic nerve fibers in the superficial
layers of the muscular coat in the region of the
curvature. Magnification, 100×. See text for details. (Reproduced with permission from Borodulya
and Pletchkova, 1973.)

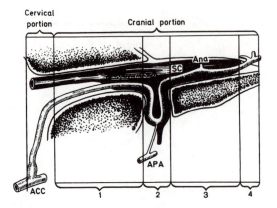

Fig. 3.32. Diagram of the topographic anatomy of the
            internal carotid artery of the dog.
            ACC is arteria carotis communis, APA
            is arteria pharingea ascendens, Ana is
            anastomosis with arteria ophthalamica
            externa, and SC is cavernous sinus.
            Various portions of the cranial part
            of the internal carotid artery are
            labelled: (1) inside the canalis ca-
            roticus; (2) the loop (curvature) of
            the artery; (3) the cavernous portion;
            (4) in the subarachnoid space. (Re-
            produced with permission from Toidze
            et al., 1983.)

curvatures of the internal carotid arteries (see below). Efferent innervation is particularly rich in the intracavernous part of this artery; the
adventitia contains a powerful plexus of bundles consisting of very thin,
nonmedullated nerve fibers. There is another plexus between the adventitia
and the media, from which thin fibrils penetrate the muscular layer, where
they form a third dense plexus.

     Detailed studies of the efferent adrenergic and cholinergic nerves
along the course of internal carotid arteries were carried out using the
Falck-Hillarp and Koelle-Gomori histochemical techniques for detection of
noradrenaline and acetylcholinesterase, respectively, in the vessel walls
(Borodulya and Pletchkova, 1973; Motavkin and Chertok, 1980). These plexuses are distributed similarly in man and many mammals (Motavkin et al.,
1981). In the cervical region of the artery, bundles of nerve fibers lying in the superficial adventitial layer are mainly parallel. The adrenergic and cholinergic fibers have never been observed to penetrate into
the muscular coat of the vessels. Apparently, most of these bundles innervate the distal parts of the internal carotid (Fig. 3.30a and Fig.
3.31a). In the intracranial part of the artery, the picture of innervation
is markedly changed. A still greater density of nerve fibers than that in
the cervical region is observed here. The number of longitudinal bundles
is reduced, the majority follow a spiral or annular course, and in deeper
adventitial layers they form a complex interlacement (Figs. 3.30b and
3.31b). The adrenergic and cholinergic nerve plexuses form a dense, multi-
layered sheath over the entire thickness of the adventitia in the intra-

cranial region. At the border of the middle sheath lies a plexus of very
thin granular fibers with varicosities which are undoubtedly neuron terminals (Figs. 3.30c and 3.31c). Terminal portions of adrenergic and cholinergic nerve fibers penetrating the middle vascular sheath and lying in the
superficial muscular bundles of the sheath can be distinctly seen in Figs.
3.30d and 3.31d. Thus, it has been noted that adrenergic and cholinergic
nerve plexuses in the cranial region of the internal carotid artery are much
denser than those in its extracranial part.

Studies of the topographic anatomy of the entire internal carotid artery in dogs (Fig. 3.32) show that the surroundings of the vessel permit it
to change its width considerably during regulation of vascular resistance
(Toidze et al., 1983). Almost two-thirds of the vessel is located in the
carotid canal of the temporal bone and continues into the cavernous sinus.
The cross section of the carotid canal is about three times larger than
that of the artery itself. The arterial wall is surrounded here by loose
fibrous connective tissue and venous plexus. Due to the low venous pressure and large lumina of the venous vessels, blood can readily be displaced
from them, as well as from the cavernous venous sinuses. Therefore, nothing
interferes with changes in the width of the cranial part of the internal carotid artery. The vertebral arteries seem to have similar characteristics.
This provides an anatomical basis for large changes of vascular width, and
thus, the resistance, of the major arteries of the brain.

Physiological Data on Neurohumoral Regulation of the Major Arteries
of the Brain. Though the majority of experimental evidence concerning the
functional behavior of the major cerebral arteries has been obtained in
experiments with rabbits and dogs, it can be assumed that this vascular
mechanism operates actively in all vertebrates. In amphibians, for instance, where the main functions of the major brain arteries are performed
by the internal cerebral arteries, a segment of this artery shows constriction in response to adrenaline and other stimuli, thereby regulating blood
inflow to the brain (Ormotsadze, 1969). On the other hand, active vasomotor responses in the internal carotid arteries have also been observed
in primates, including monkeys (Rothenberg and Corday, 1961) as well as
man (Pool, 1957; Raynor and Ross, 1960). Consequently, the role of the
major arteries of the brain in regulating cerebral blood flow is, in all
probability, the same in all vertebrates, including man. This function is
apparently also present even in those animals in which the internal carotid
arteries are almost obliterated and the cerebral hemispheres are supplied
by branches of external carotid artery and *rete mirabile*; in cats they
respond to adrenaline, as well as to strong stimulation of the cervical
sympathetic chain, increasing the pressure gradient between the aorta and
the basilar artery (Söderberg and Weckman, 1959).

Physiological stimuli regulating the vasomotor responses of the major
arteries of the brain may be of both a neurogenic and humoral nature.
Numerous investigations on the neurohumoral regulation of cerebral blood
flow have provided information about the behavior of the whole cerebrovascular bed, but they did not provide data on the differences between
functional behavior of specific vascular regions, in particular the major
arteries. The usual physiological techniques for investigating neurohumoral effects (i.e., direct exposure of the vessels to vasoactive substances or to artificial stimulation of vasomotor nerves), however,
cannot but produce disturbances of normal circulation within the brain;
thus it is difficult to obtain clear-cut results. Since the circulation
of the major cerebral arteries is provided with a considerably more refined control mechanism than elsewhere in the body, the disturbances
brought about by these experimental procedures are quickly corrected by

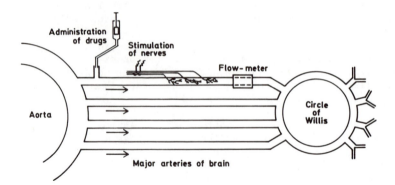

Fig. 3.33. Experimental arrangement for the study of the neural and humoral control of the internal carotid artery without significant disturbances in blood supply to the brain.

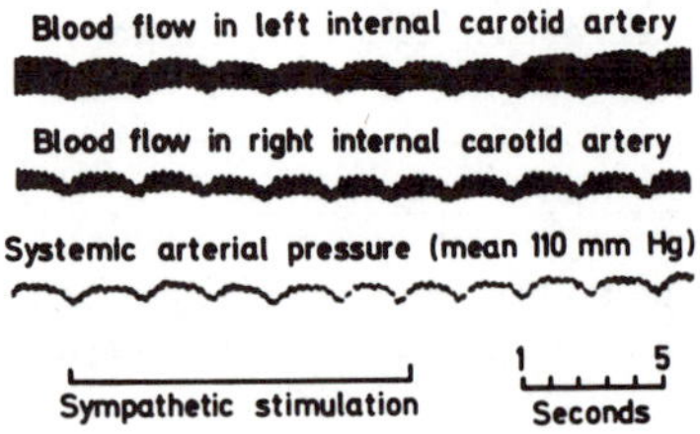

Fig. 3.34. Sympathetic vasoconstriction of the
internal carotid artery. Following
electrical stimulation (3 V) of the
left superior sympathetic ganglion,
the blood flow in the ipsilateral
internal carotid artery decreases
from 1.27 to 0.95 ml/min, while the
systemic arterial pressure and the
blood flow in the contralateral internal carotid artery remain unaltered. The blood flow has been recorded by differential manometers
and photohemotachometers. (Reproduced from Mchedlishvili, Garbulinski, et al., 1962.)

control mechanisms, while in other vascular beds these techniques provide
evidence of local vascular changes in spite of secondary circulatory disturbances. Thus, experiments on the neurohumoral regulation of cerebral
blood vessels should be carried out under conditions where the experimental procedure would not significantly disturb normal brain circulation.

Such an approach could be relatively easily applied to the major
arteries of the brain due to their anatomical peculiarity, i.e., their
parallel blood supply to the brain due to large interconnections in the
circle of Willis. Hence it is possible to affect single major arteries
without a considerable disturbance to the overall blood supply of the

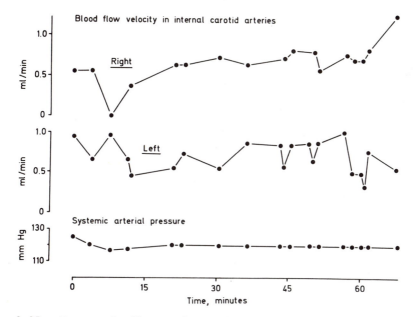

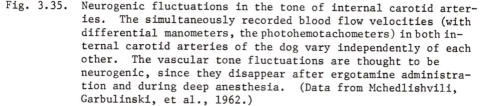

Fig. 3.35. Neurogenic fluctuations in the tone of internal carotid arter-
            ies. The simultaneously recorded blood flow velocities (with
            differential manometers, the photohemotachometers) in both in-
            ternal carotid arteries of the dog vary independently of each
            other. The vascular tone fluctuations are thought to be
            neurogenic, since they disappear after ergotamine administra-
            tion and during deep anesthesia. (Data from Mchedlishvili,
            Garbulinski, et al., 1962.)

brain (Fig. 3.33). Even small doses (0.5-1.0 µg) of adrenaline and noradrenaline considerably constrict the major arteries in dogs, whereas
acetylcholine causes significant dilatation; the blood flow rate in the
contralateral internal carotid artery remains unchanged (Garbulinski et
al., 1963). Electrical stimulation (2 V) of the ipsilateral superior sympathetic ganglia causes considerable constriction in the internal carotid
artery (the decrease in blood flow ranged from 17 to 71% of the initial
value) (Fig. 3.34). Stronger stimulation (6 V) usually causes blood flow
arrest, indicating total occlusion of the internal carotid artery lumen.
The absence of any effect upon the contralateral internal carotid artery
has suggested that neither the vessels in the circle of Willis nor the segments of peripheral cerebral vessels change their lumina significantly.
After intravenous administration of ergotamine, stimulation of the cervical sympathetic ganglia does not reduce blood flow in the internal carotid
artery over a period of 15-30 minutes (Mchedlishvili, Garbulinski, et al.,
1962). Similar results have been obtained under the same experimental
conditions in monkeys: stimulation of cervical sympathetic nerves results in a significant decrease in internal carotid blood flow measured by
an electromagnetic flowmeter (Meyer et al., 1967). However, the constrictor effects of cervical sympathetic stimulation on the basilar artery in rabbits is comparatively smaller; the pharmacological analysis has indicated
that the transmitter in this species is not noradrenaline (Bevan and
Bevan, 1977). In addition, considerable species differences in the cholinergic innervation have been found in the large arteries at the base of
the brain in rabbits, cats, and dogs (Florence and Bevan, 1979).

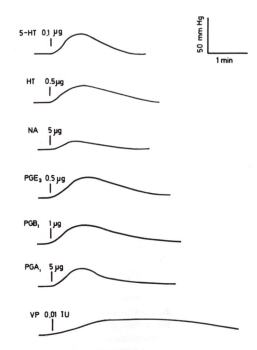

Fig. 3.36. The responses of perfusion pressure of
the isolated *in situ* internal carotid
arteries of dogs (for method see Figs.
3.19 and 3.20) to single intraarterial
administration of vasoactive substances.
5-HT, serotonin; HT, hypertensin; NA,
noradrenaline; PGE_2, PGB_1, and PGA_1,
prostaglandins E_2, B_1, and A_1, respectively; VP, vasopressin. (Reproduced
from Mchedlishvili and Ormotsadze,
1979.)

Other evidence for neurogenic regulation of the internal carotid
arteries has been observed during normal periodic fluctuations of blood
flow in these vessels; flow increases in one artery seem to cause reciprocal decreases in the other (Fig. 3.35). These blood flow fluctuations
disappear during deep anesthesia and following intravenous ergotamine administration, thus indicating a sympathetic regulation origin (Mchedlishvili,
Garbulinski, et al., 1962).

By measuring the resistance of isolated internal carotid arteries in
dogs (see p. 62-63) the effects of various physiologically active substances
(catecholamines, acetylcholine, serotonin, prostaglandins, etc.) were
analyzed (see also Chapter 5). The walls of the internal carotid arteries are very sensitive to these substances. The vessel resistance, which
reflects the vascular tone, varies within a wide range. The effects of
putative neurotransmitters, like noradrenaline and acetylcholine, are of
special interest with respect to neurogenic regulation. Evidence for the
specificity of the response of the internal carotid artery to cholinomimet-
ic drugs was shown by enhancement of their effects after inhibition of
cholinesterase by eserine and, in the case of adrenomimetics, after in-

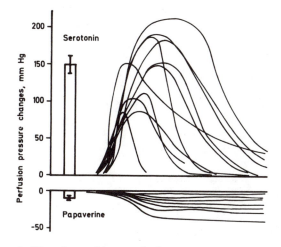

Fig. 3.37. Recordings of the comparative sizes of
constrictor and dilator responses of
major brain arteries during perfusion
pressure changes in isolated *in situ*
internal carotid artery of the dog
(for method see Figs. 3.19 and 3.20).
Constriction (increase in perfusion
pressure) induced by intraarterial administration of serotonin (0.1-0.4 µg)
is significantly greater than dilatation (decrease in perfusion pressure)
caused by intraarterial administration
of papaverine (1-2 mg). See text for
details. (Reproduced by Mchedlishvili,
Ormotsadze, et al., 1975.)

hibition of monoamine oxidase, e.g., by nialamide. On the other hand,
the dilator effects produced by cholinomimetics with muscarinic and nico-
tinic action are considerably weakened after the administration of the
specific blocking agents, while the effects of α- and β-adrenomimetics are,
as a rule, abolished by the corresponding α- and β-adrenergic blocking
drugs (Mchedlishvili, Ormotsadze, et al., 1969).

Single-dose effects of various vasoconstrictor substances on isolated
internal carotid arteries in dogs are shown in Fig. 3.36. The order of
potency of vasoactive substances has been found to be as follows: serotonin > hypertensin > prostaglandin E_2 > prostaglandin B_1 > prostaglandin A_1 > noradrenaline (Mchedlishvili and Ormotsadze, 1979). The comparatively low sensitivity of the artery to catecholamines seems to be of specific physiological importance: if the cerebral arteries readily respond
to increases in blood catecholamines (in stress, etc.), cerebral circulation
would always be affected, even when unnecessary or undesirable. But weak
responses of these arteries to catecholamines prevent such effects.

Another functional peculiarity of internal carotid responses was noted
during comparison of the effects of the most potent vasoconstrictor (relatively high doses of papaverine). It appears that constrictor responses
are approximately 15 times greater than dilator responses (Mchedlishvili,
Ormotsadze, et al., 1975), as indicated in Fig. 3.37. These results cor-

A. TRADITIONAL
MYOGENIC CONCEPT

B. POSTULATED NEUROGENIC CONCEPT

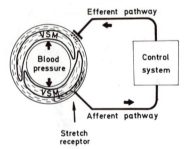

Fig. 3.38.   Two possible physiological mechanisms of cerebrovascular reactions in response to an increase in intravascular pressure that maintain constant blood flow
and pressure in brain vasculature during changes in
systemic arterial pressure.

respond to the number of vasoconstrictor nerves surrounding the internal
carotid arteries: adrenergic nerves have been found to be significantly
more abundant than cholinergic nerves (Sausa Pereira, 1979).   It can
thus be concluded that constriction is more inherent to major brain arteries than dilatation.   This functional peculiarity seems to be related to
their role in regulating the constant blood flow, pressure, and volume
within the brain, as considered in this chapter.   Thus, we come to the
conclusion that physiologically active substances circulating in the blood
stream, or originating in the nerve terminals or other structural elements
in the vascular walls, can exert considerable effects on the smooth muscle
of internal carotid arteries by causing their constriction or dilatation.

3.4.   A FEEDBACK LOOP RESPONSIBLE FOR THE ACTIVE MAINTENANCE
       OF CONSTANT CEREBRAL BLOOD PRESSURE AND FLOW

     This control of cerebral circulation is usually called "autoregula-
tion" since it was originally believed to be dependent on direct myogenic
responses of cerebral blood vessel walls to various degrees of stretch by
changing intravascular pressure.   This concept was widely recognized in
the 1950s and 1960s and still persists (Lassen, 1978).   Furthermore, experimental evidence that this regulation of cerebral blood flow is dependent on neurogenic mechanisms has steadily accumulated, implying that cerebrovascular resistance changes appropriately in response to information
from baroreceptors in the cerebral vessels (or carotid sinus) and subsequent neurogenic control.   Two possible physiological mechanisms for this
regulation of cerebral circulation, i.e., by the myogenic effect and by a
reflex involving neural pathways, are schematically presented in Fig. 3.38.
In both cases constriction or dilatation of specific brain vessels induces
changes in the cerebrovascular resistance such that the constant pressure
and flow in the cerebral vasculature are maintained within certain limits
despite alterations in cerebral perfusion pressure.

Evidence for a Myogenic Mechanism in the Control of Cerebral Blood
Flow.   The myogenic concept is actually based on studies of vascular smooth
muscle responses outside the brain (Folkow, 1962; Sparks, 1964; Johansson

and Mellander, 1975; Johnson, 1980); active contractile responses to passive stretch of isolated vascular segments have been demonstrated *in vitro*. The myogenic responses of smooth muscles in the umbilical, subcutaneous, and mesenteric arteries, as well as portal veins, are manifested in active contractions, as well as increases in their action potentials. It has been repeatedly shown that vascular smooth muscle reacts insignificantly to static stretch (when the distension of the muscles remains fixed), but the responses become evident when the stretch is dynamic (Mellander et al., 1980).

In addition, studies of blood pressure-flow relationships in isolated organs (kidney, muscles) have provided evidence that stretching vascular walls results in vasoconstriction with a respective increase in vascular resistance (Waugh, 1964; Johnson, 1980). The myogenic nature of these responses is thought to be demonstrated by the lack of effect of neural blocking agents, although it is difficult at times to reliably eliminate neurotransmission by various blockers (Bevan et al., 1980).

Pure myogenic responses have thus been attributed to cerebral blood vessels and are considered to provide adequate maintenance of constant pressure and flow within the cerebral vasculature despite changes in systemic arterial pressure. This myogenic concept of cerebral blood flow regulation actually originated during the period when brain vessels were generally believed to be deprived of neurogenic control (see p. 18).

The assumption that the myogenic mechanism is responsible for cerebral blood flow regulation was widely accepted, although convincing evidence of its actual involvement was scarce. The concept was mainly based on earlier observations in cats, where responses of pial arteries were observed despite dissection of the sympathetic, vagus, and several other nerves, as well as following application of cocaine to the vessel walls (Forbes et al., 1937; Fog, 1937, 1939). The authors believed that they had succeeded in completely depriving the cerebral arteries of neural control, but this was not true, since there are numerous other sources of nerve supply to cerebral vessels, especially in the major brain arteries (see above, p. 73).

Further evidence concerning the myogenic mechanism of cerebral blood flow "autoregulation" was obtained in dogs in which the responses of blood flow to pulsatile and nonpulsatile brain perfusion were compared (Held et al., 1969). Pulsatile flow was found to be more effective in maintaining a constant flow rate in brain vessels against changes of blood pressure level. However, the neural control of cerebral blood vessels was preserved in the above experiments and therefore the cerebrovascular responses could be myogenic as well as neurogenic.

The conclusion that "autoregulatory" responses in cerebral vessels are myogenic has been further drawn from experiments where responses are studied independent of changes in the chemical environment of cerebrovascular walls, and particularly under hypercapnic conditions (Symon et al., 1971-1972). However, since the innervation of cerebral vessels also remained intact in these experiments, the vascular responses could be both myogenic and neurogenic.

True myogenic responses of cerebral arteries have been observed with certainty only in isolated vascular segments *in vitro*. Orlov and his associates (1972) have confirmed the absence of active contractile responses of large pial arteries of cattle to static stretching. But the internal carotid and large pial arteries of dogs and human beings have been found

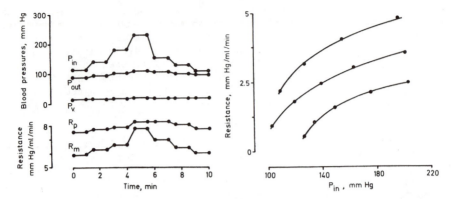

Fig. 3.39.   The response of the normally innervated internal carotid artery to changes in the inlet pressure in dogs. The inlet pressure (P_{in}, an analog of systemic arterial pressure) of the internal carotid artery (continuously perfused with autogenic
blood from the aorta) is changed by a constant-output pump,
but has little effect in the circle of Willis (i.e., the outlet pressure of the artery, P_{out}). The cerebral venous pressure, P_V, remains stable during this period. The resistance
in the internal carotid artery (R_m) changes in parallel with
the P_{in} and maintains the constancy of pressure in the circle
of Willis. To the right is a plot of the resistance in the
internal carotid artery against the inlet pressure in a series
of experiments. See text for details. (Reproduced from Mchedlishvili, Mitagvaria, et al., 1973.)

to contract in response to dynamic stretching, indicating that myogenic
effects might really occur in cerebral blood vessels under conditions of
rapid increases in arterial pressure (Orlov, 1979a). Similar results were
obtained with isolated middle and anterior cerebral arteries in the calf,
which responded to stretching (brought about by a rise in intravascular
pressure by 15 mm Hg) within the pressure range of 50-150 mm Hg (Vinall
and Simeone, 1982). As for the cellular responses in vascular smooth
muscle related to dynamic stretch, they seem to consist of depolarization
of plasma membranes resulting in muscular contraction (Johnson, 1980).

The actual problem to be solved is whether the net myogenic effect
of vascular smooth muscle could maintain constant cerebral blood pressure
and flow despite various changes in systemic arterial pressure. Comparison of experimental conditions in which the net myogenic response of vascular smooth muscles have been observed *in vitro*, with conditions where
cerebral blood pressure and flow are actually maintained at constant levels
could be helpful for solution of the problem being considered. Thorough
consideration of these conditions has been made by Mamisashvili (1979),
who drew the following conclusions. First, the stretching rate at which
the vascular smooth muscle develops a significant active response must be
very high (on the order of 20-25 mm·sec^{-1}), and is associated with a change
in intravascular pressure lasting 0.01 seconds. The cerebral blood flow
regulation being considered, however, does not depend significantly on the
rate of change in systemic arterial pressure. Second, for a significant
myogenic response, the stretching force of smooth muscle must be neither
larger nor smaller than forces occurring *in vivo*, i.e., approximately 40

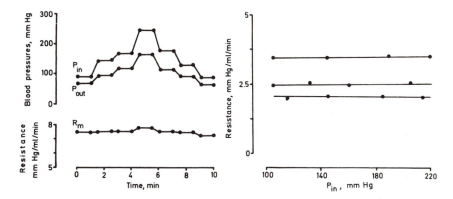

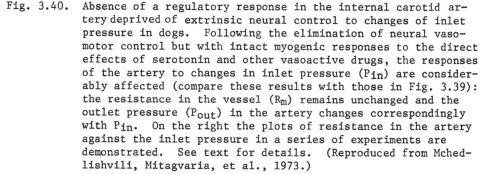

Fig. 3.40.   Absence of a regulatory response in the internal carotid artery deprived of extrinsic neural control to changes of inlet
pressure in dogs. Following the elimination of neural vasomotor control but with intact myogenic responses to the direct
effects of serotonin and other vasoactive drugs, the responses
of the artery to changes in inlet pressure (P_{in}) are considerably affected (compare these results with those in Fig. 3.39):
the resistance in the vessel (R_m) remains unchanged and the
outlet pressure (P_{out}) in the artery changes correspondingly
with P_{in}. On the right the plots of resistance in the artery
against the inlet pressure in a series of experiments are
demonstrated. See text for details. (Reproduced from Mchedlishvili, Mitagvaria, et al., 1973.)

mm Hg; the smooth muscle must be distended by 40-50% of its initial length.
However, cerebral blood flow is kept constant within certain limits of
arterial pressure changes independent of the character of these changes.
Third, the pure myogenic response of vascular smooth muscle actually lasts
1-2 minutes, while the period during which the cerebral blood flow is maintained at a constant level despite changes in systemic arterial pressure
might be very prolonged (sometimes even for years in hypertensive subjects). Therefore, it may be concluded that the net myogenic responses of
cerebral vessel walls cannot provide effective regulation of cerebral
blood flow. In all probability, cerebrovascular myogenic responses play
either a secondary role or else no role at all in maintaining constant
cerebral blood pressure and flow under conditions of cerebral perfusion
pressure changes due to alterations in systemic arterial pressure.

      Further Consideration Concerning the Role of Myogenic and Neurogenic
Responses of Major Brain Arteries in Maintaining Constant Cerebral Blood
Pressure and Flow. Identification of the effectors of the cerebral blood
flow regulation resulted in further investigation into the physiological
mechanisms responsible for vascular behavior involved in the maintenance
of constant cerebral blood pressure and flow against changes in systemic
arterial pressure. The major brain arteries have been shown (pp. 49-56)
to be the principal effectors of this type of cerebral blood flow regulation. In further experiments the functional behavior of the internal
carotid arteries in dogs during changes in inlet pressure in normally innervated arteries and those completely deprived of neural control was compared. These results are presented in Figs. 3.39 and 3.40. When the
neural control of these arteries is preserved, the stepwise changes in

pressure over a total range of 110 ± 12 mm Hg results in insignificant
changes in pressure in the circle of Willis. This is related to changes
in resistance in the internal carotid artery. The resistance changes in
the smaller blood vessels located peripherally to the circle of Willis are
negligible when the pressure changes in the latter are small and become
greater when they are more pronounced (Fig. 3.39). These experimental results permit one to conclude that the regulation of cerebral blood pressure and flow is primarily accomplished by the major brain arteries. The
smaller blood vessels (in all probability the small pial arteries) are
considered as a secondary (back-up) mechanism of regulation; they operate
when the primary mechanism (the major arteries) becomes inadequate for provision of a constant blood pressure and flow in the brain vasculature.

To analyze the feedback determining these responses in the major brain
arteries and discriminate between myogenic and neurogenic vascular responses, the neural control of the arteries had to be completely excluded.
However, since the major brain arteries (the internal carotid artery in
particular) have an abundant nerve supply from different sources (see p.
73), it was impossible to succeed in their complete surgical denervation,
though sympathectomy might decrease the regulatory responses of cerebral
blood flow (see below). To accurately deprive the arteries under investigation of an extrinsic neural control, the animals were sacrificed at a
given time (by bleeding from the femoral artery) but the perfusion of the
artery under investigation was continued with blood from a donor dog.
The muscular layer of such arteries reacted normally to vasoactive substances, particularly to serotonin, for several hours. With stepwise
variations in inlet pressure to the artery, its resistance did not change,
and hence the outlet pressure followed changes in the perfusion pressure
(Fig. 3.40). Similar results were obtained when the artery was perfused
with oxygenated Ringer-Krebs bicarbonate solution either under the same
conditions in a living muscular layer or after certain death of the arterial wall (after its prolonged perfusion with formaldehyde). These results
seem to represent substantial evidence that the feedback mechanism controlling the regulatory responses of the major arteries of the brain is of
neurogenic origin.

Further analysis of the myogenic or neurogenic responses in the internal carotid arteries in dogs to dynamic changes of intravascular pressure (simulating the "dynamic stretch") has been undertaken in an isolated
in situ artery with preserved innervation (see Fig. 3.21 on p. 63). The
artery was perfused with heated and oxygenated Ringer-Krebs bicarbonate
solution at pH 7.4. The arterial responses were investigated first under
conditions where neural control of the vessel was intact; neural control
was then deleted 15-30 minutes after killing the animal by exsanguination,
while the arterial perfusion persisted. The reactivity of arterial smooth
muscle to small doses of serotonin (0.5 µg and less) and other vasoactive
drugs remained comparable to that in the arteries before "denervation"
(Mchedlishvili and Mamisashvili, 1981; Mamisashvili et al., 1983).

These experiments indicated that during changes in intravascular
pressure the flow rate in the internal carotid artery changes considerably
less when neural control is preserved than when the vessels are denervated
(Fig. 3.41). This proves that only neurogenic feedback yields such changes
in vascular resistance and that it is this which provides a constant flow
despite changes in the perfusion pressure. This contrasts with pure myogenic effects, which cannot maintain this constancy. Comparison of arterial response in all experiments shows that normally innervated internal

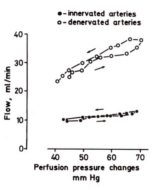

Fig. 3.41. Dependence of flow on perfusion pressure in an innervated and subsequent-
ly denervated isolated *in situ* internal carotid artery of the dog (for
method see Fig. 3.21). The artery is
subjected to uninterrupted perfusion
with heated and oxygenated Ringer-
Krebs bicarbonate solution. When the
neural control of the vessels is preserved (closed circles), a pronounced
tendency to maintain stable flow during changes in perfusion pressure is
observed. However, after complete
deprivation of extrinsic neural control to the artery (open circles), the
flow changed proportionally to pressure changes. See text for details.
(Reproduced from Mamisashvili et al.,
1983.)

carotid arteries respond at a mean rate of 5.0 ± 0.9 ml/min to changes in
perfusion pressure (approximately 50 mm Hg) (P < 0.001) but the denervated
arteries average 20.0 ± 6.8 ml/min.

Active responses in arterial walls with intact neurogenic control are
almost independent of the range of pressure changes. They have usually
been observed within ranges of 80-100 to 160-180 mm Hg. But in arteries
deprived of innervation, the myogenic effect was identified in only 25% of
tests and was detected solely during pressure changes within fairly narrow
limits of 20-30 mm Hg, e.g., from 110 to 140 mm Hg.

Vascular responses in a normally innervated internal carotid artery
are actually independent of the speed of change in intravascular pressure.
The results of the aforementioned experiments are presented in Fig. 3.42:
responses of vascular walls with intact innervation result in a constant
flow through the artery, independent of the rate of stretch. During
variations in stretch rates in normally innervated arteries, the difference between the maximal and minimal flow changes was 1.1 ± 0.6 ml/min.
However, this difference became significantly different (11.2 ± 5.3 ml/min)
in the arteries deprived of innervation (P < 0.001).

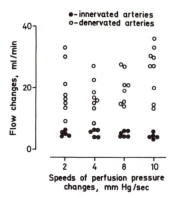

Fig. 3.42.   Dependence of flow changes on the
speed of perfusion pressure changes
in innervated and denervated internal carotid arteries (see Fig. 3.41).
When the neural control of the vessels is preserved (closed circles),
a pronounced tendency to maintain
stable flow is observed despite differences in the speed of perfusion
pressure changes. However, after
complete deprivation of neural control to the artery, the variations
in flow changes are approximately
ten times greater in the same range
of rates of perfusion pressure
changes. See text for details. (Reproduced from Mamisashvili et al.,
1983.)

Direct proof has thus been obtained that pure myogenic reactions of
specific arteries with respect to regulation of cerebral blood pressure
and flow are not sufficient for "autoregulation." They might, however,
offer a supplementary form of control of vascular responses under conditions of changes in systemic arterial pressure.

Analysis of the neural mechanism involved in the regulation of constant cerebral blood flow is difficult using standard physiological methods, although these methods have been used successfully for other vascular
beds. Dissection of nerves supplying cerebral blood vessels is difficult
since these blood vessels are supplied by different sources (see above).
In addition, the nerves are often very hard to approach surgically. Artificial stimulation of nerves containing vasomotor fibers is also difficult for the same reason. Another complication in the study of the neurogenic control system of cerebral circulation is its probable complexity
and, in particular, the presence of emergency (back-up) feedback loops,
which operate as soon as a disturbance (due to dissection or artificial
stimulation of vasomotor nerves) appears.

Although solid evidence now exists for the involvement of a neurogenic mechanism in the regulation of cerebral blood flow, experimental
data concerning the specific links of the mechanism are still poor. The

first link includes specific receptors in vessel walls that generate afferent signals which activate the whole feedback loop. The disturbance moni-
tored in this case is a systemic arterial pressure change, which immediately
causes corresponding changes in pressure and flow in the cerebral vasculature. Specific receptors that respond to blood flow velocity changes have
not as yet been identified in the cerebral vascular bed, but mechanoreceptors responding to intravascular pressure changes have been observed (Brown,
1980). Such receptors, called baroreceptors, have been identified both
morphologically and functionally throughout the cerebral vascular bed.

It might be supposed that the afferent signals involved in cerebral
blood flow regulation originate from the baroreceptors located in any part
of the systemic arterial bed. However, when considering the cerebral circulation, attention is naturally given to those baroreceptors located in the
walls of arteries supplying the brain. Such baroreceptors have been
studied in the carotid sinus. The sinus has a greater luminal diameter
than the adjacent arteries, and the vascular wall of the sinus deforms more
easily in response to intravascular pressure. The carotid sinus observes
the law of Laplace — the greater the vessel radius, the easier the wall
stretches in response to intraluminal pressure (Damask, 1978).

It is well known that the carotid bifurcation is surrounded by a
dense neural plexus that receives branches from the cervical sympathetic
chain, the glossopharyngeal, and the superior pharyngeal nerves. The
branch of the glossopharyngeal nerve, called the sinus nerve of Hering,
carries specific afferent signals from the sinus baro- and chemoreceptors.
The arterial adventitia of the carotid bifurcations contains two nerve
plexuses, a superficial and a deeper, which are considerably more dense
than those in adjacent proximal and distal arteries. The adventitial
plexuses consist of nerve bundles with both myelinated and nonmyelinated
nerve fibers, many of which have free terminals. Numerous baroreceptors,
appearing as an arborization of terminal endings of myelinated nerve
fibers and a very fine network of neurofibrils, are located exclusively
in the adventitia of the carotid bifurcation. The arborizations of the
baroreceptors may appear as more or less diffusely distributed sensitive
nerve endings among the connective tissue elements in the vascular adventitia (Borodulya, 1965; Kuprianov and Zhitsa, 1975).

Free nerve endings, structurally similar to the carotid sinus baroreceptors, were also identified morphologically along the internal carotid
and vertebral arteries, although considerably fewer receptors have been
observed in these arteries. These receptors are also formed from branchings of myelinated nerve fibers, but usually have a simpler form than
those in the carotid sinus. Only the cavernous portion of the internal
carotid artery possesses a considerably larger number of arborized receptors; therefore, this area has been considered by some to be a specific reflexogenic zone (Borodulya, 1965; Kuprianov and Zhitsa, 1975). Similar
myelinated nerve endings, morphologically comparable to the described baroreceptors, have also been found in the adventitia of branches of the
larger arteries at the base of the brain, as well as in the walls of
smaller cerebral arteries. But they usually have a small number of branchings and a relatively simple form, especially in the arteries of smaller
caliber.

Consequently, free nerve endings, which are thought to function as
baroreceptors and presumably respond to changes in intravascular pressure,
are distributed throughout the arterial bed of the brain. They receive
afferent nerve impulses and may relay signals to appropriate neuronal
areas, which in turn monitor the control system of cerebral blood flow.

Experimental data concerning the function of baroreceptors and the related physiological processes involved in the maintenance of constant cerebral blood flow, despite changes in systemic arterial pressure, are still
scant. So far only the carotid sinus baroreceptors have been studied and
in the earlier work results were rather contradictory (Bouckaert and Heymans, 1935; Cobb and Finesinger, 1932; Ask-Upmark, 1935; Gabashvili and
Mchedlishvili, 1965; Rapela et al., 1967). The inconsistency of these results may be explained by the extreme difficulty in attaining adequate experimental conditions to elucidate the function of baroreceptor reflexes
in the control of cerebral vasculature. The experimental conditions must
take into account the complexity of the cerebral vascular bed where several
sources of cerebral blood inflow and outflow are available; in addition,
cerebral blood vessels can be continuously affected from numerous baroreceptor zones. Therefore a rather complex physiological technique is necessary to elucidate the net effect of the carotid baroreceptors on cerebral
blood flow. Such a technique was formulated in experiments by Ponte and
Purves (1974), who showed that adequate stimulation of carotid baroreceptors in baboons resulted in a reduction in cerebral blood flow. These experiments provided evidence that constant cerebral blood flow during variations in perfusion pressure is controlled by the sinus baroreceptor reflex.
However, since the active changes in cerebral blood flow result from
changes in the integral cerebrovascular resistance, it was impossible to
draw any conclusions regarding which of the brain arteries actually changed
their lumina in these experiments. From experimental evidence discussed
earlier (pp. 49-56) we already know cerebral blood flow regulation is
brought about by the major brain arteries as well as by larger pial arteries. It seems reasonable, therefore, that afferent signals could reach
these vascular effectors and thus provide constant cerebral blood flow.
Other baroreceptors distributed along the major or other arteries of the
brain can, in all probability, also take part in this type of cerebral
blood flow regulation, although their physiological role has not yet been
analyzed experimentally. They may operate when the reflex from carotid
sinus baroreceptors to the major brain arteries becomes insufficient. The
hypothetical feedback loop of neurogenic regulation is schematically presented in Fig. 3.43.

Afferent impulses transmitted from the carotid or other baroreceptors
by respective pathways must reach the appropriate neural complexes, which
in turn integrate the information and monitor the whole regulatory system;
they are thus responsible for maintaining constant cerebral blood flow
against changes in cerebral perfusion pressure. However, it is not yet
known in which parts of the brain the specific centers are located, and
only a few studies have endeavored to solve this problem. Experimental
approaches to localize these neural complexes may involve either destruction or stimulation of specific structures of the brain.

The brain stem reticular formation may be involved in cerebral blood
vessel responses; this was seen in experiments with monkeys (Langfitt and
Kassel, 1968). An investigation of the effect of pyrithioxin, an acti-
vator of brain stem reticular formation, led to the conclusion that vasoconstrictor and vasodilator mechanisms within the brain stem can control
the tonus of the larger cerebral arteries (Stroica et al., 1973). But
direct evidence of an actual contribution of the brain stem to cerebral
blood flow regulation is still scarce.

The locus coeruleus has also been thought to be involved in this type
of cerebral blood flow regulation. In experiments with cats the effects
of bilateral destruction of the locus coeruleus on this regulation was investigated. The locus coeruleus influences catecholamine levels in the

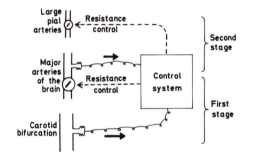

Fig. 3.43. The hypothetical reflex mechanism that
responds to central arterial pressure
changes and determines the effector
behavior of the major brain arteries
and large pial arteries, which are
directed toward maintenance of constant pressure and flow in the cerebral vasculature. The second stage of
the reflex regulation is thought to
operate when the first stage is insufficient. See text for details.

paraventricular hypothalamic nucleus, the anterior ventral nucleus of the
thalamus and the cerebral cortex, and is presumed to be involved in cerebral vasoconstriction. After experimental destruction of the locus coeruleus, however, the control of cerebral blood flow, with changes of the
systemic arterial pressure, remained intact (Bates et al., 1977). This
indicates that the locus coeruleus does not represent the center of inte-
gration of neurogenic cerebral blood flow regulation.

The efferent pathways controlling cerebrovascular resistance were
studied in the last decade. The majority of these studies were concerned
with the effects of the sympathetic system on neurogenic regulation. The
neural pathways from the cervical sympathetic chain to cerebral blood vessels have been known for many years and are easily approached for experimentation. The neurotransmitter of sympathetic nerve impulses to the
vascular effectors is noradrenaline (norepinephrine), and therefore transmission from sympathetic fibers to cerebral vessel walls can be blocked
by specific drugs. A series of experimental studies has dealt with sympathetic effects on cerebral vascular responses, and thus cerebral blood
flow, related to changes in systemic arterial pressure. Phenoxybenzamine,
a specific alpha-adrenergic blocker, was found to inhibit the constriction of cerebral blood vessels in response to increased arterial pressure
but potentiated their dilatation when the pressure dropped in patients
(Meyer et al., 1972). Furthermore, specific shifts in the curve demonstrating neurogenic cerebral blood flow regulation (see above, Figs. 3.2
and 3.3) are seen after changes in the level of sympathetic activity.
After sympathectomy and pharmacological blockade of adrenergic transmission, the lower limit of the regulatory curve is shifted toward a lower
level of systemic arterial pressure (Fitch et al., 1975). With an increase
in sympathetic activity this lower limit of the plateau of the curve
shifts in the opposite direction (Fitch et al., 1976), indicating that
cerebral blood flow regulation during decreases in arterial pressure becomes disturbed. The upper limit of the regulatory curve, on the other
hand, is even more dependent on sympathetic activity. Administration of

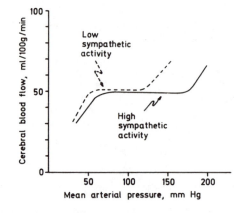

Fig. 3.44.   Shift in cerebral blood flow response
curve, i.e., increased constrictor
response, related to systemic arterial pressure changes during high sympathetic activity. See text for details. (Reproduced with permission
from Lassen, 1978.)

the adrenergic blocker, phenoxybenzamine, interferes with the maintenance
of constant cerebral blood flow at higher levels of systemic arterial
pressure (Kawamura et al., 1974; Kovách et al., 1979). There are, however, species differences — stimulation of sympathetic nerves results in
elimination of cerebral hyperemia with rising arterial pressure in rats
(Edvinsson et al., 1976) and in cats (Heistad et al., 1981), but not in
dogs (Busija et al., 1980). These experimental results may be summarized
or conceived as specific shifts of the whole pressure-flow curve, demonstrating the effects of low and high sympathetic activity on neurogenic
cerebral blood flow regulation (Fig. 3.44). Actually, the changes in
cerebral blood flow regulation during increases in sympathetic activity
were found to be analogous to those during chronic hypertension in man
(see p. 46).

It is quite probable that, in addition to the sympathetic system,
other efferent pathways may be involved in neurogenic cerebral blood flow
regulation, but they have not yet been studied.

3.5. A FEEDBACK LOOP RESPONSIBLE FOR THE CONTROL OF CEREBRAL
BLOOD VOLUME

Of the three possible physiological feedback mechanisms operating
during regulation of cerebral circulation — the myogenic, humoral (metabolic), and neurogenic mechanisms — it is only the neurogenic mechanism
that can be considered logical for volumetric regulation of cerebral blood
flow, since the information which originates from dilated cerebral veins
must reach the major brain arteries (see Fig. 3.27). Direct myogenic effects on the major arteries cannot assume a major regulatory role in this
case, since, first, the intraluminal pressure, which distends primarily
the arterial walls, cannot be considerably increased under these physiological circumstances (only a *decrease* in blood pressure in the arteries
of the circle of Willis was detected in the author's experiments); second,

myogenic effects were found to be inadequate in providing the necessary
arterial constriction even during significant rises in intravascular pressure (see pp. 84-88). Humoral effects on the major arteries of the brain
cannot be involved either: vasoactive substances would not be able to
reach the effector arteries from cerebral tissue by diffusion because of
the very great distance involved. As for the venous blood, which surrounds
the walls of the internal carotid arteries in the cavernous sinus, the metabolic substances they carry originate from cerebral tissue under conditions of deficient blood supply when humoral regulation occurs and should
cause dilatation rather than constriction of the major arteries.

During increased cerebral blood volume, regulatory feedback can originate, in all probability, from the walls of the distended cerebral veins
which are stretched by the increased venous pressure. A variety of mechanoreceptors are densely distributed on the cerebral veins (see below). Owing to the great distensibility of their walls, the cerebral veins, including their receptors, appear to be perfectly adjusted for perceiving changing blood volumes.

Evidence for a reflex from the cerebral veins to the major arteries
of the brain is still poor and generally indirect. On the one hand, there
is convincing anatomical evidence of abundant afferent innervation of the
intracranial veins (Kuprianov and Zhitsa, 1975). A nervous plexus surrounds the larger cerebral veins, and two other plexuses (a superficial
plexus and a deeper plexus) were found in the venous adventitia. The
smaller intracerebral veins are also surrounded by a nervous plexus in the
adventitial sheath, consisting of neural bundles and single fibers. The
majority of the nerve fibers are myelinated, have various diameters, and
are probably sensory in nature; there are also a small number of thin nonmyelinated sympathetic fibers. Abundant free sensory terminals of myelinated nerve fibers and other specific receptors have been detected in the
walls of cerebral veins of all calibers. The majority of the receptors
are terminal arborizations of free sensory endings with a simple or a
more complicated form (Fig. 3.45), and, in all probability, are the mechanoreceptors which respond to venous wall stretch. Specific receptor structures were also found incorporated in the pia mater, especially in the
medulla and the cisterna magna. Physiological evidence for the presence
of mechanoreceptors (baroreceptors) in the cerebral venous walls was obtained in animal experiments — an increase in pressure in venous sinuses
(and hence in the cerebral veins) results in reflex changes in systemic
arterial pressure and respiration (Vasin, 1959; Mikhailov, 1963).

On the other hand, although there is much morphological as well as
physiological evidence for the presence of efferent pathways to the major
arteries of the brain (see pp. 73-80), the experimental data on the involvement of the efferent pathways in the regulation of cerebral blood
volume are still scarce. Constriction of the major arteries of the brain
was found to be a response to a rapid increase in pressure in the cerebral
venous system (e.g., during simultaneous occlusion of all the venous
trunks in the neck or during a quick infusion of fluid into the venous
sinuses). This vascular reaction does not appear, however, when the pressure is increased in the extracranial veins of the head. Hence, the source
of information is probably from stimulated baroreceptors in the walls of
the cerebral veins, as well as those in the meninges (Mchedlishvili,
1959a; Mchedlishvili and Ormotsadze, 1962). However, in the author's
experiments, only the removal of the superior and inferior (stellate)
sympathetic ganglia in rabbits did not abolish reflex control. This indicates that other pathways may be involved in the sympathectomized animals.

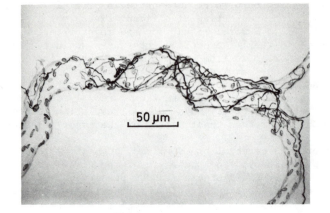

Fig. 3.45. Photomicrograph of neural plexuses in
            small cerebral veins. The free ter-
            minals of myelinated nerve fibers sur-
            rounding the walls of small pial veins
            of humans are shown after silver im-
            pregnation. Magnification, 400×. See
            text for details. (Reproduced with
            permission from Kuprianov and Zhitsa,
            1975.)

    Evidence for the involvement of the meningeal mechanoreceptors in the
constriction response of the major cerebral arteries has also been obtained
in experiments with dogs. The pressure gradient along these arteries increased significantly, by 34% over the initial value, during development
of brain edema (although the blood volume was not increased in the brain).
This effect may be interpreted as a compensatory response preventing or
restricting brain edema development (Mchedlishvili and Akhobadze, 1961;
Mchedlishvili et al., 1976).

    The input of the mechanoreceptors from the cerebral veins and meninges
must be integrated in the brain where appropriate centers monitor all factors controlling the cerebral blood volume. However, nothing is yet known
about the localization and function of neural centers involved in the control of cerebral blood volume. It is reasonable to suppose that these
neural centers may be similar to those which control the resistance in
the major arteries of the brain during changes in systemic arterial pressure, since in both cases the effectors and the vascular responses are
similar.

    Consequently, the feedback controlling the blood inflow to the brain
via the major arteries probably originates from the mechanoreceptors of
veins, and possibly small arteries of the brain, as well as from the pia
and dura mater in response to stretch. However, the localization of the
afferent pathways projecting from respective neural centers is still unclear.

3.6. SUMMARY

    Two types of cerebral blood flow regulation that maintain constant
cerebral blood pressure and flow, on the one hand, and constant cerebral
blood volume, on the other, are considered in this chapter.

Originally, it was thought that the regulation of constant cerebral blood flow, despite changes in systemic arterial pressure, was a function of the vascular smooth muscle itself. Thus, the term "autoregulation" originated. Further analysis of this physiological phenomenon, however, has clearly shown that no adequate evidence for myogenic responses of the cerebral arteries existed during the period when the concept of the myogenic nature of the regulation of cerebral blood flow was generally accepted. An important accomplishment of subsequent studies elucidated the effectors of flow regulation in the cerebral arterial system — the major brain arteries. The myogenic responses, which are characteristic of these arteries, failed to satisfy the requirements necessary to accomplish regulation of cerebral circulation. In the 1970s a large body of evidence concerning the neural control of cerebral circulation against changes in systemic arterial pressure accumulated. However, many questions still remain unsolved. In particular, little is known about which afferent neural pathways are involved, where the neural centers integrating these pathways are localized and how they function, which efferent pathways are involved, etc. All these questions require further investigation.

Another type of cerebral blood flow regulation is related to elimination of excess cerebral blood volume by restricting arterial inflow to the brain. The main vascular effectors of this regulation have also been found to be the major brain arteries. The regulation is accomplished, in all probability, by a reflex from mechanoreceptors in the cerebral venous bed and possibly from the brain meninges. The afferent and efferent pathways of the reflex, as well as the appropriate neural centers, need to be studied. The reflex constricting the major brain arteries in response to increased pressure in the cerebral venous bed is probably a specific example of the veni-vasomotor reflex described in other parts of the body (Vamada and Burton, 1954).

Both of the above-mentioned types of regulation of cerebral circulation may operate synergistically. During increased systemic arterial pressure, when both blood inflow to the brain and blood volume rise, the regulatory mechanisms considered start to operate. Resultant activation of the same effectors of regulation, i.e., constriction of the major brain arteries, maintains constant cerebral blood flow, pressure, and volume.

Chapter 4. Regulation Providing an Adequate Blood Supply to Cerebral Tissue

Adequate blood supply implies matching the flow rate in microvessels to the metabolic needs of the surrounding tissue. The metabolites present in the flowing blood, e.g., oxygen and carbon dioxide, should be at normal levels. Therefore the notion of adequate blood supply regulation includes, first, the adjustment of microvascular flow to the metabolic rate of the tissue supplied and, second, the maintenance of a constant oxygen and carbon dioxide content in circulating blood.

The activity of brain structures is closely linked with changes in their metabolism. Therefore, the blood supply to cerebral tissue must be continuously regulated to meet the varying demands of the tissue. It has been mentioned that, under resting conditions, the blood flow in cerebral microvasculature is much greater than that required to meet the metabolic needs of its tissue (Schneider, 1957). However, a marked rise in the activity of brain structures always causes an increase in microcirculation. The local blood supply regulation is, in all probability, the most reliably operating type of blood flow control in the brain. It can be investigated by measuring the actual blood flow in brain tissue under resting conditions, and then changing either the blood flow or the metabolic rate by any method, provided that the function of the appropriate regulating system has not been disturbed.

The local flow in the microcirculation, which has been measured in smaller brain regions, has not been found to be uniform throughout the brain. It varies considerably in different regions even under resting conditions, as shown by methods which provide quantitative data on the local blood flow. The ^{133}Xenon clearance method (Ingvar and Lassen, 1977b) was successfully applied for this purpose both in animal and in human cerebral cortex. It has a level of resolution of about several mm^3 of the brain tissue. A considerably higher level of resolution is provided by the autoradiographic methods that measure local cerebral blood flow and local metabolic rate in animals by the uptake of diffusible isotope tracers, e.g., ^{14}C-antipyrine and ^{14}C-2-deoxyglucose, administered in the blood (Reivich et al., 1975). This method provides a resolution of about 1 mm^3, not only in superficial brain structures but also in deeper ones. Application of these methods has shown that there is a great variability in local cerebral blood flow in different brain structures in awake rats and that a close relationship exists between the flow rate and glucose utilization. The

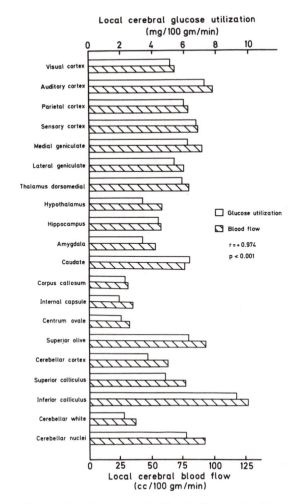

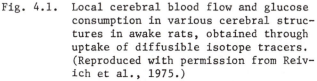

Fig. 4.1. Local cerebral blood flow and glucose
consumption in various cerebral structures in awake rats, obtained through
uptake of diffusible isotope tracers.
(Reproduced with permission from Reivich et al., 1975.)

values of local cerebral blood flow and local metabolic activity, presented
in Fig. 4.1, have been obtained in awake animals, where the natural regulation system of adequate blood flow is, in all probability, not disturbed.
The data show that local cerebral blood flow is perfectly adjusted to local
metabolic activity. In addition, the data demonstrate that the differences
in the local cerebral blood flow in various parts of the brain reflect proportional differences in the local metabolic rate, since the correlation
between these two variables is highly significant (the correlation coefficient = 0.974). Finally, the data prove that the functional state, the
metabolic activity, and the local blood flow are closely linked, i.e.,
regulated, in a way which ensures that the microcirculation is usually adequate in any part of the brain.

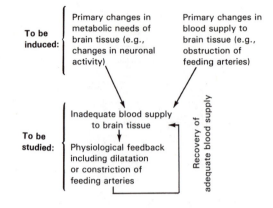

Fig. 4.2. Experimental procedures applied in in-
           vestigations of adequate blood supply
           to cerebral tissue, where regional
           blood flow in cerebral microvasculature
           is coupled to the metabolic demands of
           the tissue.

4.1. COUPLING BETWEEN BLOOD FLOW AND METABOLIC RATE IN CEREBRAL TISSUE

The regulatory system of the cerebral circulation operates to maintain conformity between the actual blood flow and the metabolic rate when-
ever it is disturbed. Hence, both deficient and excess blood flow in the
microvessels are corrected by active vascular responses involved in this
type of regulation of cerebral circulation.

Roy and Sherrington (1890) were probably the first researchers to mention the actuality of such regulation of cerebral blood flow. Since then
this coupling has become the subject of many studies, though the physiological mechanism involved in such regulation even now is not completely
understood in detail.

The standard approach to studies of this type of cerebral blood flow
regulation is to produce an inadequate blood supply to brain tissue in one
way or another. One type of experimental model involves a primary increase
in neuronal activity, and hence in metabolic needs, in cerebral tissue.
This is induced either by application of specific pharmacological agents
which evoke increased neuronal activity, like strychnine (Mchedlishvili,
1960b; Mchedlishvili, Baramidze, et al., 1967; Mchedlishvili, Ingvar, et
al., 1970), enfluorane (Myers and Intaglietta, 1976), or bicuculline
(Heuser et al., 1977; Astrup et al., 1978; Kuschinsky and Wahl, 1979), or
by stimulation of the cerebral cortex or respective peripheral pathways
(Leniger-Follert and Lübbers, 1976; Gregory et al., 1977; Leniger-Follert
and Hossmann, 1979). An increase in neuronal activity is followed by increased regional flow, which is nothing but *functional hyperemia* in cerebral tissue. Another type of experimental model involves the production of
a primary deficiency in blood supply to cerebral tissue by artificially in-
hibiting normal blood flow. The procedure may vary; either a temporary
(for a few minutes) drop in systemic arterial pressure to zero is produced
by withdrawal and subsequent reinfusion of blood (Mchedlishvili, 1960c) or
a continuous decrease in the pressure is applied to a level under the range
of regulation that would maintain sufficient blood flow in spite of a re-

duction in cerebral perfusion pressure (see Chapter 3) (Mchedlishvili, Nikolaishvili, et al., 1976); a deficient blood supply to the brain can also be produced by obstruction of individual cerebral arteries (Mchedlishvili and Ormotsadze, 1963; Hayakawa and Waltz, 1975; Molinary and Laurent, 1976; Pulsinelli and Brierly, 1979). In these experimental conditions either *postischemic (reactive) hyperemia* or intensified *collateral blood supply to cerebral tissue* is observed in the brain. These experimental procedures, which are applied in investigations of the regulation of adequate blood flow in cerebral microvessels, are schematically presented in Fig. 4.2.

These experimental models provide researchers with a tool to investigate circulatory phenomena specific for the regulation of adequate blood supply to cerebral tissue. Cerebral blood flow changes or cerebral vascular behavior under these conditions can be detected by a variety of techniques.

Coupling of Local Activity and Blood Flow. Since the 1930s, many authors have applied the above experimental models, and observed that a marked increase in neuronal activity is followed by enhancement of regional blood flow which can be measured by various methods. Thus, in response to adequate stimulation of the eye, an increased blood flow in the optic tract, in the intermediate nuclei, and in the cortical projection area has been demonstrated by several methods: by recording the temperature of the brain tissue with thermocouples (Serota and Gerard, 1938), thermistors (Cooper et al., 1966), or by thermoelectric techniques (Lugovoj, 1964); by using electroplethysmography (Antoshkina and Naumenko, 1960; Moskalenko et al., 1975); and by uptake of diffusible isotope tracers by cerebral tissue (Sokoloff, 1961). An increase in cortical activity, seen in the form of desynchronization of electrocorticograms after stimulation of the mesencephalic reticular formation, has been found to be accompanied by an increase in cortical blood flow; this had originally been shown by direct microscopic observation of the pial arterial responses (Ingvar, 1955), and later by recording blood outflow from the sagittal venous sinus draining blood from the corresponding area of the cortex (Ingvar and Söderberg, 1956). The same effect has been further demonstrated by recording cerebral blood flow with a thermoelectric technique (Krupp, 1966), by measuring blood outflow through the internal jugular vein with an electromagnetic flowmeter (Meyer et al., 1969), or by recording the tension of the hydrogen that is constantly produced electrochemically in the cortex (Leniger-Follert and Lübbers, 1976; Leniger-Follert and Hossmann, 1979). A similar increase in cortical blood flow has also been observed in awake cats; in addition to changes in the electrocorticogram, the animals' behavior (movements, orienting reactions) may also be influenced (Kanzow and Krause, 1962).

These results, demonstrating a coupling of local neuronal activity with blood flow, have been accurately corroborated in studies of neurologically normal, resting men with the use of an intra-arterial [133]Xenon technique and a 32-detector device placed over the dominant hemisphere. Different activities, including contralateral voluntary manual work and cutaneous stimulation, speech and reading, problem solving and visual activity, have been found to be accompanied by specific patterns of increased regional cerebral blood flow, which is summarized in Fig. 4.3 (Ingvar, 1975). An increase in blood supply to corresponding areas of the cerebral cortex in response to increases in neuronal activity is necessary for the maintenance of normal metabolism. Polarographic investigations have shown that at the very beginning of the period of increased cortical activity oxygen tension falls in the respective areas, but very soon, due to in-

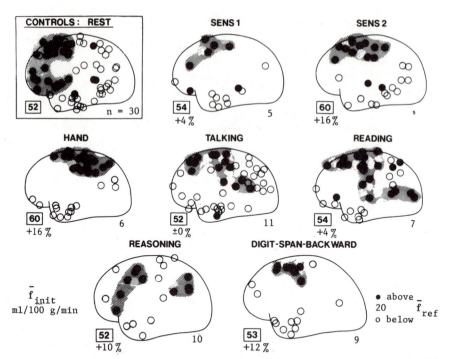

Fig. 4.3.   The effects of voluntary motor activity, sensory stimulation,
            speech, reading, memorizing, and reasoning tests on regional
            cerebral blood flow in the left hemisphere of the neurological-
            ly normal resting man. The values in boxes denote the mean ini-
            tial flow for a group; percent values below the boxes indicate
            the mean increase above resting state. The shaded areas show
            significant flow increases. Significant findings: (a) at rest
            the blood flow distribution is distinctly hyperfrontal; (b) dur-
            ing low and high intensity of contralateral cutaneous stimula-
            tion (sensory cortical areas 1 and 2) there is a precentral flow
            activation, which increases with stimulation intensity; (c) dur-
            ing contralateral voluntary manual work, the main flow increase
            takes place over the rolandic and parietal regions; (d) during
            speech and reading, a "z"-like activation pattern is induced
            over premotor, rolandic, and the sylvian regions — during read-
            ing the lower part of the "z" is especially marked; (e) problem
            solving, which includes visual activity (reasoning), augments
            the flow over the pre- and postcentral association cortex; (f)
            if visual activity is not involved in problem solving, only a
            premotor activation is observed. (Reproduced with permission
            from Ingvar, 1975.)

creased blood flow, it recovers and even exceeds its original level (Ingvar
et al., 1962). An increase in oxygen consumption in the cerebral cortex
during augmented neural activity was demonstrated (Meyer et al., 1969).
Local cerebral metabolic use of oxygen (using blood labeled with the cyclo-
tron-produced isotope ^{15}O) and local cerebral blood flow (using ^{15}O-labeled
water) were compared in humans during changes in functional activity of the
cerebral cortex. The data so obtained provide direct evidence that the regional blood flow is coupled to cerebral oxidative metabolism, as shown in
Fig. 4.4 (Raichle et al., 1976).

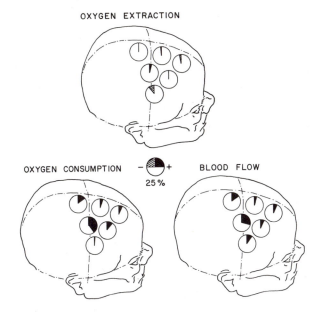

Fig. 4.4. Simultaneous changes in the regional cerebral blood
           flow and cerebral metabolic rate of oxygen in the
           right hemisphere in man during contralateral arm work
           (observed using oxygen isotope techniques). Segments
           of circles show an increase (black) or decrease
           (shaded) of the values in percent. (Reproduced with
           permission from Raichle et al., 1975.)

     The proportional relationship between local cerebral glucose utiliza-
tion and cerebral blood flow (measured using the ^{14}C-deoxyglucose and ^{14}C-iodo-
antipyrine techniques, respectively) was convincingly shown in normal, conscious rats; a very high correlation coefficient obtained (r = 0.96) demonstrated a tight coupling of the microcirculation with carbohydrate metabolism in brain tissue (Kuschinsky et al., 1981). These experimental results
are presented in Fig. 4.5.

     An opposite state has been observed in patients with comas of differ-
ent origin (post-anoxic, post-traumatic, etc.). Their cerebral oxygen uptake is significantly decreased and cerebral blood flow is consequently reduced due to loss of consciousness (Lassen, 1959; Baldy-Moulinier and
Frèrebeau, 1969).

     The coupling of regional cerebral blood flow with the functional and
metabolic activities in brain tissue has been convincingly demonstrated by
many investigators. The following sequence of events is apparent: enhanced neuronal activity in any region of the brain results in an increased
metabolic rate and an augmented energy production by oxidative glucose
utilization, which is necessary for increased ion pumping in membranes and
for transmitter synthesis in the respective brain structures. This is inevitably coupled with an increased blood supply to these tissue regions.
Thus, the same sequence of events occurs in the brain that occur in other
tissues, such as muscles and glands, where enhanced function is always
coupled with an increased rate of microcirculation.

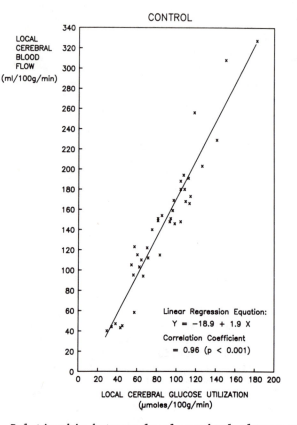

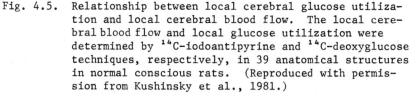

Fig. 4.5. Relationship between local cerebral glucose utiliza-
          tion and local cerebral blood flow. The local cere-
          bral blood flow and local glucose utilization were
          determined by ^{14}C-iodoantipyrine and ^{14}C-deoxyglucose
          techniques, respectively, in 39 anatomical structures
          in normal conscious rats. (Reproduced with permis-
          sion from Kushinsky et al., 1981.)

     The regulation of adequate blood supply to cerebral tissue may thus
be visualized as a relationship in which regional cerebral blood flow is
proportionally related to brain tissue function and metabolism (Fig. 4.6).
The link between local activity and hence the metabolic needs of tissue,
on the one hand, and rate of microcirculation in the tissue, on the other,
cannot occur without a feedback loop relating these two local functions.
This means that information from the tissue metabolism must be transmitted
to the blood vessels about the actual demand in the blood supply, and the
microcirculation must always be immediately adjusted by these control signals to the actual metabolic needs. This feedback loop, which maintains
adequate regional blood flow regulation, is schematically represented in
Fig. 4.7. There might also be a feedforward mechanism linking the neuronal activity with the rate of microcirculation (Kuschinsky, 1982-1983). In
this case the signals initiating the increased neuronal activity (with respectively enhanced metabolism) reach both the neurons and the appropriate
feeding arteries simultaneously (Fig. 4.7). In this case the increase in
microcirculation occurs at the same time as the increase of neuronal activity.

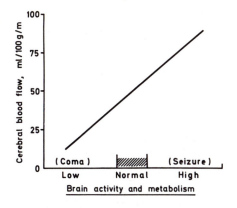

Fig. 4.6.   Dependence of regional cerebral blood
            flow on brain activity and metabolism.
            (Reproduced with permission from Lassen,
            1978.)

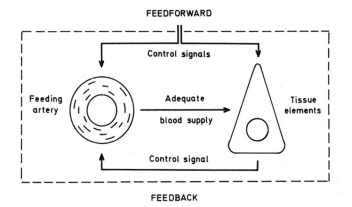

Fig. 4.7.   Feedback control of adequate blood supply occurring in
            regulatory mechanisms that couple neuronal activity
            and blood supply to the tissue. The feedback control
            signals originate in the tissue and reach the feeding
            arteries. The feedforward control signals which cause
            an increase in neuronal activity simultaneously reach
            the feeding arteries and result in appropriate changes
            of microcirculation within the tissue. (Reproduced
            from Mchedlishvili and Baramidze, 1984.)

     The flow rate in a microvascular region, irrespective of its size
(i.e., the whole brain or a single microvessel), is ultimately dependent
upon the general principle of flow, already mentioned on pp. 6 and 44 of
this book, i.e., $F = \Delta P/R$, where F is blood flow, ΔP is perfusion pressure,
and R is vascular resistance. This means that the enhancement of blood
flow, related in this case to increases in tissue metabolic demands, must
be dependent either on increases in perfusion pressure (e.g., caused by a
rise in the systemic arterial pressure) or on decreases in local vascular
resistance.

As in Chapter 2 (p. 18), both physiological experiments and observations in humans have repeatedly shown that systemic arterial pressure, and hence cerebral perfusion pressure, do not increase in response to a deficient blood supply to cerebral tissue, except in the specific regions related to systemic arterial pressure regulation. Thus far, it has been proved that any increase in cerebral blood flow related to the degree of neuronal activity is due to dilatation of the vessels in the brain itself, and can occur even if the perfusion pressure level has been either stabilized artificially or does not increase naturally. Therefore it is the decrease in local cerebrovascular resistance that should be considered as the physiological mechanism responsible for enhanced cerebral blood flow while the metabolic demands of the cerebral tissue have been increased.

Vascular Effectors of the Physiological Regulation System That Adjust Local Cerebral Blood Flow to Tissue Metabolic Needs. Without identifying the vascular effectors it is hardly possible to efficaciously investigate the physiological mechanisms regulating cerebral blood vessel behavior when the coupling of regional blood flow with functional and metabolic activities of brain tissue is fulfilled. However, the problem of identifying which cerebral blood vessels are actually involved in regulating adequate blood supply to cerebral tissue was not considered before the 1960s.

In the earliest studies carried out with rabbits, the functional state of the major and pial arteries has been compared under conditions of increased cortical activity (caused by local application of strychnine to the cerebral surface). The arterial pressure in both the aorta and the circle of Willis remained unchanged, thus indicating that the resistance in the major arteries of the brain (the internal carotid and vertebral arteries) had been unaffected. In contrast, the pial arteries were found to be dilated under these conditions (Mchedlishvili, 1960b). The areas of strychnine application, of the spike discharges in electrocorticograms, and of dilatation of the pial arteries have been found to coincide in the cerebral cortex. Further, it has been revealed that the smaller the caliber of the pial arteries, the greater is their dilatation; thus, arteries with an initial diameter smaller than 75 μm dilate twice as much as the wider vessels (Fig. 4.8). The relationship between the degree of vasodilatation and the initial vascular diameter is shown in Fig. 4.9. The local blood flow in the cerebral cortex, estimated from the hydrogen clearance technique, is considerably increased (by 50-100%) under these conditions. The pial vasodilatation and the enhanced blood flow in respective cerebral regions in these experiments are due to increased activity in the cerebral cortex, but these vascular effects are independent of the direct effect of strychnine on pial vessel walls. The latter result was then ruled out since the direct microapplication of the drug to pial arteries does not cause their dilatation, and can even result in vasoconstriction (Mchedlishvili, 1963), similar to strychnine's usual effect on arteries outside the brain. Regular dilatation of the pial arteries following the application of other convulsive drugs — enflurane, pentylenetetrazole, and bicuculline — to the cerebral cortex of cats has also been observed in more recent studies (Myers and Intaglietta, 1976; Kuschinsky and Wahl, 1979). The calcium channel blocker — nifedipine — causes pial vasodilatation,* and the smaller arteries show, in this case, considerably more diameter changes than the larger vessels (Brandt et al., 1979).

---

*The intrinsic processes in arterial smooth muscle connected with vascular tone changes definitely involve calcium ions.

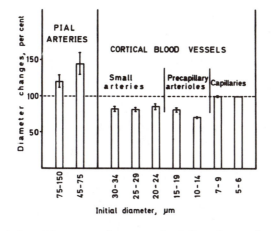

Fig. 4.8. Diameter changes of pial and cortical
           blood vessels during increased metabolic
           activity in the cortex of rabbits. The
           pial arteries undergo regular dilatation;
           smaller vessels are more dilated than the
           larger ones. In contrast, the luminal
           diameter of parenchymal vessels in the
           cerebral cortex (small arteries and
           arterioles) has usually decreased due to
           contraction; the diameter of the true
           capillaries is unchanged. (Reproduced
           from Mchedlishvili, Baramidze, et al.,
           1967.)

     Similar changes in the major and pial blood vessels have been found
to occur in the postischemic state when cerebral blood flow is regularly
increased compared to the preischemic period, which serves as the control.
In the postischemic state, following 1-2 minutes of stoppage of cerebral
blood flow (caused in rabbits by dropping the systemic arterial pressure
to zero by exsanguination), the blood flow increases by approximately 123%,
as estimated by the hydrogen clearance technique (Mchedlishvili et al.,
1974). The pressure difference between the aorta and the circle of Willis,
reflecting the resistance in the major arteries (internal carotid and
vertebral arteries), increases by a mean of 177%. This is evidence that
the major brain arteries do not dilate in the postischemic period but, on
the contrary, undergo constriction, and are therefore not involved in the
postischemic hyperemia of brain tissue. The reestablishment of the initial state of resistance in the major arteries takes place within 20-30
minutes after the recovery of cerebral blood flow from ischemia (Mchedlishvili, 1960c). Similar results have been obtained during the postischemic period in dogs, when cerebral ischemia has been produced either
by a complete drop in systemic arterial pressure or by a significant increase in intracranial pressure. Under these circumstances the pressure
gradient in the major cerebral arteries rises by 60% and 64%, respectively.
The conclusion that the major brain arteries constrict under these conditions has been further corroborated in experiments where flow resistance
through circulatory isolated internal carotid arteries has been measured
(Mchedlishvili, 1972).

     In contrast to this constrictor response in the major arteries, the
pial arteries show dilatation in the postischemic state of the brain. The

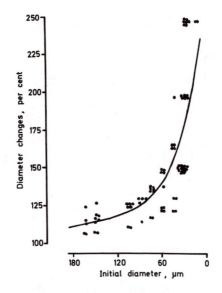

Fig. 4.9.   Relationship between resting diameter of
pial arteries and degree of dilatation
of the arteries during increased cerebral cortex activity by strychnine application to the cerebral surface. Pial
arteries with smaller resting diameters
(under 100 µm) dilate more than vessels
larger than 100 µm. (Reproduced from
Mchedlishvili, Baramidze, et al., 1974-
1975.)

vessels with a smaller initial diameter are dilated to a greater extent
than the larger vessels (Fig. 4.10). The dependence of the degree of pial
arterial dilatation on the initial diameter of the blood vessels is shown
in Fig. 4.11. An analogous relationship between pial arterial dilatation
and the resting diameter of the blood vessels has been shown during vasodilatation produced by a deficient blood supply to the cerebral cortex resulting from a considerable decrease in systemic arterial pressure (Mchedlishvili, Nikolaishvili, et al., 1971, 1976; MacKenzie et al., 1979).
This pial arterial response is shown in Fig. 3.8 on p. 51.

Consequently, enhanced cerebral blood flow during functional and postischemic hyperemias is related to a significant dilatation of the pial
arteries, especially those of smallest diameter. The major arteries of
the brain, on the contrary, do not dilate appreciably; moreover, during
postischemic hyperemia in the whole brain they even exhibit an obvious
vasoconstrictor response (this response has been considered in detail on
pp.66-67 in Chapter 3). These peculiarities in cerebrovascular behavior provide evidence that the smallest pial arteries are, in all probability, the
vascular effectors involved in the regulation of adequate blood supply to
cerebral tissue, in contrast to the major arteries, which certainly do not
fulfill this function.

As for the terminal arterial ramifications plunging into the cerebral
cortex, their functional behavior remains an unsolved problem. Evidence

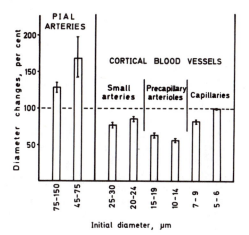

Fig. 4.10. Diameter changes of pial and cortical blood vessels during the postischemic state in the brain. After temporary stoppage of cerebral blood flow in rabbits, the pial arteries, especially those with a larger resting diameter, dilate, while the internal diameter of microvessels in the depth of the cortex decreases. (Reproduced from Mchedlishvili, Baramidze, et al., 1967.)

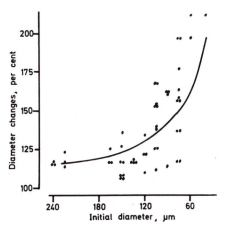

Fig. 4.11. Dilatation of pial arteries of various resting diameters during the post-ischemic state in the brain. Following a 1-2 minute stoppage of cerebral blood flow in rabbits, a predominant dilatation of the smaller pial arteries is observed. Figure 4.9 shows the same relationship during increased activity in the cerebral cortex. (Reproduced from Mchedlishvili, Baramidze, et al., 1974-1975.)

for vasomotor responses in these vessels is still rather poor since, in contrast to the pial arteries, they are still inaccessible for direct *in vivo* observations. The cortical arteries enter the cerebral cortex almost perpendicular to its surface and are then called radial arteries. Along the course of these vessels, minute arteriolar offshoots undergo further ramifications, and finally form the cortical capillary network.

The middle coat of the cortical arteries is composed of a few, gradually decreasing number of smooth muscle cell layers. *In vivo* fixation by perfusion of the cerebral vasculature with formaldehyde solution under standard conditions shows that the parenchymal arterial muscle cell nuclei become significantly shortened and thickened during functional and asphyxic hyperemias in the cortex compared to control conditions (Baramidze and Mchedlishvili, 1970). These changes in the arterial smooth muscle of cerebral parenchyma are comparable to those detected in mesenteric arteries constricted by adrenaline (Van Citters et al., 1962; Lang, 1965).

Further evidence for the weak vasomotor activity in the cortical (parenchymal) arteries is the sparse efferent vasomotor nerve supply to their walls. In this respect, the cortical arteries differ considerably from the adjacent pial arteries, and are more like the cortical capillaries (Harper et al., 1972; Cervós-Navarro, 1977). The nerve fibers accompanying the cerebral vessel walls originate from the central noradrenergic system (the locus coeruleus) and are thought to be related to the permeability of the vessel walls (Raichle et al., 1975).

The chemical composition of intracerebral (parenchymal) arterial walls, in this respect, is more comparable to the walls of the cerebral capillaries than to other arteries. The arterial walls contain enzymes (in particular, nucleotide phosphatases) which are known to be involved in the transport of substances across vascular walls (Torack and Barrnett, 1964; Baramidze and Zelman, 1974). Convincing evidence for the contribution of the cortical arteries to blood-brain-barrier function is the presence of a sparse network of capillaries surrounding the cortical arteries (Fig. 4.12), thus indicating that the surrounding tissue is fed directly from these arteries (Cervós-Navarro and Rozas, 1978).

The distinctive patterns of pial and cortical arterial behavior correspond to their topographical anatomy. As we have already mentioned (p. 14), the pial arteries are located on the cerebral surface inside the relatively wide canals of subarachnoid space and are surrounded by cerebrospinal fluid (Fig. 4.13). This fluid is under a relatively low pressure and is readily displaced in the subarachnoid canals. Therefore, the pial arteries can change their width over a wide range without mechanically affecting the cerebral cortex. The smaller arteries lying within the cortex are covered from the outside by connective tissue and glial structures; there is no free space around their walls (Luse, 1962; Pease and Schultz, 1962). Therefore, if dilatation of these vessels does occur, it would exert mechanical pressure on the surrounding structures of cerebral tissue. These anatomical characteristics of the pial and cortical (parenchymal) arteries are schematically shown in Fig. 4.14.

The results of the very few direct investigations of the vasomotor responses of the cortical arterial branches carried out are more contradictory than complementary. In experiments performed at the author's laboratory, the parenchymal arteries of the cortex were investigated in histological slices following *in vivo* fixation of the vessels walls by perfusion of formaldehyde under standard conditions. During strychnine application to the cortical surface, the number of active capillaries (with

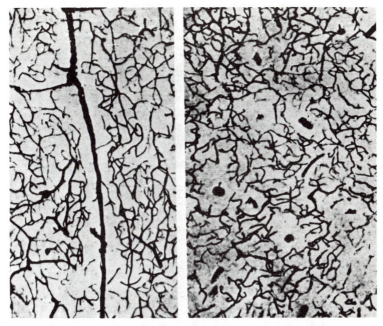

Fig. 4.12.   Photomicrographs of the sparse capillary network (containing
             India ink) surrounding arterial branches in the depth of the
             human parietal cortex. The tissue surrounding the radial ar-
             tery is devoid of capillaries, thus proving that the tissue is
             fed directly by these arteries. (Reproduced with permission
             from Cervós-Navarro and Rozas, 1978.)

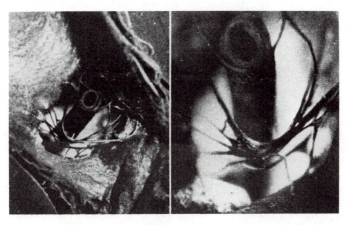

Fig. 4.13.   Photomicrograph of a pial artery suspended from a channel wall
             in the cerebrospinal space on chordae, which stabilize the
             position of the artery in the channel. Right: high-power
             view of the same artery. The comparatively large space sur-
             rounding the arterial walls allows for considerable diameter
             changes of the vessels without mechanically affecting the
             cerebral tissue. (Reproduced by permission from Arutiunov et
             al., 1974.)

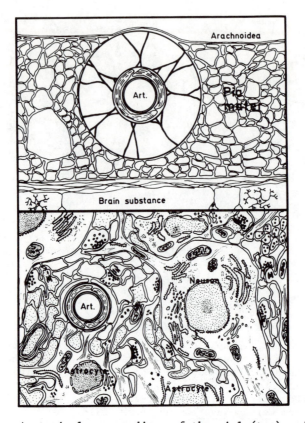

Fig. 4.14. Anatomical surroundings of the pial (top) and the
            cortical (parenchymal) (bottom) arteries. The posi-
            tion of the pial arteries inside large channels in
            the subarachnoid space allows for diameter changes
            within large limits without affecting brain tissue
            (which is actually far from the vessel walls). In
            contrast, the parenchymal arteries of the cerebral
            cortex are closely surrounded by tissue structures
            and have no free space in which to expand.

an open lumen and filled with red cells and plasma) per unit of cortical
tissue volume increases by one-third compared to the contralateral (control) hemisphere (Mchedlishvili, 1956b). A thorough examination of the
diameter of the cortical arterial branches has demonstrated that under
various conditions of increased blood flow in the cortex (functional and
postischemic hyperemias, primary deficiency of blood supply, and asphyxia)
the external diameter of the cortical arteries does not increase and, on
the contrary, shows a tendency to decrease somewhat. At the same time,
the internal vascular diameter, and hence the lumen, of the small cortical
arteries and particularly of the precapillary arteries, decreases (Fig.
4.15). When convulsive activity in the cerebral cortex due to strychnine
application lasts longer, the luminal contraction of the cerebral arteries
exhibits a uniform tendency to continue (Fig. 4.16). This is related to a
decrease in cortical blood flow to levels even lower than the initial blood
flow (Mchedlishvili, Baramidze, et al., 1970b). Experimental results,
which disagree with these data, were obtained under conditions of hyper-

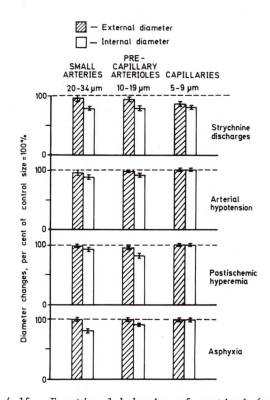

Fig. 4.15. Functional behavior of cortical (parenchymal) arterial ramifications and diameter of capillaries during increased
cerebral blood flow. The external diameter of the cortical arteries of rabbits
does not change significantly, and the
luminal diameter even has a tendency to
decrease when cortical blood flow increases. (Reproduced from Mchedlishvili,
Ormotsadze, et al., 1975.)

and hypocapnia (Sadoshima et al., 1980), and will be discussed while considering the vascular effectors involved in the regulation of cerebral
blood flow related to blood gas level changes in cerebral blood flow and
tissue (see p. 120). Dacey and Duling (1982) succeeded in investigating
the muscular reactivity in isolated rat intracerebral arteries. The vessels were found to respond to changes of pH within the range of 8.0 to
6.85 and to dilate following the administration of adenosine. Such reactions of vascular smooth muscle seem natural. But the obtained results do
not necessarily show how the intracerebral arteries behave when the microcirculation is regulated in the brain under normal physiological conditions.

From the above data we may conclude that under conditions of increased
metabolic demand in the cerebral cortex, the feeding arterial branches vary
considerably in response: the small pial arteries show maximum dilatation
while the larger vessels dilate far less. The absence of distinct dilatation in the parenchymal arterial branches does not interfere with a de-

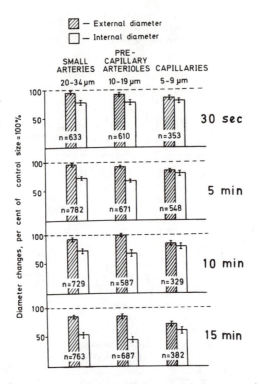

Fig. 4.16. A tendency toward luminal narrowing of
            cortical blood vessels in the course
            of convulsive activity of the cortex.
            A 15-minute period of convulsive activ-
            ity in the cerebral cortex of rabbits
            (caused by strychnine application to
            the cerebral surface) results in a pro-
            gressive narrowing of the cortical
            arteries, arterioles, and capillaries,
            hence leading to a gradual reduction in
            blood flow, which had initially been
            enhanced. (Reproduced from Mchedlish-
            vili, Ingvar, et al., 1970.)

crease in net cerebrovascular resistance during functional and postischemic hyperemias, as seen in direct determinations of regional blood flow
rate in the brain by clearance techniques (see above). In view of the
contradiction between the absence of dilatation of the parenchymal brain
arteries and the widely accepted physiological concept that changes in the
microcirculation throughout the body are primarily determined by diameter
changes in the smallest precapillary arteries, this assertion is hard to
believe. However, the experimental evidence for no dilatation is convincing.

    Two problems in examining the role of different cerebral arteries in
regional blood flow regulation can be distinguished: first, the contribution of each type of vessel to cerebrovascular resistance *under conditions
of rest* and, second, the actual effect of dilatation or constriction of
particular arteries on the *changes of this resistance during naturally occurring regulation* of cerebral blood flow.

While considering the contribution to the cerebrovascular resistance
of various parts of the arterial bed supplying the cerebral cortex with
blood, one can assume that at rest the resistance is probably greater in
the cortical (parenchymal) arteries than in the pial arteries. This conclusion can be drawn from Poiseuille's law, according to which the resistance is inversely proportional to the fourth power of luminal diameter
(which is certainly smaller in cortical arteries) and directly proportional to the first power of both flow velocity and vessel length (both of which
are greater in the pial arteries than in the cortical arteries). However,
differences in the resistance at rest between these two types of vessels,
if they actually exist, must be partly reduced due to the Fahraeus-Lindqvist rheological phenomenon, i.e., the smaller the vessel caliber the
smaller the apparent viscosity of flowing blood (Fahraeus and Lindqvist,
1931; Isenberg, 1953; Haynes and Rodbard, 1962).

Different *changes in the resistance* occur in the various vascular
beds feeding the cerebral cortex with blood. The experimental evidence
considered above shows that an increase in the diameter of the smallest
pial arteries is very significant under conditions of functional and postischemic hyperemias, while the diameter changes of the cortical (parenchymal) vessels are relatively small and have no definite direction. This appears to be convincing evidence for the dominant role of the pial arteries
as the vascular effectors of the regulation of adequate blood supply to the
cerebral cortex. The problem of vascular effectors determining adequate
blood flow in other parts of the brain remains uninvestigated.

As mentioned in Chapter 2 (p. 37), the natural selection of the
vascular effectors for every type of cerebral blood flow control achieved
in the evolutionary process always appears to be optimal. In the case of
regulation of the adequate blood supply to cerebral tissue, i.e., coupling
between the blood flow and metabolic rate, this event is local in nature.
Therefore, neither changes in the systemic arterial pressure level, nor
changes in the resistance of the major cerebral arteries feeding the entire
brain, are ideal from the viewpoint of efficiency of this regulation. The
anatomical peculiarities of the parenchymal brain arteries (including the
absence of interarterial anastomoses for blood redistribution between individual regions and the absence of free space surrounding the vessel walls
for their expansion during vasomotor responses) do not provide the best opportunity for their active and efficient involvement in this regulation.
The pial arteries, however, are both anatomically and functionally designed
to carry out the function of vascular effectors in this type of cerebral
blood flow regulation.

4.2. REGULATION OF OXYGEN AND CARBON DIOXIDE LEVELS IN CEREBRAL
      BLOOD AND TISSUE

The amount of oxygen and carbon dioxide circulating in blood is very
important for normal cerebral metabolism. A significant amount of oxygen
is continually consumed by brain tissue and utilized for oxidative phosphorylation. Energy required for preservation of the cerebral structure
is then produced. Carbon dioxide, the principal end product of cerebral
metabolism, must constantly be removed by the blood stream from the brain.

Oxygen and carbon dioxide are readily diffused through biological
membranes and hence their concentration in the cerebral blood and the surrounding tissue has a tendency to be in equilibrium. Both gases must be
maintained in the blood circulating in the cerebral vasculature at a constant, essential level.

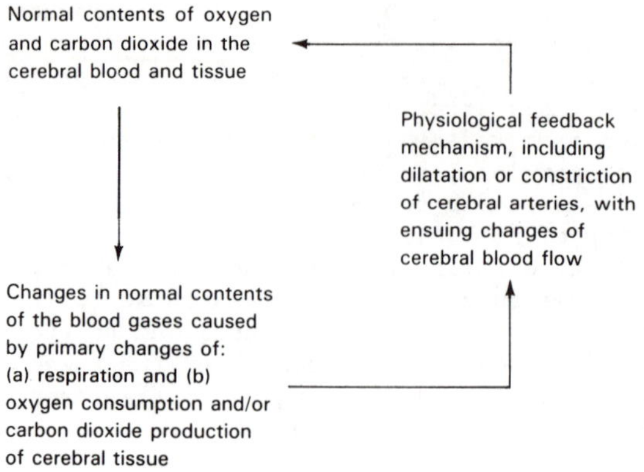

Normal contents of oxygen
and carbon dioxide in the
cerebral blood and tissue

Physiological feedback
mechanism, including
dilatation or constriction
of cerebral arteries, with
ensuing changes of
cerebral blood flow

Changes in normal contents
of the blood gases caused
by primary changes of:
(a) respiration and (b)
oxygen consumption and/or
carbon dioxide production
of cerebral tissue

Fig. 4.17. Automatic control of constant respiratory
gas content, O_2 and CO_2, in cerebral
blood by its flow rate in brain vasculature.

The content of oxygen in cerebral blood vessels is the difference between the amount of gas brought in by the bloodstream from the lungs and
the amount consumed by the brain tissue. The content of carbon dioxide in
cerebral blood is the sum of the amount circulating in the blood and
the amount produced by brain tissue from where it continuously diffuses
into the blood vessels. The parameter usually used to measure the contents of both gases in the cerebral blood and tissue is their tension, i.e.,
P_{O_2} and P_{CO_2}, respectively. The tension gradient of these gases between
blood and tissue is the force that determines diffusion between the two
media; this tension is the main transport mechanism that distributes gases
between the blood and tissue (for oxygen) and the tissue and blood (for
carbon dioxide).

The regulation of oxygen and carbon dioxide contents in cerebral
blood is accomplished in two different ways. One way is by controlling
the effectiveness of lung respiration; this function is not considered in
the present book. The other way of maintaining a constant level of blood
gases in the cerebral blood and tissue is by regulation of the rate of
cerebral blood flow, which will be considered here. This regulatory mechanism is schematically presented in a simple way in Fig. 4.17.

Coupling of Oxygen Content in Cerebral Blood (and tissue) to Cerebral
Blood Flow. In the arterial blood transporting oxygen from lungs to the
brain the P_{O_2} averages 94 mm Hg under normal conditions (Spector, 1956).
The diffusion of oxygen through cerebral capillary walls into the interstitial space is driven by the P_{O_2} gradient between the blood and tissue
compartments, where the P_{O_2} is about 25-35 mm Hg, but can be much higher
or lower (Lübbers, 1968). The brain tissue elements — the nerve and glial
cells and their processes — consume oxygen that reaches the interstitial
space.

Oxygen utilization by the brain has been determined by many authors
since the 1940s. It amounts to about 64 ml per minute for the whole human
brain and 3.3-4.2 ml per 100 g of brain tissue per minute. This means
that almost 15-20% of the oxygen taken up from the atmospheric air is
utilized by the brain (Kety and Schmidt, 1948). The higher the metabolic

rate of the brain tissue, the higher is the oxygen uptake by its tissue elements. Therefore, different brain structures utilize varying amounts of oxygen: the gray matter of the cortex consumes almost five times more oxygen than the white matter. The mean oxygen consumption of the brain can be increased up to 7.8 ml oxygen per 100 g tissue per minute (Opitz and Schneider, 1950).

As a result of oxygen uptake by cerebral tissue, the venous blood outflow from the brain contains significantly less oxygen than the arterial blood: the venous P_{O_2} of the brain amounts to approximately 34-36 mm Hg under normal conditions. It drops considerably if the oxygen content in the arterial blood has primarily decreased or the oxygen uptake by the tissue has significantly increased. A drop in the cerebral venous P_{O_2} level to 18 mm Hg was found to be related to disturbances in brain function and even to damage to its structural elements (Meyer et al., 1965). A drop in the brain venous P_{O_2} to 12 mm Hg is related to irreversible tissue damage (Hirsch and Schneider, 1968).

The P_{O_2} in cerebral tissue varies considerably in different areas. The O_2 level is dependent on both the microcirculation rate in various brain areas and the local oxygen uptake. As determined by microelectrodes in different areas of the brain, the cerebral tissue P_{O_2} was found to range from 0 to 90 mm Hg (Leniger-Follert et al., 1975).

The relationship between the oxygen content in the arterial blood and the actual cerebral blood flow has been investigated for many years by many authors. The experimental procedures usually applied to identify this relationship involve changing the oxygen content in the arterial blood by changing respiration (for instance, by occluding the trachea and hence inducing asphyxia) or by altering the oxygen content in the inspired air. After a change in arterial P_{O_2}, cerebral blood flow changes can be investigated by a variety of methods. To evaluate whether the altered arterial blood P_{O_2} affects the cerebral blood vessels and cerebrovascular resistance directly, the systemic arterial pressure must be controlled, since significant changes in blood oxygen content can affect the arterial pressure level by the chemoreceptor reflex.

Regardless of the method applied to estimate the cerebral blood flow, its rate has always been enhanced by considerable decreases in arterial P_{O_2} both in animals and man. The converse is also true — the cerebral blood flow regularly decreases in response to considerable increases in the P_{O_2} of arterial blood (Kety and Schmidt, 1948; Cohen and Alexander, 1967; Kogure et al., 1970).

Animal studies reveal that cerebral blood flow increases, albeit insignificantly, as soon as the arterial P_{O_2} starts to drop below normal values (Opitz and Schneider, 1950; Borgström et al., 1975). But further decreases in blood oxygen content cause the cerebral blood flow to start increasing significantly: this occurs as soon as the arterial P_{O_2} reaches approximately 50 mm Hg (Courtice, 1941; Opitz and Schneider, 1950; Kogure et al., 1970). The blood oxygen-cerebral blood flow relationship (Fig. 4.18) correlates perfectly with a decrease in cerebral venous P_{O_2} to 25-28 mm Hg (Noell and Schneider, 1942). A decrease in arterial P_{O_2} to 20 mm Hg induces a twofold increase in cerebral blood flow (Hamer et al., 1976).

An opposite change in cerebral blood flow occurs with increasing arterial P_{O_2}. When the oxygen content in the inspired air increases from the normal 20% to 100% (i.e., when the animal breathes pure oxygen) the

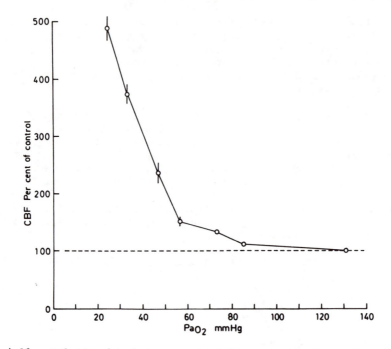

Fig. 4.18.   Relationship between arterial oxygen tension and cerebral blood
             flow (CBF).   (Reproduced with permission from Borgström et al.,
             1975.)

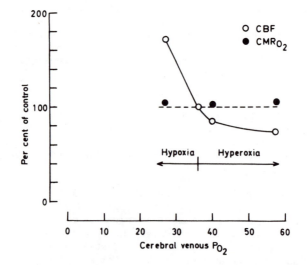

Fig. 4.19.   Influence of hypoxia and hyperoxia on cerebral blood
             flow and oxygen consumption rate in man. The cere-
             bral blood flow (CBF) changes independently of the
             cerebral metabolic rate (CMR) of oxygen, which re-
             mains unchanged during both hypoxia and hyperoxia.
             The values of CBF and CMR_{O_2}, given in percent of the
             normoxic control, are related to cerebral venous P_{O_2}.
             (Reproduced with permission from Sjesjö et al.,
             1979.)

cerebral blood flow increases by about 13%. When the arterial P_{O_2} rises even higher during respiration of pure oxygen under high atmospheric pressure (3-4 atmospheres), cerebral blood flow decreases to about 25% of the initial values (Kety and Schmidt, 1948; Lambertsen et al., 1953).

Consequently, the existing experimental data demonstrate an inverse correlation between the level of arterial oxygen tension and the rate of cerebral blood flow. The effect of changing arterial oxygen tension on cerebral blood flow is seen despite the fact that the cerebral metabolic rate of oxygen remains unchanged (Fig. 4.19). This proves that the effect of arterial P_{O_2} on cerebral blood flow is accomplished not through changes in cerebral tissue metabolism, but by a direct influence on the regulation of cerebral blood vessel diameter.

The Relationship between Carbon Dioxide Content in Cerebral Blood (and Tissue) and Cerebral Blood Flow. The responses of cerebral blood vessels to changes in blood carbon dioxide levels are usually estimated when the P_{CO_2} is primarily changed in the arterial blood (by altering the lung ventilation rate or the carbon dioxide content in the inspired air), and the cerebral blood flow is then measured by any feasible method. An increase in P_{CO_2} in blood above the normal levels causes striking increases in cerebral blood flow: in healthy humans, hypercapnia induced by respiration with a gas mixture containing 5-7% CO_2 results in cerebral blood flow increases by about 75-100% (Lennox and Gibbs, 1932). Even slight hypercapnia induces a substantial enhancement of cerebral blood flow if it is combined with arterial hypoxia (Quint et al., 1980). Hypocapnia, on the contrary, causes a reduction in cerebral vascular tone: hyperventilation, which decreases blood P_{CO_2} below 26 mm Hg, results in a decrease in cerebral blood flow by 35% (Kety and Schmidt, 1948; Patterson et al., 1955). This was confirmed repeatedly by many researchers both in animal and human experiments (for references see reviews by Hirsch and Schneider, 1968; and Purves, 1972). Thus both hyper- and hypocapnia result in a pronounced change in cerebral blood flow.

The effect of carbon dioxide tension changes on cerebral blood flow has been found within the range of about 15-20 to 70-80 mm Hg (Noell and Schneider, 1944). The relationship between the degree of arterial P_{CO_2} change and the cerebral circulation rate has a sigmoid shape (Fig. 4.20), but within the range of normal blood P_{CO_2} (approximately 40 mm Hg) the relationship is almost linear. The curve is steepest in this range: the blood flow changes by approximately 6% when the blood P_{CO_2} changes by 1 mm Hg (Harper, 1965). When the arterial P_{CO_2} reaches about one-half of its normal value, i.e., approximately 20 mm Hg, cerebral blood flow stops decreasing (Reivich, 1964; Harper and Glass, 1965). This P_{CO_2} response in brain vessels is thought to be dependent on the secondary, and independent, effect of a deficient blood supply to the brain tissue on cerebral blood flow (see above). The validity of this interpretation was confirmed by estimating the cerebral venous P_{O_2}, which decreased below 19-21 mm Hg, from this lowered arterial P_{CO_2}; this decrease in venous P_{O_2} prevented further reductions in cerebral blood flow (Hirsch and Schneider, 1968).

Vascular effectors that regulate steady oxygen and carbon dioxide content in cerebral blood and tissue have not yet been conclusively established. This problem has not even been considered in the numerous studies in which the effect of the blood gases on cerebral blood flow was investigated. The researchers have nonetheless believed that the vascular effects are brought about by changes in the cerebral vessel diameter and respective changes in cerebrovascular resistance. However, the problem of determining which blood vessels of the brain are actually involved in this

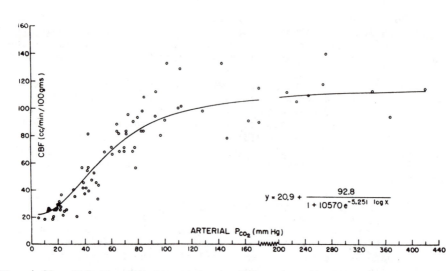

$$y = 20.9 + \frac{92.8}{1 + 10570\,e^{-5.251\ \log x}}$$

Fig. 4.20.   Relationship between arterial carbon dioxide tension and cere-
             bral blood flow in monkeys. (Reproduced with permission from
             Reivich, 1964.)

regulation of cerebral blood flow was not considered in the majority of
studies until recently.

     The problem of identifying the vascular effectors in this type of
cerebral blood flow regulation cannot be solved without comparative studies
of cerebral blood vessels of different sizes which may respond specifically
to changing oxygen and carbon dioxide tension in blood. However, identification of the vascular effectors would not necessarily elucidate the vasomotor mechanism responsible for the vessel's behavior. This could be from
a direct effect of changes in oxygen and carbon dioxide tension in circulating blood on vascular walls, or a complicated vasomotor control mechanism
operating, at least partly, outside the vessel wall, similar to neurogenic
vasomotor regulation.

     It seems certain that in the cerebral vascular bed only the arteries,
not the capillaries or veins, are the vascular effectors of this type of
cerebral blood flow regulation (see Chapter 1). Among the cerebral arteries the following vascular segments may be involved in this regulation:
the major arteries of the brain (the internal carotid and vertebrals), the
larger and smaller pial arteries, and the intracerebral (parenchymal) minor
arteries and arterioles. Complex effects of both blood gases, i.e., carbon
dioxide and oxygen, have been observed in studies carried out during systemic asphyxia produced by occlusion of the trachea; this resulted in both a
deficiency of oxygen and an accumulation of carbon dioxide in the circulating blood.

     As early as the middle of the 19th century Donders (1851) found that
10 seconds after closure of the mouths and noses of rabbits the brain surface turned red; using microscopy the author observed that previously invisible small vessels became visible on the brain surface. The volume of
blood in the pial vessels began decreasing within 2 minutes after recovery of respiration, but it was still elevated 15 minutes later. Subsequent investigations of the pial vessels employing photomicrography confirm early observations that, following tracheal occlusion, the diameter

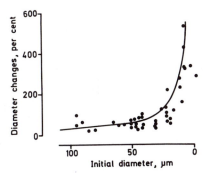

Fig. 4.21. Dilatation of pial arteries of various
resting diameters during hypercapnia.
During respiration of hypercapnic gas
mixtures in cats, the same regularity
of predominant dilatation of smaller
pial arteries occurs as seen during
functional and postischemic hyperemias
in rabbits (see Figs. 4.8 and 4.10).
(Modified with permission from Auer
and Johansson, 1980.)

of all pial vessels increases considerably. These hitherto invisible vessels, normally 10-20 µm in diameter, appear on the brain surface; the pial
dilatation lasts about 20 minutes after the recovery of respiration (Klosovsky, 1951). The vasodilatation of pial arteries (the vessel diameter
increases by about one-third of the initial value) is an active vascular
response, since it occurs independent of the systemic arterial pressure,
i.e., even when the pressure does not rise because of artificial stabilization (Mchedlishvili, 1960b).

In response to increased carbon dioxide tension in the blood, the pial
arteries, which have various resting diameters, undergo a variable dilatation: the smaller vessels (13-40 µm in diameter) dilate on average by
47.7%, while the larger vessels in cats (41-90 µm in diameter) dilate by
29.5% (Raper et al., 1971). Plots of the degree of pial arterial dilatation against the resting vascular caliber (Fig. 4.21) has revealed that the
smallest pial arteries exhibit the highest degree of dilatation (Auer and
Johansson, 1980; Wei et al., 1980). Similar results have also been obtained during arterial hypoxia when animals inhale air containing 8% oxygen (Jenett and Craigen, 1981). The higher responsiveness of smaller pial
arteries to hypercapnia and hypoxia are in full agreement with the experimental results obtained during functional and postischemic hyperemias in
the cerebral cortex (see above, pp.104-107).

In contrast to the pial arterial branches on the cerebral surface, the
behavior of the minor intracerebral (parenchymal) blood vessels remains
less investigated. The existing experimental data are rather poor and contradictory. The inaccessibility of these blood vessels for direct *in vivo*
investigations necessitates performing studies *post mortem*. These microvascular responses have been investigated in unstained microscopical sections of rabbits' cerebral cortex after *in vivo* fixation of the vessel
walls and surrounding tissue by perfusing the cerebral vessels with formaldehyde under standard conditions. Measurement of the external and internal diameters of a large number of cortical arteries of various calibers

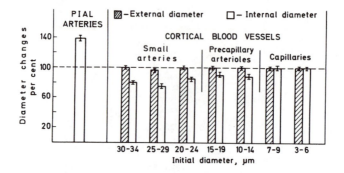

Fig. 4.22. Diameter changes of pial and cortical vessels during
            asphyxic hyperemia in the rabbit brain. Pial arter-
            ies dilate, but cortical (parenchymal) vessels be-
            have differently; the external diameter remains un-
            changed, while the luminal diameter of the small
            arteries and arterioles may even decrease, despite
            increases in the blood flow rate. See text for de-
            tails. (Reproduced from Mchedlishvili, 1972.)

have shown that during hypercapnia the lumina of the cortical microvessels
contract slightly compared to the control, while the diameter of the capillaries remains unchanged (Fig. 4.22). These results have been obtained
following inhalation of gas mixtures containing up to 20% carbon dioxide
(Mchedlishvili and Baramidze, 1965), as well as 1-2 minutes following occlusion of the trachea (Mchedlishvili, Ormotsadze, et al., 1967b). Distinct results have been obtained more recently in a study in which cerebral cortices in intact rats were fixed by freezing. Measurements of the
internal and external vascular diameters in stained microscopical sections
of the cerebral cortex have indicated that the responses of parenchymal
arteries are comparable to those of the pial vessels, i.e., they dilate
during hypercapnia and constrict during hypocapnia. The degree of dilatation of cortical arteries was smaller, but their constriction was, on the
contrary, more pronounced than in pial arteries (Sadoshima et al., 1980).
Thus, a tendency of the cortical arteries to constrict (in contrast to the
pial arteries, which tend to dilate) is evident in this case, similar to
that seen during increased activity of the cerebral cortex (see pp. 108-
112). However, due to insufficient experimental results we cannot yet
ascertain the functional behavior of the intracerebral (parenchymal) vessels under these conditions.

     Experimental data related to responses of the major arteries of the brain
(internal carotid and vertebral arteries) are not sufficient either to
draw definite conclusions as to how they actually behave in response to
changing oxygen and carbon dioxide contents in blood. The vascular responses of these vessels have been studied during asphyxia, which was complicated and produced drastic effects. Therefore, asphyxiation experiments
cannot be considered in the analysis of the vessels' behavior during normal
regulation of constant blood gas contents in cerebral blood and tissue.

     The functional behavior of the major brain arteries during asphyxia
has been studied since the 1960s, i.e., since the physiological role of the
vessels in the control of cerebral blood flow attracted attention. By ap-
plying the two principal techniques of *in vivo* estimation of arterial response, i.e., measurement of the pressure gradient in the arteries and the

resistography of isolated internal carotid arteries in dogs, it has been shown that the arteries undergo regular constriction during asphyxia (Mchedlishvili, 1960b, 1962; Mchedlishvili, Ormotsadze, et al., 1967b). Resistance in the major arteries is increased simultaneously with decreasing resistance in the arteries located peripherally to the circle of Willis (see Chapter 3, p. 66). However, the constrictor response of the major brain arteries during asphyxia seems not to be dependent on the direct effect of drastic hypoxia and hypercapnia but is, in all probability, the manifestation of another type of cerebral blood flow control, i.e., blood flow control directed at preventing excessive cerebral blood volume, which increases significantly due to total pial vasodilatation (see Chapter 3, pp. 64-69). Under these conditions, despite constriction of the major arteries (and a possible slight constriction of the intracerebral arteries; see above), dilatation of the pial arteries is so pronounced that there is a decrease in total cerebrovascular resistance. The cerebral blood flow and volume increase during asphyxia even before the systemic arterial pressure starts to rise.

However, when the tension of O_2 or CO_2 is changed separately, e.g., in dogs breathing either hypercapnic (10% CO_2) or hypoxic (10% O_2) gas mixtures, the resistance in the major arteries of the brain decreases considerably. Hypocapnia due to hyperventilation results in a decrease in vascular resistance (Heistad et al., 1978).

Hence, the actual experimental results show that the pial arteries, especially the smaller vessels, uniformly increase cerebral blood flow during decreased oxygen and increased carbon dioxide tension in the blood. The opposite, i.e., constrictor, responses of the pial vessels during significant rises in oxygen and drops in carbon dioxide contents in the blood have not been the subject of much research. The major arteries of the brain can respond in two ways: they constrict if the cerebral blood volume has increased considerably (due to very pronounced pial vasodilatation) and dilate during hypercapnia or hypoxia.

Consequently, it seems reasonable to conclude that the pial arteries are the main vascular effectors of this type of cerebral blood flow regulation. In drawing this conclusion, we take into account that oxygen and carbon dioxide tension in brain tissue is closely related to its metabolism and remember that only the minor pial arteries are the principal vascular effectors responsible for the regulation of blood flow and metabolism coupling (see pp. 104-113). However, it appears that the major brain arteries also play a part in this form of cerebral blood flow regulation when there are systemic changes in oxygen and/or carbon dioxide content in blood. Proceeding from these considerations, we may put forward a tentative hypothesis to explain this phenomenon. The responses of the major arteries and the pial arteries are related to different physiological control mechanisms of cerebral blood vessels. The former, a systemic control mechanism, which includes the carotid chemoreceptors, is probably related to the active behavior of the major arteries, while a local regulatory mechanism causes the pial arterial responses (see p. 173). This dual mechanism involving the major and pial arterial participation in blood gas level regulation is schematically shown in Fig. 4.23. The simultaneous and coincidentally directed responses of the major and pial arteries under the conditions being considered (so long as the cerebral blood flow control related to excessive blood volume accumulation in cerebral vasculature is not simultaneously operating) may explain why the effects of oxygen and carbon dioxide on cerebral blood flow are so pronounced that they were easily revealed in numerous animal studies beginning from the 1930s and widely applied in clinical practice (for references see Purves, 1972; Olesen, 1974).

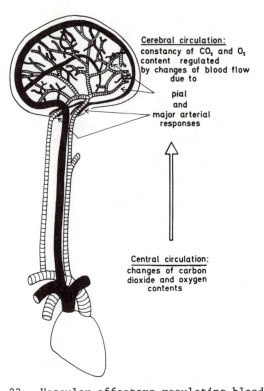

Fig. 4.23.   Vascular effectors regulating blood gas
             levels in cerebral blood and tissue by
             changing cerebral blood flow. Changes
             in carbon dioxide and oxygen contents
             in systemic blood induce respective
             changes in cerebral blood flow (direct-
             ly correlated with carbon dioxide and
             inversely correlated with oxygen levels)
             by active responses in the pial and
             major arteries that maintain constant
             blood gas levels.

4.3. ORGANIZATION OF PIAL MICROVASCULAR EFFECTORS

From evidence cited above it has been concluded that the pial arterial system represents the vascular effectors of regulation of adequate
blood supply to the cerebral cortex (Mchedlishvili, 1960b, 1964). The
pial vessels originate from the anterior, middle, and posterior cerebral
arteries. They branch consecutively, have numerous anastomotic interconnections, and thus form a complex network on the brain surface (Figs. 1.8
and 1.9). The terminal branches of the pial arterial bed bend and enter
the cerebral cortex almost perpendicularly to its surface (Fig. 4.24).

The pial arterial system's provision of adequate blood supply to cerebral tissue is very sensitive. This is due to the following reasons: (a)
they feed the cerebral tissue elements which are especially sensitive to
oxygen and nutritient deprivation, and (b) they respond mainly to local
changes in the activity of cerebral tissue, especially the cortex (in contrast to most other brain tissues), under physiological conditions. The
latter peculiarity of cerebral microcirculation has been clearly shown by

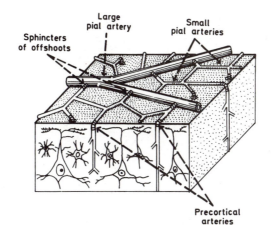

Fig. 4.24.   Diagram of the pial arterial network on
             the brain surface. There are two types
             of vessels: the larger branches and
             the network of minute arteries which
             possess active microvascular segments
             (sphincters at offshoots from larger
             trunks and precortical arteries). The
             terminal branches, as radial arteries,
             penetrate the cerebral cortex and feed
             the gray and white matter. See text
             for details.

the mapping of human cortical functions and regional blood flow (see pp. 99–
100). Hence, the microcirculation in the cerebral cortex usually undergoes
changes in small areas. These changes may be related to a rapid redistribution of blood among microvascular areas, which occurs without disturbing
the blood supply to the neighboring areas (like the "steal phenomenon,"
see p. 30). Therefore, the control of microcirculation in the cerebral cortex should be extremely reliable, especially during pathological disturbances in blood supply caused, e.g., by microemboli in individual pial
arterial branches, etc. Thus the regulatory function of the pial microvascular system with respect to an adequate blood supply to cerebral cortex should, in all probability, be nearly perfect and consequently be an
exciting subject for investigations in this field.

    As we shall see on pp. 129–135, the pial microvascular system has
gradually evolved to become so complex that it is difficult to properly
ascertain its structural and functional peculiarities in highly developed
animal species. Therefore, the best subjects for investigations are species which have obtained all the principal features of the definitive system in the course of phylogeny, but still have not become so complex as to
create difficulties in experimentation. The pial microvascular system
reached this optimal degree of developmental complexity in rabbits, in
which all the elements in the systems of more highly developed animals
(probably including humans) are present but in a rather simplified form.
Therefore, rabbits have been used as subjects in the majority of studies
concerned with the organization of the pial microvascular effectors regulating adequate microcirculation in the cerebral cortex.

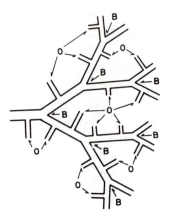

Fig. 4.25. Two types of pial arterial ramifications
on the brain surface: the offshoots (0)
of smaller arterial branches from larger
trunks and bifurcations (B) into vessels of approximately identical sizes.
Both kinds of arterial ramifications
have different functional significance.
See text for details.

We will next consider the organization of the pial microvascular system to ascertain how and whether it can function as the effector of regulation of microcirculation in such a highly differentiated tissue as the
cerebral cortex.

Anatomical and Functional Significance of Pial Arterial Bifurcations.
A careful consideration of the pial arterial network shows that it possesses two main types of blood vessels that differ from each other not only in
diameter but also in their mode of branching. The anatomical peculiarities of these blood vessels can be well distinguished in microscopic preparations of comparatively large pieces of pia mater after *in situ* fixation.
The pial arterial network in rabbits comprises blood vessels having a
caliber from 300-400 μm (the first portions of the anterior, middle, and
posterior cerebral arteries) to 15-50 μm (the terminal branches) (Mchedlishvili, Baramidze, et al., 1974-1975). Two types of branching can be
distinguished in this arterial network: (a) bifurcations of the arterial
trunks into two branches with average diameters 0.84 ± 0.09 and 1.0
units, and with angles between the trunk and the branches in the range
of 25° to 80° and (b) offshoots of smaller arterial branches from the
larger trunks at approximately right angles (Fig. 4.25).

The spacing of bifurcations of the pial arteries between the circle
of Willis and the smallest branches becomes progressively smaller with decreasing arterial caliber; this relationship is linear (Fig. 4.26). The
angles between the trunk and the branches are also dependent on vascular
caliber: the smaller the vessel diameter the greater the angle. This relationship is nonlinear: in larger pial arteries an increase in branching
angle is negligible, while in arteries with a diameter smaller than 80-100
μm it is considerable (Fig. 4.27). Thus, the pial arteries with smaller
diameters show more frequent branching and greater angles between trunks
and branches.

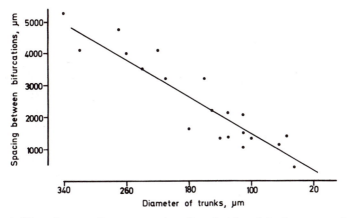

Fig. 4.26.   Inversely porportional relationship between the fre-
             quency of bifurcations and the resting diameters in
             the pial arterial bed of rabbits. (Reproduced from
             Mchedlishvili and Mamisashvili, 1974.)

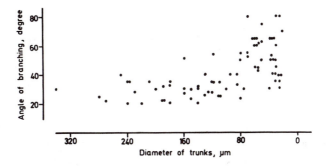

Fig. 4.27.   Relationship between angles of branching from trunks
             at bifurcations and resting diameter of pial arter-
             ies in rabbits. The angles of branching are almost
             similar in all the larger pial arteries, but notice-
             ably increase in smaller vessels with a resting
             diameter under 100 μm. See text for details. (Re-
             produced from Mchedlishvili and Mamisashvili, 1974.)

     In animals without hyperemia in the cerebral cortex the cross-section-
al areas of the vascular lumina after bifurcations of the pial arteries
show a rather strict regularity. While the total cross-sectional area of
the branches is generally greater in the larger branch vessels compared to
their trunks, in arteries under 100-80 μm in diameter this ratio always becomes smaller (Fig. 4.28). Hence, according to the law of conservation of
mass the rate of blood flow in the smallest pial arterial branches should
be greater than in their respective trunks before branching under normal
conditions. The author does not know whether such a peculiarity of the
microvascular bifurcations is seen elsewhere in the circulatory bed, but
it certainly does play a significant functional role in the present case
with respect to control of cerebral microcirculation (see below).

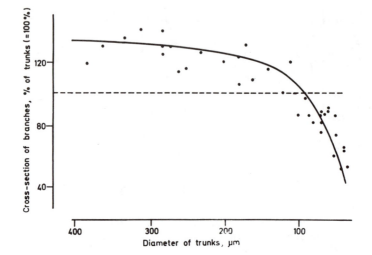

Fig. 4.28. Relationship between cross-sectional areas of pial vessels
            formed at arterial bifurcations and trunk diameter in rabbits.
            In larger pial arteries the cross-sectional area of branches
            compared to the trunks increases at every bifurcation, while
            at the bifurcations of smaller pial arteries (with resting
            diameters under 100 μm) the area becomes smaller and therefore
            the flow velocity increases proportionally during rest. See
            text for details on the functional significance of this phe-
            nomenon. (Reproduced from Mchedlishvili and Mamisashvili, 1974.)

     It follows from these considerations that within the pial vascular sys-
tem the smaller pial arteries, under 100-80 μm in diameter, should have the
greatest resistance at rest. This should be the case because, in addition
to the small diameter, these pial arteries branch most often, have the
largest angles of bifurcation from the parent vessel, and have a relatively
high rate of blood flow (compared to the respective parent vessels). The
vascular walls, consisting mainly of smooth muscle cells that determine
vascular tone, are relatively thicker in the pial arteries under 100 μm in
diameter (Fig. 1.10 on p. 11).

     As soon as increased metabolic demands arise in an area of the cortex,
however, it is the smaller pial arteries with a diameter under 80-100 μm
that undergo the most pronounced dilatation (Figs. 4.8-4.11). Determination of the total luminal cross-sectional area of pial arterial branches
has shown that in rabbits the ratio of the net area of the smaller arterial branches to the luminal area of the feeding middle cerebral artery is
3:1 at rest. But this ratio becomes 12:1 as soon as the pial arteries dilate in response to a deficient blood supply to the brain. The deficiency
was caused in this case by a mean decrease in the level of systemic arterial pressure from 101 to 41 mm Hg following partial exsanguination. These
data are presented in Fig. 4.29. Similar results have been obtained during
functional and postischemic hyperemias (Mamisashvili et al., 1975, 1977).
Thus, in the pial arterial system it is the smallest vessels, which have
the maximum resistance at rest, that undergo the greatest dilatation as
soon as metabolic demands arise from the cerebral cortex.

     At a given pressure, the blood flow rate in arteries is determined by
their resistance. Since Poiseuille's law cannot be applied to minute ves-

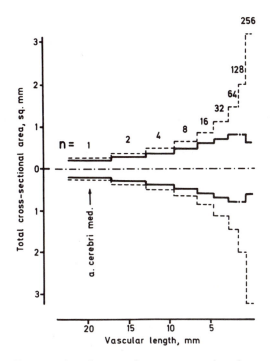

Fig. 4.29.   Changes in the total cross-sectional area along the
             ramifying pial arteries of rabbits, starting from
             arteria cerebri media and proceeding to the small-
             est vascular branches, both under resting condi-
             tions (solid lines) and during arterial hypotension
             (the mean arterial pressure was approximately 40 mm
             Hg) caused by partial exsanguination (dotted lines).
             n = the number of bifurcating branches. (Repro-
             duced from Mamisashvili et al., 1977.)

sels comparable in caliber to the small pial arteries under study (Haynes
and Burton, 1959; Wayland, 1965), an attempt has been made to derive a
quantitative relationship between the radius and resistance in the pial
arterial bed. In the derivation of the formulas some principles of ideal
behavior are considered (Rosen, 1967). When fluid is flowing through a
system of tubes, the work to be performed is determined by the hydro-
dynamic resistance in the system. The smaller the resistance, the greater
is the effectiveness, or optimality, of the system from the point of view
of energy loss. The relationship between the radii of the pial arterial
trunks and their respective branches is shown in Fig. 4.28:

$$cr_0^2 = r_1^2 + r_2^2,$$

where r_0 is the radius of the trunk and r_1 and r_2 are those of the
branches, while c is a constant for $r_0 > 100$ μm and a function of r_0 for
$r_0 < 100$ μm.

   Suppose that within the ramifying system of pial arteries the relationship of radii ($cr_0^2 = r_1^2 + r_2^2$) is optimal from the point of view of
energy loss, and then consider the evaluating function which was proposed
by Rosen (1967):

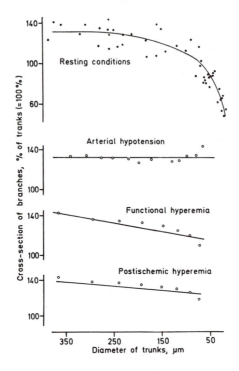

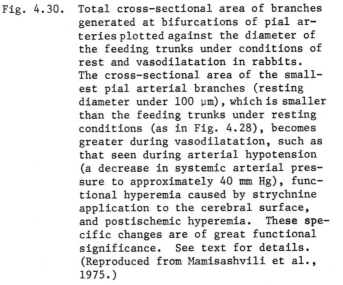

Fig. 4.30. Total cross-sectional area of branches
generated at bifurcations of pial arteries plotted against the diameter of
the feeding trunks under conditions of
rest and vasodilatation in rabbits.
The cross-sectional area of the smallest pial arterial branches (resting
diameter under 100 μm), which is smaller
than the feeding trunks under resting
conditions (as in Fig. 4.28), becomes
greater during vasodilatation, such as
that seen during arterial hypotension
(a decrease in systemic arterial pressure to approximately 40 mm Hg), functional hyperemia caused by strychnine
application to the cerebral surface,
and postischemic hyperemia. These specific changes are of great functional
significance. See text for details.
(Reproduced from Mamisashvili et al.,
1975.)

$$P = Q^2R + K\pi r^2L,$$

where P is dispersion of power, Q is flow, R is resistance, r is the vessel radius, L is the vessel length, and K is a dimensionality coefficient.

The expression calculated by Rosen (1967) on the basis of the optimality principle shows good agreement with the mentioned experimental data
only for pial arteries having a diameter over 100 μm. For smaller pial
arteries, with a diameter under 100 μm, this optimality principle is not

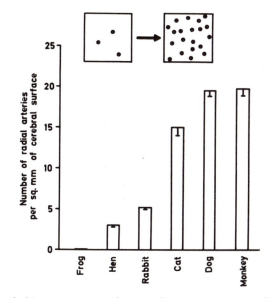

Fig. 4.31. Density of radial arteries in different
            species. The number of terminal branch-
            es in the pial arterial bed per 1 mm² of
            brain surface gradually increases in an
            evolutionary sequence from zero (in the
            amphibia). Thus, a progressively small-
            er mass of cerebral tissue is fed by in-
            dividual arterial branches in more high-
            ly developed species.

valid during rest (Fig. 4.30). This probably could be explained in the
following way: the smallest pial arteries represent the main regulator of
the blood supply to the cerebral cortex. Thus, it is not the minimum dissipation of power, but rather the regulation of blood flow to the cortex, that
is to be assumed as an optimality criterion for the blood transport in
these arteries. That is why the optimality principle cannot be applied to
these arteries under conditions of rest. However, when there is a deficient blood supply, and hence an increased metabolic demand in the cerebral cortex, the relationship of the total cross-sectional areas of the
smaller pial vessels under 100 μm in diameter actually shifts in a way
that optimality of blood transport is provided from the point of view of
the minimum dispersion of power (Fig. 4.30).

The Basic Structural Units of the Pial Arterial System. The terminal
branches of the pial microvascular bed are the precortical arteries, which
turn into the radial arteries and penetrate the cerebral cortex. These
arteries are the only vessels that feed the deep areas of cortical tissue,
since interarterial connections are not present in the deep cortex (Klosovsky, 1951; Gannushkina, 1973). Therefore, no possibility of blood redistribution from one tissue area to another exists at the periphery of
the pial arterial bed.

We have calculated the number of radial arteries per unit of cortical
surface area in various species (frog, bird, rabbit, cat, dog, monkey) and
have found that their density steadily increases in the evolutionary

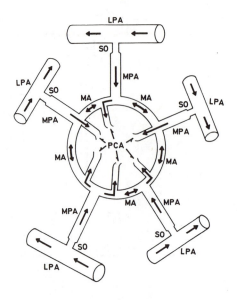

Fig. 4.32.   The typical structure of an arterial
             circle in the terminal pial vascular bed
             formed by: the larger pial arteries
             (LPA), sphincters at offshoots of small-
             er arterial branches (SO), minor pial
             arteries (MPA), interarterial micro-
             anastomoses (MA), and precortical arter-
             ies (PCA). The arrows indicate the pre-
             sumable direction of blood flow in the
             microvessels. See text for details.
             (Reproduced from Mchedlishvili and Kur-
             idze, 1984.)

sequence (Fig. 4.31). We can thus conclude that the pial arterial system
has evolved to regulate blood supply in progressively smaller areas of the
cerebral cortex. In the human brain, the number of radial arteries is
four times greater than radial veins (Duvernoy et al., 1981). It follows
from these considerations that the distribution of blood between individual radial arteries is a main function of the pial arterial system.

     The basic structural unit providing for this blood distribution is
the vascular circle formed by consecutive branches and anastomotic interconnections of medium and small pial arteries. These arterial circles are
distributed throughout the surface of the cerebral hemispheres. Their
regular appearance in the network of larger pial arteries has been mentioned earlier (Klosovsky, 1951; Gannushkina, 1973). However, the anatomical peculiarities of the arterial circles at the smallest pial vessel
branches, as well as their functional significance in the regulation of
blood supply to the cortex, has not yet been studied.

     Investigation of the arterial circles in microscopic preparations of
the pia mater (Mchedlishvili and Kuridze, 1984) showed that every arterial
circle in the terminal vascular network is fed by several arterial branches;
other minor vessels arising from the circles enter the cortex as radial
arteries. The arterial circles formed by consecutive ramifications and

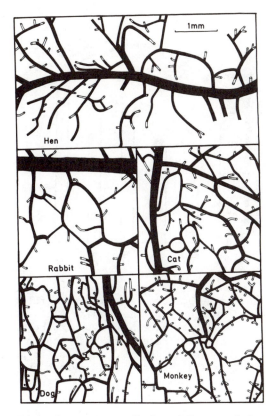

Fig. 4.33.   Typical patterns of the pial arterial networks in
             different species: hen, rabbit, cat, dog, monkey.
             The scale for all drawings is given in the top
             right-hand corner. See text for details. (Repro-
             duced from Mchedlishvili and Kuridze, 1984.)

interconnections in pial vessels in the terminal microvascular bed are
schematically presented in Fig. 4.32 as a typical arterial circle with all
its components labeled.

    Mapping of the pial arterial circles in different species has shown
how they appeared and developed in the evolution of vertebrates (Fig.
4.33). Consideration of this process can contribute to a better understanding of the changes in the anatomy of the pial arterial circles that
provide for an increasingly refined and precise regulation of the cerebral
microcirculation in the more highly developed vertebrates.

    The amphibians, whose forebrain surface is not generally provided
with a pial arterial system, have no pial arterial circles, as expected.
Pial arterial circles are preferentially formed in the larger arteries in
birds. Most of the larger pial arteries form pial arterial circles in
lower mammals, such as rabbits. But the circles are mostly built from
smaller pial arteries in more highly developed mammals — cats, dogs, and
monkeys (Fig. 4.34). As mentioned on pp. 124-129, the smaller pial arteries, having diameters under approximately 100 µm, are better fitted to
regulate vascular resistance. Thus the arterial circles formed by the

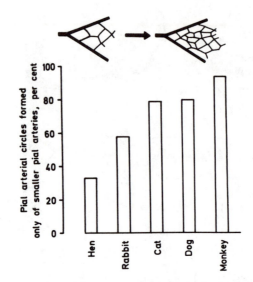

Fig. 4.34. The number of pial arterial circles
formed only by the smaller pial arteries (which have been shown to be more
fitted for regulating the blood flow
than the larger pial vessels) is progressively increased in more highly developed animals. See text for details.

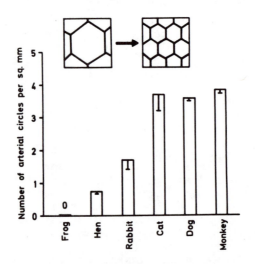

Fig. 4.35. The amount of pial arterial circles per
mm² cerebral surface area gradually increases from the lower to higher animal
species, but in cats, dogs, and monkeys
the number reaches a saturation point,
almost similar in these animal species.
(Reproduced from Mchedlishvili and Kuridze, 1984.)

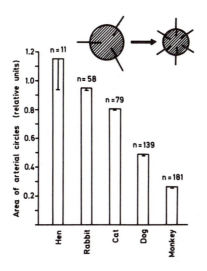

Fig. 4.36. The area occupied by individual pial
arterial circles in various animal species gradually decreased during evolution from amphibia, to birds, and then
to various mammals. n = the number of
arterial circles studied.

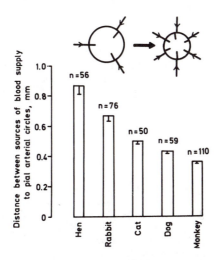

Fig. 4.37. The density of arterial branches supplying pial arterial circles in various
animal species. During evolution, the
pial arterial circles have been progressively better supplied with blood,
since the distances between single
sources of the blood supply gradually
decreased. n = the number of the
arterial circles studied. (Reproduced
from Mchedlishvili and Kuridze, 1984.)

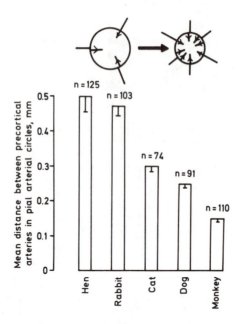

Fig. 4.38. The density of terminal arterial branches
arising from pial arterial circles in
various animal species. During evolution, the distance between the terminal
branches arising from the pial arterial
circles and entering the cerebral cortex gradually decreased, demonstrating
an increase in their density (compare
Fig. 4.31). n = the number of arterial
circles studied. (Reproduced from
Mchedlishvili and Kuridze, 1984).

smallest pial vessels should be better able to adjust the microcirculation
in minor cortical areas to the metabolic needs of the surrounding tissue.

The number of pial arterial circles per mm² of cortical area increases
from zero (in the amphibian) to much greater amounts in birds, rabbits, and
cats. It is almost similar in cats and in dogs and monkeys (Fig. 4.35).
Estimates of the cortical area occupied by individual arterial circles show
that the area becomes progressively smaller in more complex animals (Fig.
4.36). This seeming discrepancy in the data between the number of arterial circles per unit cortical area and the area occupied by the individual
circles can be explained by the complex form of arterial circles in higher
species. Thus, in the evolutionary process the individual pial arterial
circles regulate a progressively smaller mass of cerebral tissue.

In spite of the fact that the pial arterial circles gradually decrease in size during the evolution of vertebrates, the number of the
arterial branches which feed every circle with blood steadily increases.
This has been shown by determinations of the distance between the feeding
vessels of the pial arterial circles in various animal species (Fig.
4.37). On the other hand, the number of terminal arterial branches arising from every circle, i.e., the precortical arteries, also progressively

increases despite the smaller size of each circle (Fig. 4.38). This is comparable to the data presented in Fig. 4.31 concerning the density of radial arteries supplying the cerebral cortex with blood.

Thus it becomes clear that during the evolution of vertebrates, the organization of the specific structural units of the pial arterial bed, i.e., the pial arterial circles, has progressed. In higher vertebrates the pial arterial circles are formed mostly from the smaller pial arterial branches which represent the pial vascular segments most active in the regulation of blood supply to the cerebral cortex. Another anatomical peculiarity of the pial arterial system is that in higher animals each of the pial arterial circles occupies a smaller area of the cerebral surface and, therefore, it steadily supplies a progressively smaller mass of cortical tissue; this is independent of blood supply to the neighboring areas; because of this the pial arterial system can better adjust the blood flow in the cortex to the metabolic rate of its tissue. This is necessary both during increased metabolic demands in the tissue and during obstructions of blood flow in individual pial arteries.

The terminal pial vessels entering the cerebral cortex (i.e., the precortical arteries) can thus be supplied with blood from several sources in more highly developed mammals. The number of blood sources increases with increasing development. The pial arterial microanastomoses are located at the terminal branches, i.e., close to the precortical arteries. This provides various routes of blood supply to the smaller areas of the cortex and, in particular, distribution of blood between neighboring microvascular regions. Because of this, the smallest cortical areas can normally be supplied with blood even under circumstances when blood flow in individual, or even in several, pial arterial branches has become disturbed by thrombi, emboli, etc.

If we compare the anatomy of the pial arterial bed to microvascular beds in other organs, we can conclude that, on the whole, the principle of dichotomy is common for all of them. Besides a "vertical structure," the pial arterial bed has acquired during evolution a well-developed "horizontal structure," i.e., numerous anastomoses at several levels. This provides an opportunity to increase the sources of blood supply and distribute blood among neighboring microvascular regions. Probably only the cerebral cortex in man has gained such a high level of opportunities to regulate blood supply to its smallest regions.

Specific vascular portions of the pial arterial bed have been discovered both in microscopic preparations following *in vivo* fixation of the pia mater (Mchedlishvili, Baramidze, et al., 1974-1975; Baramidze and Mchedlishvili, 1977; Baramidze and Gordeladze, 1980; Baramidze et al., 1982b) and in the course of *in vivo* examination of pial arterial behavior in rabbits (Mchedlishvili, Baramidze, et al., 1978; Baramidze and Gordeladze, 1980; Baramidze et al., 1983) and Wistar rats (Jokeleinen et al., 1982). Active vascular portions that have been identified in the minor pial arteries are: the sphincters at the offshoots of smaller microvessels from the larger trunks, the precortical arteries, and the interarterial microanastomoses (Figs. 4.39 and 4.40).

The morphological characteristics of these active microvascular portions in rabbits are as follows. The *sphincters at the offshoots* of pial arteries are located at the initial portions of the smaller pial arteries branching at approximately right angles from the larger vessels (but never at arterial dichotomies) (Figs. 4.39 and 4.40). The diameter of the branches with sphincters usually varies from 20 to 90 µm, but can be larger.

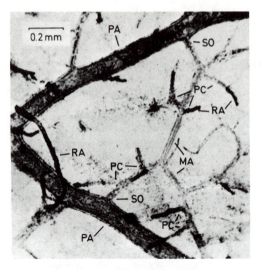

Fig. 4.39. Photomicrograph of the pial arterial
            microvessels on the cerebral surface,
            showing the different microvessels form-
            ing the pial arterial system on the
            cerebral surface in rabbits. PA — the
            comparatively large pial artery; SO —
            the sphincter at offshoots of smaller
            arterial branches; PC — the precorti-
            cal arteries that are the terminal
            branches of the pial microvascular bed;
            RA — the radial arteries entering the
            cerebral cortex (only the first portions
            are visible); MA — the microanastomoses
            between the terminal branches of the
            pial arterial system.

They represent short vascular segments ≈10–20 μm long, with moderately narrowed lumina where the side branches leave the larger pial vessels. In
fixed tissue *in situ*, as well as in photomicrographs *in vivo*, the segments
usually appear narrower, by about 10–15%, compared to the distally located
parts of the same arterial branch. Under resting conditions the degree of
constriction at the sphincters differs considerably throughout the cerebral cortex (Fig. 4.41). The amount of smooth muscle in the media of the
sphincters usually does not exceed that of the adjacent arterial portions.
However, the longitudinal axis of the muscle cells, which is primarily
transverse to the vascular axis, becomes arranged obliquely at the
sphincters.

    The *precortical arteries* represent the terminal branches of the pial
arteries (Figs. 4.39 and 4.40) and merge into the radial arteries that
enter the cerebral cortex after bending at a right angle with respect to
the brain surface. The caliber of the precortical arteries varies from
15 to 55 μm in rabbits. Three types of the precortical arteries have been
identified. They are schematically presented in Fig. 4.42: (a) A side
offshoot of the pial arteries, bending at an approximately right angle,
penetrates the cerebral cortex perpendicular to its surface. This is the
most common type of precortical artery, since it was detected in almost

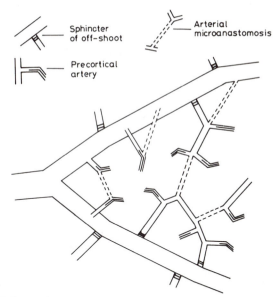

Fig. 4.40. Schematic representation of the pial arterial micro-
            vessels on the cerebral surface in the rabbit, com-
            parable to the photomicrograph presented in Fig.
            4.39. See text for details. (Reproduced from Bar-
            amidze et al., 1982b.)

90% of 200 randomly selected blood vessels. The length of precortical
arteries of this type (from the point of their branching off from the pial
arteries to the site of their entering the cerebral cortex) is 124 ± 15 µm
(M ± SD). (b) The precortical arteries, which offshoot from the cortical
side of pial arteries, penetrate directly into the cerebral cortex. If
the parent artery is comparatively large, the first portion of the precortical artery, as a rule, has a thicker muscular layer. This type of
precortical artery was observed in only 7% of all the blood vessels studied. (c) The precortical arteries, which are similar to the previous type,
but offshoot from smaller pial arteries. This type was found only in 4%
of the blood vessels studied. The luminal diameter of the precortical
arteries is especially variable throughout the cerebral hemispheres (Fig.
4.42).

     The *pial arterial microanastomoses* are located at the smallest
branches of pial arteries (Figs. 4.39 and 4.40). In rabbits they usually
connect either two precortical arteries, or one of them with the smallest
pial arterial branch, or most rarely two small pial arteries under 100 µm
in diameter. The diameter of the lumina of the anastomotic vessels is
usually smaller than that of the microvessels which they connect.

     The behavior of the pial arterial microanastomoses is characterized
by several peculiarities. First, their lumina usually remain open and
undergo smaller changes than those of the adjacent microvessels which they
connect. Second, blood flow in the microanastomoses is very changeable:
it readily changes its direction of response. This is a significant functional difference between the microanastomoses and the microvessels con-

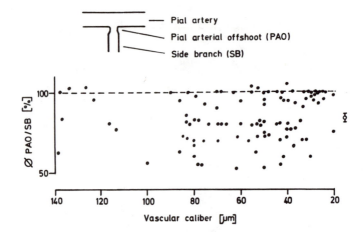

Fig. 4.41.   The functional state of sphincters at offshoots of
             pial arterial branches under resting conditions can
             be determined by the graph of the degree of luminal
             contraction of the sphincters at pial arterial off-
             shoots (PAO) of side branches (SB) from larger pial
             arteries (presented in percent of the lumina of re-
             spective side branches taken as 100%) plotted
             against the resting caliber of respective side
             branches.   The data are obtained from microscopic
             preparations of rabbit pia mater following *in vivo*
             fixation during resting conditions.   (Reproduced
             from Mchedlishvili, Baramidze, et al., 1974-1975.)

nected by them (Fig. 4.43).   In addition, the red cell:plasma ratio in the
microanastomoses undergoes considerable changes compared to the rich red
cell content in the blood in the adjacent blood vessels.   The anastomotic
arterial vessels turn into plasmatic ones, deprived of red cells, for
short or long periods of time, in spite of the fact that the lumina of the
microanastomoses remain unchanged along their course (Fig. 4.44).   This
latter phenomenon depends on the separation of red cells and plasma at the
bifurcations and is related to the difference of flow rates in two branches
(for details of this phenomenon see pp. 274-291 in Chapter 6).   On this
basis we can assume the following function of the pial arterial microanastomoses: they provide secondary distribution (redistribution) of
blood between the adjacent microvascular regions of cerebral cortex that
is beneficial both under the physiological and pathological conditions.
Under physiological conditions this occurs when the blood supply to any
cortical region has been altered.   Due to the scarcity of diameter changes
in microanastomoses, blood is readily redistributed toward the adjacent
microvascular regions in two cases.   The first case is the moderate increase in metabolic demands of the tissue which induces dilatation of only
the precortical arteries.   In this case, blood flow in the microanastomoses become directed toward these precortical arteries, hence contributing to blood supply to the respective area of tissue.   The other case involves an extensive increase in metabolic demands from the cortex resulting in dilatation of the precortical arteries along with the larger feeding
arteries.   In this case, the blood flow in the microanastomoses become
directed from these vessels toward the neighboring precortical arteries
and respective tissue areas.   This protects them from the "steal phenom-

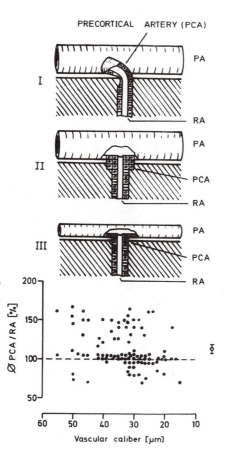

Fig. 4.42. Three types of precortical arteries in
the pial arterial bed in rabbits with
different patterns of localization of
muscle cell nuclei in their walls.
PA — pial arteries, PCA — precortical
arteries, RA — radial arteries. Below:
the functional state of the precortical
arteries of different resting caliber,
expressed as the ratio of the internal
diameter to that of the respective
radial arteries under resting conditions. (Reproduced from Mchedlishvili
and Baramidze, 1971.)

enon," i.e., redistribution of blood into the microvascular region with
considerably increased blood flow. Under pathological conditions the
blood flow in microanastomoses is even more important, since it maintains
blood supply to those microvascular areas whose feeding arteries (the minute pial branches) have been obstructed by an embolus, thrombus, etc.
Thus, the pial arterial microanastomoses increase the reliability of the
regulatory mechanisms of blood supply to the smallest microvascular regions when the microvascular blood flow has moderately or extensively increased, or some minute pial vessels have been cut off from circulation.

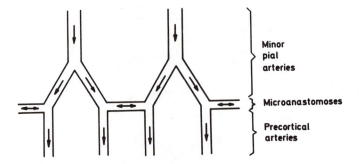

Fig. 4.43. Typical patterns of blood flow directions
            in the terminal ramifications of pial
            arteries. The direction of blood flow in
            the minor pial arteries and in the pre-
            cortical arteries is usually constant,
            while the blood flow in the microanastom-
            oses readily changes its direction.

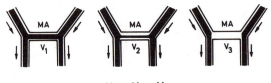

$$V_1 > V_2 > V_3$$

Fig. 4.44. Dependence of red cell:plasma ratio on
            flow velocity in microanastomoses. In
            contrast to the minor pial and precorti-
            cal arteries, the red cell:plasma ratio
            in blood flowing in the microanastomoses
            is changeable and is, as a rule, direct-
            ly correlated with the velocity of flow
            in them (in comparison with the feeding
            arterial branches). See text for de-
            tails.

     By investigating the shortest route of blood flow from the larger pial
arteries to individual precortical arteries (and thus to radial arteries
entering the cerebral cortex) in rabbits, the number of microvascular effectors along these routes has been determined (Baramidze et al., 1982b).
In the majority of cases (66% of those randomly selected) three effectors,
i.e., a sphincter at offshoots, a precortical artery, and a microanastomosis, are present; in 24% of cases there are two of them, i.e., a sphincter
and a precortical artery; and in the remaining 10% of cases more than three
microvascular effectors are detected (one of the effectors is doubled).

     Consequently, all the blood vessels forming the pial arterial bed may
be divided into two types, from a structural and functional point of view.
The larger pial arteries mainly perform the transport function; these are
the dichotomizing larger pial arteries, which possess less potential to
regulate the blood supply to smaller areas of brain tissue. The minute

pial arteries primarily perform a control function: these minor pial
arteries with a characteristic mode of bifurcation (see pp. 124-129) possess specific active vascular portions along their course, with specific
wall structure, innervation, and vascular responses (see below).

Peculiarities of pial vasomotor responses are related to their anatomy and functional characteristics. From the anatomical point of view the
pial arterial bed differs from arterial beds in other organs. Only in the
brain are the overwhelming majority of feeding arteries located on its surface, i.e., outside the brain substance. The major arteries (the internal
carotid and vertebral arteries) regulating several important parameters of
cerebral circulation (see Chapter 3) are located partly outside the cranial
cavity. Their branchings, including the large vessels at the base of the
brain which branch into the anterior, middle, and posterior cerebral arteries, form the pial arterial network, down to the minor arteries 20-50 µm
in diameter, located on the cerebral surface. In other parts of the body
the arterial ramifications supplying the microvascular bed branch successively, down to the smallest arteries, inside the mass of the organ.

This peculiarity of the pial arterial network probably did not appear
randomly during the millions of years of the evolution of vertebrates. In
the process the structure of the cerebral arterial network adapted to the
function performed by the vessels, i.e., the efficient regulation of blood
supply to the cerebral tissue. This function of the pial arteries is manifested in changes of vascular resistance due to vasodilatation or vasoconstriction, which can easily occur since all pial arteries are inside the
comparatively large canals of the subarachnoid space on the brain surface.
The pial vessels are attached to the walls of the canals by thin chords
(Figs. 4.13 and 4.14 on pp. 109 and 110). This allows changes in the
arterial width without exerting any mechanical effect on the cerebral tissue. The cerebrospinal fluid surrounding the vessel walls can be readily
displaced in the canals during dilatation or constriction of the arteries;
in addition, the pial arteries pass above the veins on the brain surface
(Klosovsky, 1951; Duvernoy et al., 1981); hence arterial diameter changes
do not affect the blood flow in individual veins.

In accordance with the main function of the pial arterial network,
i.e., the regulation of an adequate blood supply to cerebral tissue, the
inherent pial vascular responses have been elucidated under experimental
conditions when either the demands for blood arising from the cerebral tissue become inadequate or primary changes in the oxygen and/or carbon dioxide content in the cerebral blood, and hence cerebral tissue, is seen. As
has already been shown (pp. 105-107 and p. 119), the pial arterial responses are correlated with their resting vascular caliber. In rabbits
the minor pial arteries with a resting diameter smaller than ≈100 µm show
considerably greater changes than the larger vessels; the relationship is
nearly exponential. This correlation is especially evident during the
dilatatory vascular responses (Figs. 3.8, 4.9, 4.11, and 4.21) first discovered in the 1970s when the pial arterial responses (usually dilatation)
were plotted against the initial vascular diameter (Betz et al., 1974;
Mchedlishvili, Baramidze, et al., 1974-1975; Brandt et al., 1979;
MacKenzie et al., 1979; Auer and Johansson, 1980).

Another characteristic of pial arterial responses is the priority
of dilatation over constriction. Although these blood vessels, similar
to other muscular arteries of the body, can constrict and dilate,
they have a greater ability to dilate. Both constriction and dilatation
can be produced by a comparable degree of reciprocal changes in blood supply to the cerebral cortex. By increasing and decreasing brain perfusion

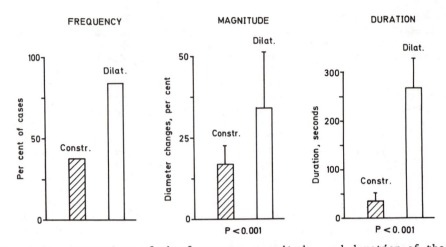

Fig. 4.45.   Comparison of the frequency, magnitude, and duration of the
              constrictory and dilatatory responses (M ± SD) of pial arter-
              ies in rabbits to comparable stimuli. The vasodilatation was
              produced by a primary decrease in cerebral blood flow following
              a drop in systemic arterial pressure by 59 ± 26 mm Hg (ex-
              sanguination), and the vasoconstriction occurred in response
              to excessive cerebral blood flow following elevation of sys-
              temic arterial pressure by 68 ± 3 mm Hg due to intravenous in-
              fusion of noradrenaline. (Modified from Mchedlishvili,
              Ormotsadze, et al., 1975.)

pressure to the same extent (the changes being outside the limits of regulation) it has been found (Mchedlishvili, Ormotsadze, et al., 1975) that
the frequency and size of the dilatatory responses of pial arteries were
almost twice as great as vasoconstriction, and the duration of the dilatation was approximately eight times longer (Fig. 4.45). This provides evidence that the pial arteries are more prone to dilatatory than to con-
strictory responses.

    This peculiarity of pial arterial responses is, in all probability,
related to their inherent behavior when regulating the adequate blood
supply to cerebral tissue. Indeed, among the two possible kinds of blood
inadequacy, deficient blood supply seems to be more frequent and more
dangerous for cerebral tissue than excessive blood flow.* The characteristic behavior of pial arteries is important from another point of view.
As will be shown below (see p. 183 in Chapter 5), the pial arteries are
considerably less likely to develop vasospasm than the major arteries of
the brain (whose function is not related to the regulation of sufficient
blood supply to cerebral tissue). Thus, in all probability, the functional behavior of pial arteries is rarely involved in causing a deficiency in
blood supply to cerebral tissue.

    Consequently, the behavioral peculiarities of the pial arteries include
significantly greater vascular responses in smaller pial arteries than

---

*Excessive blood flow is dangerous during significant rises in systemic
arterial pressure if the pial arteries are pathologically dilated (see
Chapter 5), but this disturbance is usually compensated for by constriction of the major brain arteries (see Chapter 3).

larger vessels to natural stimuli. A considerable preference of dilatation
over constriction is also seen in pial arteries.

The functional heterogeneity of pial arterial responses involved in
the regulation of adequate blood supply to minor cortical areas is now obvious. Heterogeneity, an important feature of the previously described anatomical and functional characteristics of the pial arterial system, aids
in the regulation of adequate blood supply to neighboring cortical areas.

A suitable experimental approach for elucidating the specific response
patterns of various pial arteries (Baramidze et al., 1983) is an experimentally produced increase in cortical activity with simultaneous investigation of the pial microvascular responses upon its surface. However, a
drastic increase in cortical activity is hardly a suitable experimental
approach for this purpose, since it immediately produces dilatation of the
whole pial arterial network, which would yield a faulty analysis of the
sequences and magnitude of vascular responses of various segments of the
pial arterial bed. Therefore, other experimental conditions should be applied. For example, a relatively mild and uniform increase in cortical
activity on a large area can be produced, e.g., by application of drugs
such as strychnine in relatively low concentration to the cerebral surface, and simultaneous investigation of the responses of all terminal portions of the pial arterial bed carrying blood to cerebral tissue can be
executed. Such a microvascular bed includes the following consecutively
traced vascular segments: (a) a relatively larger pial arterial trunk,
(b) the sphincter at the offshoot of a minor arterial branch from the
trunk, (c) the minor pial branch itself carrying blood to the terminal
branches, and (d) these terminal branches, i.e., the precortical arteries
that bend, turn into radial arteries, and enter the cerebral cortex (Figs.
4.39 and 4.40). Rabbits, as experimental animals, are ideal for such an
investigation of the functional behavior of the pial arterial system, since
their system has already obtained all the specific features in higher
animals, but yet is not too complicated (see p. 123).

Figure 4.46 shows that it is the precortical arteries that dilate
most regularly and with the greatest degree in response to a mild increase
in cortical activity. The other microvascular segments of the pial arterial bed dilate less constantly and to a considerably smaller degree. The
sphincters at offshoots either do or do not respond, and this has a considerable influence on the degree of precortical arterial response: if
the sphincters remain silent (the first group on the left in Fig. 4.47),
the dilatation of the precortical arteries is considerably greater than in
cases when the sphincters undergo dilatation (the second group on the
right in the same figure).

Figure 4.48 demonstrates the latent periods of the dilatatory responses of different pial arterial segments. With a mild increase in
neuronal activity of the cortex the precortical arteries dilate with the
shortest latent period. The sphincters at pial arterial offshoots and the
peripheral minor pial arteries either respond or do not respond, and dilatation of the sphincters usually appears earlier than in the minor pial
arteries. Dilatation of the minor pial arteries may be an additional tool
for increasing blood supply to the cerebral cortex. The larger pial
arteries may play a role in the regulation of blood supply to the cerebral
cortex; these arteries respond with the least frequency and the longest
latent period.

An important problem is the determination of the boundary of dilatatory responses in the pial arterial network. This problem can be solved

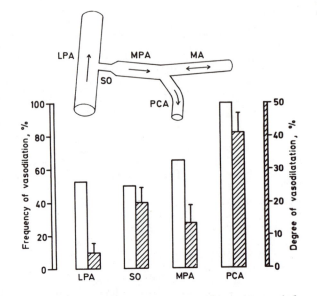

Fig. 4.46.   Dilatatory responses of various pial
microvascular segments to a mild increase in cortical activity in the rabbit. The frequency of vascular responses (white columns) is expressed as
percent of all the experiments (=100%),
and the degree of dilatation (hatched
columns) is expressed as percent of
their initial diameter (=100%). LPA —
large pial arteries, SO — sphincters at
offshoots, MPA — minor pial arteries,
PCA — precortical arteries, MA — a
microanastomosis. (Reproduced from
Baramidze et al., 1983.)

in experiments in which an increase in cortical activity appears locally,
e.g., from the application of a small crystal of strychnine (approximately
30- to 50-μm large) to the cerebral surface. Figure 4.49 shows that the
distribution of dilatation in the adjacent segments of the feeding pial
arteries is similar to the above-mentioned patterns. However, in rabbits
whose pial microvascular network still possesses numerous narrow microanastomoses (in contrast to higher species) the spread of dilatation always stops at the anastomatic level. Hence, the precortical arteries
located on the other side of the microanastomosis do not respond at all,
regardless of the distance from the dilated pial microvessels. Hence, the
narrow microanastomoses in the terminal pial arterial network of rabbits
represent those microvessels that connect the lumina of pial terminal
branches. At the same time, they segregate the responses of pial arterial
microvessels and thus restrict them to the routes by which blood flows to
the appropriate cortical areas under normal conditions.

     Concluding Remarks on the Contribution of the Pial Arterial System to
the Regulation of Microcirculation in the Cerebral Cortex. The structural
and functional peculiarities of the pial arterial bed provide for excel-
lent regulation of blood supply to minor microvascular areas of the cerebral cortex. The capacity to perfectly regulate the local microcirculation

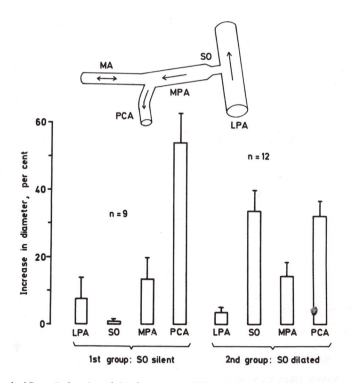

Fig. 4.47.   Relationship between dilatation of sphincters at off-
             shoots and precortical arteries during mild increases
             in cortical activity in the rabbit. The absence of
             dilatation of the sphincters at pial arterial off-
             shoots (1st group, on the left side) is related to a
             considerable dilatation of precortical arteries. But
             when the sphincters respond, the dilatation of pre-
             cortical arteries is considerably reduced (2nd group,
             to the right side). LPA — large pial arteries, SO —
             sphincters at offshoots, MPA — minor pial arteries,
             PCA — precortical arteries, MA — a microanastomosis.
             See text for details. (Reproduced from Baramidze et
             al., 1982.)

accurately is especially important in the brain, where activity changes
occur primarily in local regions under physiological conditions. The pial
microvascular system provides an adequate blood supply to local as well as
widespread tissue areas in the brain. This is possible since the pial
arterial regulation system adapted to the development of the cerebral cortex in the evolutionary process. Thus, the pial arterial system evolved
to regulate adequate microcirculation on gradually smaller tissue areas in
the course of the evolutionary process of vertebrate species.

     Since the purpose of the pial microvascular regulation system is to
satisfy the continuously changing metabolic demands arising from individual small areas of the cerebral cortex, the organization of the pial vascular effectors must provide, primarily, a rapid adjustment in local blood
flow to the metabolic needs of respective areas of the cerebral cortex and,
second, it must protect cerebral tissue against various negative physiological effects from neighboring tissue areas (e.g., due to a sudden increase

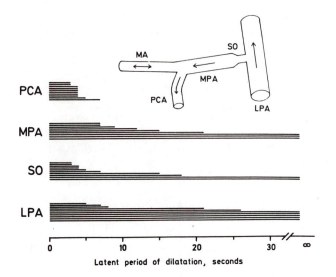

Fig. 4.48.   The duration of latent periods of dila-
             tatory responses of various pial micro-
             vascular segments to mild increases in
             cortical activity in the rabbit. PCA —
             precortical arteries, MPA — the minor
             pial arteries, SO — the sphincters at
             their offshoots from LPA, the large pial
             arteries. ∞ means that no vascular re-
             sponse appeared in the course of the ex-
             periment. (Reproduced from Baramidze et
             al, 1983.)

in their activity and blood supply) and against disturbances in blood flow
in individual microvessels.

   The arrangement of the pial arterial bed, discussed above, furnishes
some assurance of a sensitive regulation of blood supply to the larger and
smaller areas of the cerebral cortex, all the way down to those supplied
by single radial arteries, i.e., those of approximately 0.05-0.2 mm² of
its surface. The terminal branches of the pial arterial network entering
the cerebral cortex, i.e., the precortical arteries, can be supplied with
blood from several sources. The number of these sources is greater in the
more highly developed vertebrates. The microanastomoses are close to the
precortical arteries, and therefore are able to redistribute blood among
the adjacent microvascular beds. Thus, blood supply to the smallest areas
of the cerebral cortex by way of the precortical arteries protects against
cases in which the lumen of an individual, or even several, minor pial
arterial branches become obstructed and the blood flow is disturbed (e.g.,
because of thrombosis or embolism).

   There are usually two active microvascular effectors of regulation
along the blood flow to individual precortical arteries: sphincters at
offshoots and precortical arteries. It may be assumed that local changes
in vascular diameter in active effectors are more advantageous for the
organism than if the diameter changes appear all along the microvessels,
since the former probably operates with less energy cost. To provide ade-

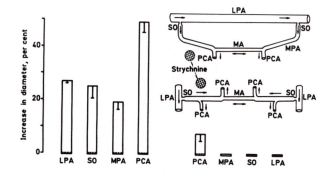

Fig. 4.49. Local pial arterial dilatation during in-
            creases in the activity of the cerebral
            cortex. Following local application to
            rabbits' cerebral cortex of a small crys-
            tal of strychnine (≈50 μm in diameter)
            causing increase in its activity (see the
            schematic design of two patterns of pial
            arterial branches in the top right corner),
            the respective precortical arteries (PCA)
            and the feeding vessels [i.e., the minor
            pial arteries (MPA), sphincters at off-
            shoots (SO), and large pial arteries
            (LPA)] dilate almost similarly to the pat-
            terns shown in Fig. 4.46 (left group of
            columns). The dilatation is absent, how-
            ever, on the other side of the micro-
            anastomoses (MA) (right group of columns).
            See text for details. (Reproduced from
            Mchedlishvili, Baramidze, et al., 1984.)

quate blood supply to the smallest areas of cerebral cortex during increased activity and metabolic needs, dilatation of precortical arteries
appears most often. Subsequently similar vascular responses of the adjacent pial arterial branches and sphincters occur at their offshoots from
larger vessels. Vasodilatation is usually restricted to the arterial
branches feeding only the respective cortical areas. Blood flow in the
microanastomoses is usually directed toward the adjacent vascular regions.
This protects the neighboring cortical areas from the "steal phenomenon,"
which entails deficiency of blood supply to the tissue if blood is redistributed only in the dilated precortical artery.

     Thus, as soon as the neuronal activity of the cerebral cortex increases
(even in very small areas of the cortex relative to individual precortical
arteries, i.e., to 0.05-0.06 of 1 mm² of the cortical surface in more
highly developed mammals), the regulatory signals spread to the feeding
precortical arteries as well as to the adjacent minor pial arteries and
sphincters at their offshoots from larger vessels (Fig. 4.50). The larger
the cortical area with increased activity and high metabolic rate, the
more widespread is the dilatation of the pial arterial branches.

     Consequently, the organization of the pial arterial system provides
adequate blood supply to the cortical areas where metabolic needs have
been changed. Furthermore, it provides adequate blood supply to the ad-

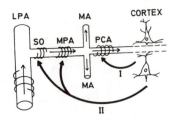

Fig. 4.50. Feedback controlling pial arterial dil-
            atation in response to neuronal activ-
            ity. When the metabolic needs of the
            cerebral cortex increase insignificant-
            ly, the feedback reaches only the pre-
            cortical artery (PCA) to produce dil-
            atation (I). But when the needs are
            greater, then the regulatory signals
            are also spread toward the feeding minor
            pial arteries (MPA) and the sphincters
            at their offshoots (SO), to cause their
            dilatation (II). The blood then flows
            via the microanastomoses (MA) to the
            adjacent microvascular regions, thus
            protecting them from "steal" of blood
            supply. See text for details. (Repro-
            duced from Mchedlishvili and Baramidze,
            1984.)

jacent tissue areas by preventing redistribution of blood flow from them
to the areas with increased metabolic demands.

4.4.   FEEDBACK CONTROLLING ADEQUATE BLOOD SUPPLY TO CEREBRAL
       TISSUE AND CONSTANT RESPIRATORY GASES IN BLOOD

     The feedback associated with the coupling of cerebral blood flow,
metabolic rate, and constant oxygen and carbon dioxide content is one of
the most complicated key problems concerning physiological mechanisms of
cerebral blood flow regulation. Two possible feedback mechanisms may control cerebral blood vessel diameter during regulation: humoral and neurogenic effects, which are responsible for adequate local microcirculation.
It is quite possible that both mechanisms operate concomitantly and com-
plement each other. But from a physiological point of view the actual involvement of the regulatory mechanisms must be analyzed.

     The humoral feedback mechanism implies a direct effect of any vaso-
active agent, including metabolites and blood gases, on vascular smooth
muscle. Some agents, like oxygen and carbon dioxide, can affect vascular
walls from the lumina. Others, for instance hydrogen and potassium ions,
adenosine, etc., affect vascular smooth muscle from outside, after reaching the arterial walls by diffusion through surrounding tissue. Up to the
1960s, when the neurogenic control mechanism of cerebral blood vessels was
completely rejected by the physiologists, the humoral mechanism was the
dominating concept concerning the physiological control of adequate blood
supply to, and blood gases content in, brain tissue. It still represents

the preferred concept of cerebral blood flow regulation. However, considerable difficulties arise when the direct effects of endogenous vasoactive
substances are investigated *in vivo*, since the dissection of cerebral vascular nerves does not cause a total deprivation of neural control in blood
vessels. Previously, researchers thought that evidence for pure humoral
control (without neural involvement) could be obtained while investigating
isolated vascular strips or smooth muscle cells *in vitro*. However, this is
complicated by the fact that even after such isolation some intramural
neural structures are preserved. The intramural elements could cause specific metabolic disturbances in the muscle cells such as the breakdown of
adenyl nucleotides, changes in ionic composition of cytoplasm, etc.

The neurogenic mechanism of vascular effects on blood gases or tissue
metabolic changes on cerebral blood vessels implies that the feedback regulating the vascular lumina includes neural pathways. But this does not
rule out the possibility that the pathways are in turn affected by some
humoral (including metabolic) substances originating from blood or tissue
or that some humoral neurotransmitters are involved in neurogenic effects
on vascular smooth muscle.

However, when the cerebral blood flow has increased in an intact
animal or man following inhalation of gas mixtures with increased carbon
dioxide levels, both direct humoral and neurogenic effects on the arteries
may occur. Hence, such experimental conditions cannot demonstrate either
direct or neurogenic effects of a humoral agent on cerebral blood vessels.
Despite a great number of published experimental results concerned with
cerebral blood flow regulation, only a few studies contain evidence contributing to solution of the problem of how the humoral and neural mechanisms operate in such cases.

As mentioned earlier (p. 102) the neurogenic feedback mechanism can
operate simultaneously with the neurogenic feedforward mechanism. The latter implies that the control signals that activate some neural structures
during brain function simultaneously evoke a vasomotor dilatatory effect
on the feeding arteries of the same neuronal structures. In this case an
increase in their blood supply occurs almost simultaneously with the increased neuronal activity and metabolism without a delay, which is characteristic for any feedback mechanism.

The majority of studies of the problem under consideration are concerned with the blood supply to the cerebral cortex, the most easily approachable part of the brain; only a few are concerned with subcortical
structures, the brain stem, and the cerebellum. However, the generaliza-
tion of the results obtained in some particular brain areas and to various
animal species is in principle incorrect, since the physiological mechanisms regulating adequate blood supply to every brain portion have evolved
independently and may be somewhat diverse. Our current level of knowledge
does not yet allow us to consider such diversity in the regulatory mechanisms in all parts of the brain.

The Possibility of Direct Effects of Carbon Dioxide and Oxygen on
Cerebral Vessel Walls. When the responsiveness of cerebral blood flow to
the blood gas content changes were revealed, most researchers considered
this to be a direct, i.e., purely humoral, effect on vascular smooth
muscle. The effect of changes in oxygen content within physiological
ranges has been found to be comparatively small, while that of carbon dioxide is considerably more potent.

The direct vasodilator effect of carbon dioxide on cerebral vessels was considered in the 1940s and 1950s as the crucial event in regulation of cerebral blood flow for the following reasons: first, carbon dioxide was known to be one of the most potent physiological agents affecting cerebral blood vessels (Novack et al., 1953; Meyer et al., 1962); second, carbon dioxide, being the natural end-product of cerebral metabolism, was thought to be the messenger regulating coupling of regional blood flow with metabolic rate in the brain (Ingvar, 1958; Meyer and Gotoh, 1961); third, carbon dioxide has a very high diffusion coefficient in cerebral tissue, about $3.3 \cdot 10^{-6}$ cm^3 per second at 37°C (Sjesjö and Thews, 1962), and, therefore, it could readily reach the vascular walls by diffusion from surrounding tissue within a few seconds and thus cause a change in cerebral blood flow.

However, experimental data have gradually accumulated that the vasodilator effect of carbon dioxide on cerebral blood vessels is not as simple as had been supposed by earlier investigators. In particular, it was shown that carbon dioxide does not affect vascular smooth muscle directly, since the latency of the "intravascular" and "extravascular" effects has been found to be surprisingly different: 15–30 and 60–90 seconds, respectively (Mayer and Gotoh, 1961).

The problem of whether the carbon dioxide effect on cerebral vessel walls is direct or not was studied in isolated vessels. In the earlier studies of Shalit et al. (1967), the *in situ* perfusion of middle cerebral arterial branches in dogs with their own blood showed that an increase in P_{CO_2} in the blood from 29.9 to 65.0 mm Hg results in a significant reduction in flow. This proved that a vasoconstrictor effect rather than a vasodilator effect of carbon dioxide occurs, similar to other parts of the body. Later studies, however, have demonstrated dilatation of the same artery, isolated *in vitro*, when the P_{CO_2} increases from about 38 to 87 mm Hg in the perfusion fluid (Steinbock et al., 1976).

Many investigators have concluded that carbon dioxide affects cerebral blood vessels indirectly, and that this effect is mediated by hydrogen ions. The ions appear in the fluid surrounding the vessel walls from the hydration reaction of carbon dioxide: $CO_2 + H_2O \rightarrow H^+ + HCO_3^-$. This reaction is catalyzed by the enzyme carbonic anhydrase, which is present inside both red blood cells and the surrounding tissue. This reaction probably takes place mostly outside the blood vessel walls, i.e., in the surrounding tissue, where the carbon dioxide content is readily equilibrated owing to its high diffusion ability. Hydrogen ions so produce their "extravascular" dilator effect on cerebral arteries. Evidence for such a mechanism has been obtained in experiments with the blockade of carbonic anhydrase by acetazolamide which abolishes the vasodilator effect of carbon dioxide (Meyer and Gotoh, 1961; Azin, 1981). The sequence of events resulting in vasodilatation brought about by increasing carbon dioxide in the blood is schematically demonstrated in Fig. 4.51.

The indirect effect of carbon dioxide on the pial arteries has been demonstrated in the experiments with cats by perfusing the space under the cranial window with mock cerebrospinal fluid containing various amounts of carbon dioxide; the vessel diameter changes in proportion to the gas level and to respective changes in the pH of the fluid. The pial vascular responses have been proven to be the effect not of carbon dioxide but of pH changes, since the arteries do not respond to changes in the P_{CO_2} if the pH of the fluid has been held constant (Kontos et al., 1977a, 1977b). These experiments show that it is not carbon dioxide per se, but rather hydrogen ions, which are responsible for vasodilatation, but whether this

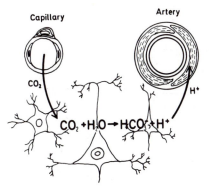

Fig. 4.51.   The hypothetical humoral effect of increased blood carbon dioxide on cere-
bral arterial smooth muscle.   According
to this view, the hydrogen ions originate by hydration of carbon dioxide outside the vessels, in the brain tissue,
via catalysis by carbonic anhydrase
which is present in the tissue.

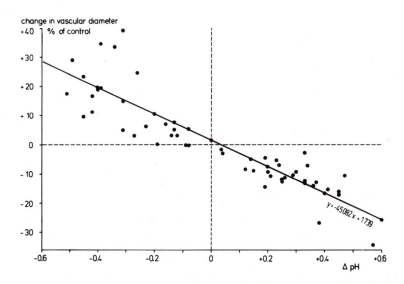

Fig. 4.52.   Correlation between changes in perivascular pH and diameter
changes of pial arteries in cats after the microapplication of
mock cerebrospinal fluid with varying pH on vessel walls from
the outside.   (Reproduced with permission from Kuschinsky,
1982.)

is a *direct* effect of hydrogen ions on vascular smooth muscle requires more
detailed investigation.

A far more convincing line of evidence for the direct dilator effect
of hydrogen ions on pial vessel walls was obtained with microapplication

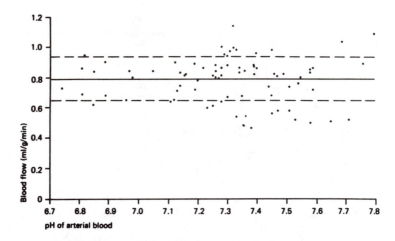

Fig. 4.53.   Cortical blood flow during changes of blood pH in dogs. This
graph demonstrates the absence of changes in cerebral blood
flow, and hence cerebrovascular responses, to alterations of
blood pH produced by administration of lactic acid and sodium
bicarbonate. (Reproduced with permission of Harper and Bell,
1963.)

techniques: the pial arteries in cats dilate within seconds after the
start of injection of mock cerebrospinal fluid with different pH into the
perivascular space (Kuschinsky et al., 1972; Schneider et al., 1977). The
proportional relationship between the pH of applied fluid and the pial
arterial diameter is shown in Fig. 4.52. Thus, it is generally accepted
that the effect of carbon dioxide on cerebral vessels is mediated by changes
in the hydrogen ion concentration, with which the blood P_{CO_2} is readily
equilibrated in the vessel wall medium.

However, certain difficulties arose in explaining the direct humoral
effect of hydrogen ions on cerebral vessels, since no actual effect on
cerebral blood flow was seen when H^+ concentration was primarily changed
in the blood by lactic acid or sodium bicarbonate administration (Fig.
4.53) (Harper and Bell, 1963; Pannier et al., 1974). This is difficult to
understand from the viewpoint of the direct effect of hydrogen ions on vascular smooth muscle, since these solutions can also readily penetrate, although to a lesser degree than carbon dioxide (Meyer et al., 1961), through
endothelium layers in the arteries to reach the vascular muscle cells. In
all probability, the physiological mechanism of carbon dioxide and hydrogen ion effects on cerebral blood flow is not as simple as had been supposed initially. Summarizing the existing experimental data, Plum (1978)
remarked, "...the more we have learned, the harder it has become to regard
carbon dioxide or the hydrogen ion as the universal messenger that links
increased tissue metabolism to the relaxation of cerebral smooth muscle"
(p. 6).

Although oxygen has a potent effect on vascular smooth muscle, significant complications were encountered in attempts to show that cerebrovascular responses during oxygen deficiency in cerebral tissue are due to the
direct vasomotor effect of oxygen on the cerebrovascular smooth muscle.
This was even more difficult to study in the brain than in other organs
where the effects of oxygen on arterial smooth muscle can be analyzed much

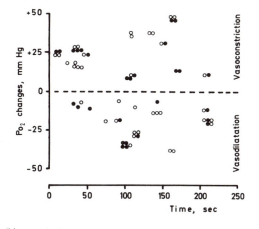

Fig. 4.54. Pial arterial constriction and dilata-
            tion in the rabbit cerebral cortex re-
            lated to P_{O_2} changes at variable levels
            as well as following different latent
            periods. The changes in cerebral blood
            flow have been produced by changes in
            the perfusion pressure of the brain:
            the vasoconstriction was related to
            arterial hypertension (systemic arteri-
            al pressure rose by ≈70 mm Hg) and the
            vasodilatation occurred in response to
            arterial hypotension (systemic arterial
            pressure dropped by ≈60 mm Hg from the
            normal range). White circles denote
            pial arteries having initial diameter
            over 100 μm, and black circles denote
            an arterial diameter under 100 μm.
            (Modified from Mchedlishvili et al.,
            1976.)

more easily (Sparks, 1980). Compared to arteries outside the brain, no
convincing evidence has yet been obtained which might indicate that changes
in oxygen tension of arterial blood or cerebral tissue control the cerebrovascular diameter directly under natural conditions. Careful studies of
cerebral vascular responses to hypoxia have shown that vasodilatation cannot result from the oxygen deficiency affecting the blood vessel walls
either directly or by way of metabolic changes (lactacidosis) in the brain
tissue (Borgström et al., 1975). An analogous conclusion has been drawn
from examining pial arterial diameter changes (Mchedlishvili, Nikolaishvili, et al., 1976) and studying the NAD/NADH redox state and vascular
volume in the cerebral cortex (Dóra and Kovách, 1982). These studies were
carried out during primary changes in blood supply to cerebral tissue due
to significant arterial hypo- and hypertension. No correlation was observed between the P_{O_2} of cerebral cortex and the onset of pial arterial
response (Fig. 4.54). Other evidence that it is not oxygen causing direct
cerebrovascular responses has been obtained under conditions of functional
hyperemia: when the increased neuronal activity results in augmented regional blood flow to the cerebral cortex, P_{O_2} regularly rises (but does not
drop) in the cortical tissue due to increased blood supply (Leniger-Follert
et al., 1977). Thus, oxygen tension changes *per se* do not seem to directly
affect the pial arterial walls and provoke their vasomotor response when
the gas content has changed in cerebral blood and tissue.

Although the possibility has not been excluded that both carbon dioxide and oxygen can directly affect the vascular smooth muscle, no convincing evidence has been obtained which proves that cerebrovascular responses are primarily determined by the effect of blood gases on cerebral vessels and blood flow. We can only speculate that the direct effect of carbon dioxide and oxygen on cerebral vessel walls is a secondary mechanism, which operates when the main physiological regulating mechanism becomes insufficient. Further studies are necessary for clarification of the physiological mechanism in which changes in blood gas levels are coupled with the cerebral blood flow.

The Effects of Humoral Agents Related to Tissue Metabolism on Cerebral Vessel Walls. Hydrogen and potassium ions, as well as adenosine, have been examined as the most feasible candidates responsible for coupling metabolism and local blood flow in the brain.

Hydrogen ions can form in cerebral tissue when simple acidic by-products of carbohydrate metabolism, such as lactic and pyruvic acids, accumulate in the brain. An excess accumulation of these acids is usually related to a deficiency in blood supply and, in particular, oxygen in the blood. Accumulated hydrogen ions can travel a considerable distance in cerebral tissue because of their relatively high diffusion rate.

Since hydrogen ions have been assumed to affect the cerebral vessel walls directly (see above), they were considered as important messengers responsible for functional hyperemia (Betz, 1972; Lübbers, 1972; Purves, 1972). However, serious doubt arose concerning the validity of this since there is firm evidence that vasodilatation and increases in local cerebral blood flow appear much earlier during regulation than the accumulation of hydrogen ions in the tissue. Thus, the local blood flow increases two times after regulation begins in the visual cortex, i.e., within 5-7 and 10-15 seconds, while a decrease in pH in the cortex occurs only during the second wave of blood flow increase (Moskalenko et al., 1975). Similar results have been obtained in a series of further studies. During epileptic seizures caused either by bicuculline intravenous administration (Heuser et al., 1977; Astrup et al., 1978), or direct electrical stimulation of the cerebral cortex (Urbanics et al., 1978), as well as during somato-sensory stimulation (Gregory et al., 1977), functional hyperemia appears in the cortex much earlier than the accumulation of hydrogen ions. The vasodilatation is actually related to decreases (but not to increases!) in the hydrogen ion concentration. The latter change is probably caused by an increased washout of carbon dioxide from cerebral tissue by increased blood flow. Further evidence against hydrogen ions acting as specific triggers of vasodilatation is the absence of correlation between the vascular responses and the acidic shift of pH in the cerebral cortex observed during hypoxia (Borgström et al., 1975) and deficient blood supply to the brain (Mchedlishvili, Nikolaishvili, et al., 1976). The pH can be increased and decreased under these conditions, and the latent period of vascular response has been found to be highly variable, i.e., from 36 to 250 seconds (Fig. 4.55).

The experimental results cited above provide evidence that hydrogen ions cannot be responsible for the onset of vasodilatation, and hence hyperemia, in cerebral tissue under conditions of increased activity and metabolic rate. Some authors assumed (Urbanics et al., 1978; Astrup et al., 1978) hydrogen ions maintain hyperemia in the brain, provided that its production is stimulated by some other effect on the cerebral vessel walls. Hydrogen ions can be assumed to be responsible for prolonged hyperemia in cerebral tissue during ischemia when a considerable amount of lac-

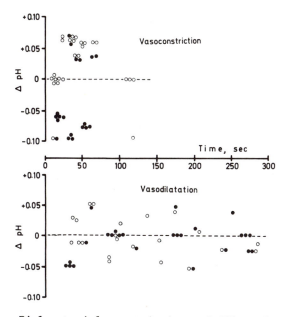

Fig. 4.55. Pial arterial constriction and dilatation in the rabbit cerebral cortex related to pH changes occurring
at different latent periods. The arterial constriction occurred in response to an increase in systemic
arterial pressure (by ≈70 mm Hg), and the vasodilatation was due to a decrease in the arterial pressure
(by ≈60 mm Hg). White circles denote larger pial
arteries having an initial diameter over 100 μm, and
black circles denote vessels with an initial diameter under 100 μm. (Modified from Mchedlishvili,
Nikolaishvili, et al., 1976.)

tate accumulates in the tissue. However, experimental data obtained by
direct measurement of the pH in the cerebral cortex show that no actual
correlation exists between the concentration of hydrogen ions and vasodilatation: following 15 minutes of incomplete cerebral ischemia the
acidification of the tissue lasts much longer than hyperemia does (Mchedlishvili, Nikolaishvili, et al., 1974; Mchedlisvili, Antia, et al., 1974).
Although the direct relaxing effect of hydrogen ions on the cerebral vascular smooth muscle is evident, their role as a specific trigger of functional and postischemic vasodilatation, and hence hyperemia, in the brain
under conditions of increased metabolic demand in cerebral tissue causes
some doubt.

Another substance thought to be a messenger linking tissue functional
activity with local blood flow is the *potassium ion* (Sparks, 1980) found
in the cell bodies of brain tissue. As is generally known, these ions are
located chiefly intracellularly because of their steady active transport
across the plasma membranes to intracellular spaces. Increases in neuronal activity are generally related to prompt and transient redistribution
of potassium ions, resulting in extracellular concentration increases.
Thus, potassium ions can spread during neural activation by diffusion
along the interstitial spaces and reach the walls of the feeding arteries.

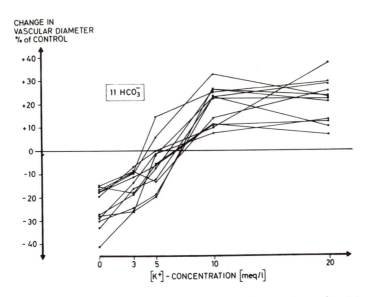

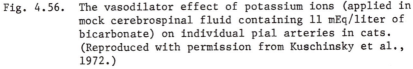

Fig. 4.56. The vasodilator effect of potassium ions (applied in
            mock cerebrospinal fluid containing 11 mEq/liter of
            bicarbonate) on individual pial arteries in cats.
            (Reproduced with permission from Kuschinsky et al.,
            1972.)

The increase in potassium ion concentration close to cerebral arterial
walls results in a decrease in their tone, similar to other arteries in the
body (Sparks, 1980). The direct dilatory effect of potassium ions on pial
arterial walls has been observed in studies with microapplication techniques. Figure 4.56 shows that mock cerebrospinal fluid containing 5 mM
potassium applied to vascular walls does not produce significant dilatation, but higher concentrations of the ions (10-12 mM) result in an evident dilatation of the pial arteries (Kuschinsky et al., 1972). An increased concentration of potassium ions has been discovered on the brain
surface during epileptic seizures caused by intravenous administration of
bicuculline (Heuser et al., 1977). An especially great increase in potassium concentration occurs under ischemic conditions when the active transport mechanism of the ions in the cellular plasma membranes is impaired
(Branston et al., 1977).

The vasodilator mechanism of potassium ions may be related, on the one
hand, to alterations in the membrane potential of vascular smooth muscle
cells associated with sodium and calcium fluxes and, on the other hand,
to a reduced noradrenaline release from nerve endings (Sparks, 1980).

However, certain difficulties arise in explaining functional vasodilatation solely by the direct effect of potassium ions on cerebral blood
vessel walls because of time discrepancies between the vascular responses
and the changes in potassium ion concentration in the tissue. The duration
of the potassium vasodilator effect is relatively short, and no correlation
has been found between the time course of cerebral blood flow changes and
concentration of potassium ions in the medium surrounding the vascular
walls (Mutsuga et al., 1976). Vasodilatation has been detected within 1-2
seconds after the onset of arterial hypoxia in the cerebral cortex while

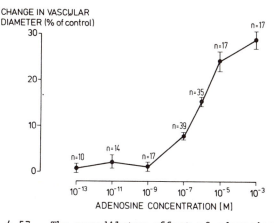

Fig. 4.57.   The vasodilator effect of adenosine (applied in mock cerebrospinal fluid) on
pial arteries in cats. n = the number
of vessels tested. (Reproduced with
permission from Wahl and Kuschinsky,
1976.)

the potassium ion concentration is still unchanged (Zeuthen et al., 1979).
A similar time discrepancy was found in the rat brain during the postischemic period. The normal potassium ion concentration was actually recovered in cerebral tissue within 4 minutes after the onset of ischemia
(10 minutes long), but the cerebral blood flow undergoes a maximal increase
at just this time (Hansen et al., 1980). It can be concluded that potassium ions are responsible for only the initial increase in cerebral blood
flow, but not for the whole course of functional or ischemic vasodilatation.

Another difficulty arises in explaining pial vasodilatation, especially in specific segments of the pial arterial bed (see pp. 135-144),
that occurs on the cerebral surface within seconds. To directly affect
these vessels, the potassium ions, which originate in the deeper layers of
the cerebral cortex, must diffuse along a path about 1.5-2 mm long. This
cannot occur within the few seconds that separate the onset of increased
activity and the onset of vascular responses; it definitely requires a considerably longer period.

The *cyclic AMP system* is activated by adenosine, as well as calcium
ions, which are normal constituents in the contraction-relaxation process
of the vascular smooth muscle (see pp. 221-226). Therefore they probably
play a significant part in vasomotor responses irrespective of their cause,
e.g., release by a direct action of some humoral factor or by vasomotor
nerve impulses. In addition, adenosine, as well as ATP, can be produced
from specific purinergic nerves and thus affect the vascular smooth muscle
as a neurotransmitter (Burnstock, 1975). In several studies with microapplication techniques (Rehncrona et al., 1977; Wahl and Kuschinsky, 1977)
an increase in adenosine in the perivascular space resulted in dilatation
of the pial arteries. Adenosine produces vasodilatation beginning at a
concentration of 10^{-7} M (Fig. 4.57).

During epileptic seizures caused by intravenous administration of bicuculline, hyperemia appears in the cerebral cortex almost simultaneously

with changes in the electrocorticogram (Meldrum and Nilsson, 1976). However, the adenosine content increases in brain tissue considerably later (Nilsson et al., 1978). In another study the adenosine content in cerebral tissue was found to be increased within 10 seconds after the onset of seizures (Winn et al., 1980). Adenosine has been further found to increase 2.5-fold in the brain within seconds during profound ischemia (Winn et al., 1979) when the pial arteries undergo considerable dilatation; this proves adenosine is involved in the vascular response.

However, there are some experimental conditions, for instance hypoglycemic seizures, where an increase in cortical activity and in blood flow occur simultaneously without any changes in the concentration of potassium ions, hydrogen ions, and adenosine (Astrup et al., 1978). Therefore, functional vasodilatation in the brain may occur simultaneously without participation of the humoral factors considered above, including adenosine. Another factor that interferes with the understanding of the concept of adenosine as a messenger causing the functional vasodilatation is that it antagonizes the effects of potassium and hydrogen ions on pial arterial smooth muscle (Wahl and Kuschinsky, 1977; Boisvert et al., 1978).

From the foregoing we may conclude that different humoral vasoactive agents like hydrogen and potassium ions, as well as adenosine, *can* affect the cerebral vascular smooth muscle and therefore *may* be involved in the control of adequate blood supply to cerebral tissue. But the problem of whether the mentioned humoral agents are usually involved in functional vasodilatation cannot be solved. Humoral agents of endogenous origin can certainly affect the vascular walls not only separately, but in various combinations differing both in timing and in concentration.

Serious conflicts arise when we try to understand the presently known behavior of the pial arterial bed, i.e., the most probable vascular effectors of this type of cerebral blood flow regulation. If the vasodilator effect during regulation of adequate blood supply to the cerebral cortex were brought about only by diffusion of potassium or hydrogen ions or any other vasoactive substance from the cortex, then how could the regulatory portions of the pial vascular system behave so specifically (see pp. 135–144)?

When considering humoral coupling factors in cerebral blood flow regulation, the same principles should be applied as those employed for ascertaining the role of neurotransmitters (Purves, 1979b). This means that experiments should demonstrate that activated neurons release the substance into extracellular fluid and that its concentration rises despite the buffering action of glial cells; that the substance causes dilatation of the respective blood vessels and that there is a correlation between the time course of the rise in substance concentration and changes in local blood flow; and that the effect of the proposed substance upon the blood flow can be mimicked by local application. All this requires sophisticated techniques and a high level of technical experience. But until this is done, the question of how local metabolism and blood perfusion are matched will not be completely solved.

Consequently, despite the relatively simple experimental models needed to investigate the direct effect of different humoral vasoactive agents on vascular smooth muscle, nobody has been able to prove so far that the mechanism linking tissue metabolic processes with local blood flow is primarily accomplished by the direct effect of blood gases and/or tissue metabolic substances on cerebral vessel walls. Nevertheless, this humoral vasomotor effect may operate in the organism as an accessory tool

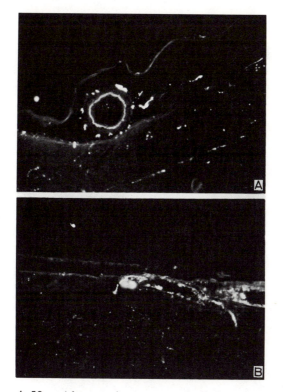

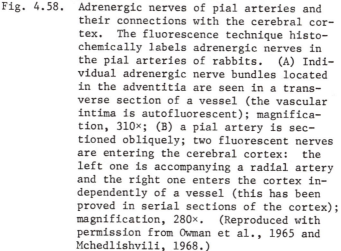

Fig. 4.58. Adrenergic nerves of pial arteries and their connections with the cerebral cortex. The fluorescence technique histochemically labels adrenergic nerves in the pial arteries of rabbits. (A) Individual adrenergic nerve bundles located in the adventitia are seen in a transverse section of a vessel (the vascular intima is autofluorescent); magnification, 310×; (B) a pial artery is sectioned obliquely; two fluorescent nerves are entering the cerebral cortex: the left one is accompanying a radial artery and the right one enters the cortex independently of a vessel (this has been proved in serial sections of the cortex); magnification, 280×. (Reproduced with permission from Owman et al., 1965 and Mchedlishvili, 1968.)

when the principal physiological mechanism is deficient for any reason. Therefore the involvement of a regulatory neurogenic mechanism must be considered.

Adrenergic and Cholinergic Nerves Regulating Pial Arterial Behavior.
As previously mentioned, neurogenic control of cerebral circulation was neglected until the 1960s. Two findings were essential in bringing about the conceptual shift in physiological understanding of this problem. The first was the discovery of the role of the pial arteries as the effectors of regulation of adequate blood supply to the cerebral cortex (see pp.

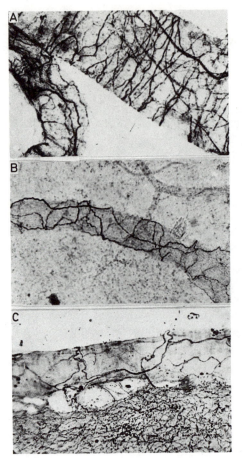

Fig. 4.59. Cholinergic nerves of pial arteries and
            their connections with the cerebral cor-
            tex. The cholinesterase is histochem-
            ically identified in the nerve plexuses
            in the pial arteries of rabbits. (A)
            The posterior cerebral artery, 600 μm in
            diameter, with a branch; magnification,
            80×; (B) a smaller pial artery, 200 μm
            in diameter; magnification, 100×. A and
            B are total preparations of the pial
            mater. (C) Cholinergic nerve bundles,
            which connect the perivascular plexus of
            the pial artery, 200 μm in diameter, with
            the cerebral cortex in transverse sec-
            tion; magnification, 80×. (Reproduced
            with permission from Pletchkova et al.,
            1969.)

104–113). The second was the visualization of adrenergic and cholinergic
nerves in pial walls along with the gradual accumulation of experimental
evidence for neurogenic control of these arteries.

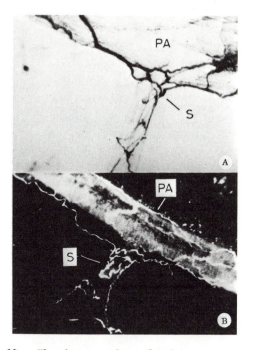

Fig. 4.60.   The innervation of sphincters at pial ar-
             terial offshoots. The photomicrographs
             show the cholinergic (A) and adrenergic (B)
             nerve supply of sphincters (S) at offshoots
             of small pial arterial branches from larger
             pial arteries (PA) in rabbits; magnifica-
             tion 100× and 80×, respectively. (Repro-
             duced with permission from Baramidze et al.,
             1982.)

    Pial arterial adrenergic (Falck et al., 1965; Owman et al., 1965,
1966) and cholinergic nerves (Lavrentieva et al., 1968; Pletchkova et al.,
1969) were first seen in rabbits (Figs. 4.58 and 4.59). Since then many
studies have shown abundant adrenergic and cholinergic innervations in
pial arteries in various animals and man (Nielsen and Owman, 1967; Motavkin and Dovbish, 1970; Iwoyama et al., 1970; Edvinsson et al., 1972; Motavkin and Osipova, 1973; Owman et al., 1974; Denn and Stone, 1976; and many
others). Thus, the walls of the pial arteries are surrounded by plentiful
adrenergic and cholinergic nerve fibers forming plexuses in the vascular
adventitia and accompanying the blood vessels all along their course down
to their smallest branches on the brain surface. The distribution of the
vascular adrenergic and cholinergic nerves in different cerebral territories is variable; this is related to diversity in vascular responses
(Cervós-Navarro, 1977; Owman and Edvinsson, 1979).

    The density of pial arterial nerves is relatively high in large ves-
sels and gradually decreases as the vascular caliber becomes smaller. The
density of nerves containing cholinesterase, which was investigated morphometrically in rabbits, was found to decrease almost proportionally with
the decrease in the vascular caliber; this density decreases faster in
transverse nerves than in longitudinal nerves (Lavrentieva et al., 1968).

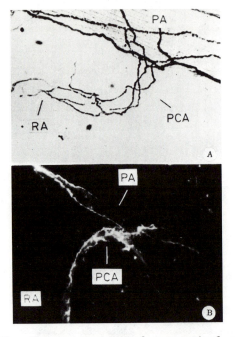

Fig. 4.61.   The innervation of precortical arteries.
The photomicrographs show the cholinergic
(A) and adrenergic (B) nerve supply of
precortical arteries (PCA) adjacent to
the small pial arteries (PA) of rabbits.
Single nerve fibers are running along the
radial arteries (RA) entering the cerebral
cortex; magnification, 100× and 80×, respectively.   (Reproduced with permission
from Baramidze et al., 1982.)

However, the specifically active vascular segments of the minute pial
arterial ramifications have a particularly rich supply of adrenergic and
cholinergic nerves.

The sphincters at the offshoots of smaller pial arteries from the
larger trunks contain plentiful cholinergic and adrenergic nerve fibers,
often with varicosities; these fibers are rarely encountered in the walls
of the neighboring pial arteries (Fig. 4.60).   The comparative density of
the nerve fibers at the sphincters and at the adjacent arterial segments
has been determined morphometrically and is shown in Fig. 4.62.   The density of adrenergic and cholinergic nerves has also been found to be high
in the precortical arteries, although they have the smallest caliber in
the pial arterial bed (Fig. 4.61).   In microscopic preparations it is possible to follow a single nerve fiber which originates from the plexus of
the precortical arteries and runs along the radial arteries into the cortex (Fig. 4.61).   Figure 4.62 shows the density of cholinergic and adrenergic nerve fibers surrounding the precortical arteries in comparison to
the adjacent pial arterial branches and the radial arteries inside the
cerebral cortex.

The plentiful cholinergic and adrenergic nerves at the sphincters of
pial arterial offshoots and of the precortical arteries are related to the

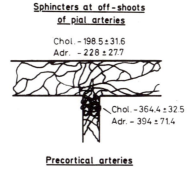

**Sphincters at off-shoots
of pial arteries**

Chol. - 198.5 ± 31.6
Adr. - 228 ± 27.7

Chol. - 364.4 ± 32.5
Adr. - 394 ± 71.4

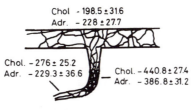

Precortical arteries

Chol - 198.5 ± 31.6
Adr. - 228 ± 27.7

Chol. - 276 ± 25.2
Adr. - 229.3 ± 36.6

Chol. - 440.8 ± 27.4
Adr. - 386.8 ± 31.2

Fig. 4.62. The comparative density of innervation
[cholinergic (Chol.) and adrenergic (Adr.)
nerves] of sphincters at the offshoots of
pial arteries and of precortical arteries
in rabbits. The numbers represent M ± SD.
The differences are statistically significant (P < 0.0001). (Reproduced with permission from Baramidze et al., 1982.)

most active changes in vascular lumina during the regulation of adequate
blood supply to the cerebral cortex (see pp. 135-141). The coupling of
abundant nerves with varicosities to extensive diameter changes in blood
vessels is evidence of an active neurogenic control (Cerrós-Navarro, 1977).
Other evidence for neurogenic control of these microvessels includes their
independent response compared to adjacent portions of the pial microvessels (see pp. 143-144), in spite of the fact that no considerable morphological and histochemical differences have been detected in these walls
(Baramidze et al., 1981).

The nerve supply of the pial arterial microanastomoses near the precortical arteries or the neighboring smallest pial arterial branches is
relatively poor. In rabbits the walls of the microanastomoses usually
possess only one or two cholinergic and adrenergic nerve fibers running
along the microvessels; only the larger microanastomoses possess more
nerve fibers in their walls (Baramidze et al., 1982).

The interrelationship between nerve terminals and the vascular smooth
muscle cell membranes has been studied by electron microscopy. The synaptic cleft in the pial arterial walls of cats is 80-100 nm wide and two
populations of synaptic vesicles were found: granular vesicles, which are
most likely adrenergic, and clear vesicles, which are probably cholinergic
(Nelson and Rennels, 1970). Investigations with both electron microscopy
and histochemical methods have revealed nonmedullated axons with synaptic
vesicles in the walls of the pial arteries of rats near their contact with
smooth-muscle cells. Some of these neural structures, which disappear

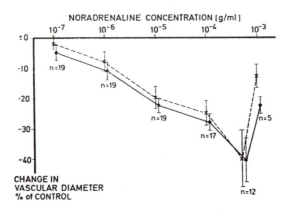

Fig. 4.63. The effect of noradrenaline (applied in a
mock cerebrospinal fluid containing 11
mEq/liter bicarbonate, which itself has almost no vascular effect), on the pial arteries of cats. Black circles = noradrenaline + HCO_3; x = noradrenaline — HCO_3. The
curve shows M ± SE; n is the number of vessels tested. (Reproduced with permission
from Wahl et al., 1971–1972.)

after sympathectomy and administration of reserpine, are adrenergic; others
are evidently cholinergic nerve fibers. Both have been found in close
proximity to vascular smooth-muscle cell membranes (Iwoyama et al., 1970).
The neuromuscular cleft in rat intracerebral arteries is also at least 80
nm wide, and three groups of terminals have been detected: those with
large vesicles, with small vesicles, or without vesicles (Cervós-Navarro
and Matakas, 1974). However, distribution of nerve terminals containing
agranular and granular vesicles in the pial arterial walls is dissimilar
in cats and rabbits (Lee, 1981).

Anatomical proximity of adrenergic and cholinergic nerves has been
found within the same nerve trunks in pial vessels; this is presumed to indicate that an interaction might take place between adjacent terminals
(Edvinsson and Owman, 1976). However, no vesicles accumulated at specific
sites in the membranes at axoaxonal contacts or the neuromuscular contacts. This indicates the possibility that synaptic activity may occur
"at a distance" from the actual contact (Cervós-Navarro, 1977).

It is important that pial vascular nervous plexuses have been found
in direct connections with the cerebral cortex located close to the vascular wall: connecting nerve bundles, both adrenergic (Owman et al., 1965)
and cholinergic (Pletchkova et al., 1969), have been found which are presented in Figs. 4.58b and 4.59c. These findings were subsequently corroborated by Edvinsson et al. (1973). Thus it might be concluded that
pial arterial nerves are connected with various areas in the cerebral cortex by two kinds of neural pathways: first, by those which follow the
arterial branches entering the cerebral cortex and, second, by nerve fibers
separated from the vessel walls that penetrate the superficial layers of
the cortex.

The adrenergic nerves in pial arteries were found to originate from
the cervical sympathetic ganglia, since their removal results in the dis-

appearance of noradrenaline fluorescence in the vascular nerves (Owman et al., 1965; Edvinsson et al., 1972). In cats the superior cervical sympathetic ganglion has been found to supply the middle cerebral and posterior communicating arteries bilaterally (Marin et al., 1980).

The origin of most vascular cholinergic nerves is far from clear. Investigation of the cholinergic pathways is restricted since they are encased in bone and are far less accessible for manipulation than the adrenergic nerves. It has long been known that cerebral vasodilator nerves run in the facial nerve, through the geniculate ganglion and the greater superficial petrosal nerves, since electrical stimulation of these nerves produced dilatation of the pial arteries; this stimulation was abolished after atropine was given (Chorobsky and Penfield, 1932; Cobb and Finesinger, 1932; Pinard et al., 1979). Physiological evidence for the involvement of these nerves in cerebral vasodilatation was subsequently corroborated (Meyer et al., 1971; Salanga and Waltz, 1971; Ponte and Purves, 1974). However, section of the petrosal nerves does not cause (even within four months) a significant loss of cholinesterase in the adventitial plexus of pial arteries or a considerable ultrastructural degeneration in the nerve terminals (Purves, 1979a). This indicates that most of the vascular cholinergic nerves originate from some source other than the petrosal nerve.

The central cholinergic and adrenergic structures related to pial periarterial nerve plexuses are almost unknown; experimental evidence is still very scarce. Brainstem stimulation has been found to cause dilatation of cerebral vessels, thus indicating the existence of a neural center which controls cerebral blood flow (Molnár and Szántó, 1964). Further evidence has cast doubt as to whether there is only one center in the brain controlling the blood flow in all regions. Ganglionic formations containing cholinesterase have been described in the anterior cranial fossa. These structures may be post-ganglionic parasympathetic fibers related to the cholinergic nerves of pial vessels of the fronto-parietal region, but the origin of the preganglionic fibers remains unknown (Licata et al., 1975). Stimulation of the fastigial nucleus in rats results in widespread vasodilatation in the cerebral cortex independent of cortical metabolic changes (Nakai et al., 1981). The adrenergic innervation of cerebral arteries has been thought by some to originate in the locus coeruleus (Hartman et al., 1972; Raichle et al., 1975). However, further investigations did not completely corroborate this assumption (Heistad, 1981). On the other hand, catecholaminergic neurons in the brainstem have also been thought to innervate cerebral arteries (Itakura et al., 1977).

Identification of the central pathways of cerebral vascular nerves by stimulation of brain structures in physiological experiments may be complicated by the difficulty in ascertaining the mechanism of vasodilatation; it may be a result of primary activation of the respective neuronal groups in the cortex related to the blood vessels or a result of a direct vasomotor neural effect on the blood vessel wall. The findings of adrenergic and cholinergic nerves in pial arterial walls agree well with the results of neurotransmitter studies affecting arterial smooth muscle. Using microapplication techniques (Wahl et al., 1971-1972), adrenaline and noradrenaline have been shown to produce vasoconstriction of pial arteries (Fig. 4.63). This response is blocked by a specific alpha-adrenergic blocker, phentolamine (Nielson and Owman, 1971; Wahl et al., 1971-1972).

However, the pial arteries are considerably less sensitive to noradrenaline than arteries in other parts of the body. This has been shown in cats, rabbits, and goats. Not only is a higher concentration of noradrenaline required to activate the alpha-adrenergic receptors of the pial arteries, but the maximum responses are much smaller than those due to

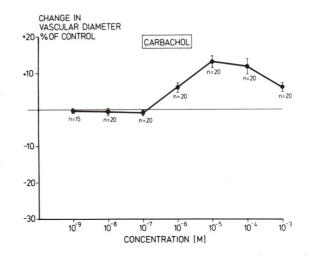

Fig. 4.64. The effect of carbachol on pial arteries of
cats. The curve shows M ± SE; n is the
number of vessels tested. (Reproduced with
permission from Kuschinsky et al., 1974.)

other agents (Bevan et al., 1980). The alpha-adrenergic receptors in the
pial arteries are specifically activated (Duckles and Bevan, 1976; Lee et
al., 1976; Bevan and Bevan, 1977). A certain diversity in the alpha-
adrenergic receptors has been found in the pial arterial smooth muscle responses of dogs and sheep (Duckles, 1979).

On the other hand, acetylcholine and carbachol cause a dose-dependent
dilatation of pial arteries (Fig. 4.64) which is blocked by atropine
(Kuschinsky et al., 1974; Lee et al., 1975). The pial arterial receptors,
however, respond specifically to acetylcholine (Toda, 1979). The cerebral
arterial walls have been found to contain high levels of choline acetyl-
transferase and acetylcholine; the latter is released upon activation of
the intramural nerves (Bevan et al., 1981a). However, only part of the
neurogenic dilator response is atropine-sensitive; a possible transmitter
for the atropine-resistant component is vasoactive intestinal peptide
(VIP) (Bevan et al., 1981b).

These results suggest that there are alpha-adrenergic as well as
cholinergic receptors in the media of the pial arteries, although these
receptors have some differences compared to those in other blood vessels
in the body.

Physiological Evidence for the Involvement of a Neural Mechanism in
the Effect of Blood Gases on Cerebral Blood Flow. Evidence gradually accumulated indicating that a neurogenic vasomotor effect is involved in
cerebral blood flow responses to changes in oxygen and carbon dioxide content in the blood. Probably the first evidence of this kind is a close
relationship between changes of oxygen tension in the venous (but not in
the arterial!) blood and cerebrovascular responses, as demonstrated by
Schneider and his associates (Opitz and Schneider, 1950). In this case
feedback to the cerebral arteries evidently arises from the veins or the
surrounding cerebral tissue (it cannot be a direct effect of oxygen on
the arterial walls) and it may be neurogenic in nature. Another fact
pointing to an involvement of neurogenic mechanisms in cerebral vasodil-

atation in response to oxygen deficiency in blood is the very short latent period of the cerebral blood flow response: it starts within 1-2 seconds when no significant metabolic changes occur in the brain (Zeuthen et al., 1979). The increase in cerebral blood flow appears during hypoxemia and hypercapnia when the extracellular pH is still unchanged (Nilsson et al., 1975) and the content of adenosine has not been altered (Nilsson et al., 1978). In addition, the effect of high P_{CO_2} in blood on cerebral vessels has been found to cease in ischemic brain regions as a result of occlusion of the middle cerebral artery (Waltz, 1970). This, in turn, seems to indicate that the carbon dioxide effect is neurogenic, since neurons are considerably more sensitive to a blood supply deficiency than vascular smooth muscle cells.

The involvement of a cholinergic mechanism in cerebral vasodilatation caused by a carbon dioxide increase in blood was demonstrated by blockage of the response with atropine (Rovere et al., 1973) and by enhancement of the response with physostigmine, a cholinesterase inhibitor (Scremin et al., 1982). The adrenergic nerves also seem to participate in responses of the cerebral blood vessels to carbon dioxide. Alpha-adrenergic blockers significantly change the cerebrovascular responses to hyper- and hypocapnia (Meyer et al., 1977). The responsiveness of large vessels of the circle of Willis to carbon dioxide is significantly decreased in chronically sympathectomized monkeys (Stone and Raichle, 1975). The influence of catecholaminergic neurons on the cerebrovascular response to carbon dioxide has been further corroborated (Berntman et al., 1979).

It is well known that chemoreceptors highly sensitive to arterial oxygen and carbon dioxide levels are located in specific parts of the arterial bed, i.e., in the aortic arch and the carotid sinus. These chemoreceptive areas — the aortic and carotid bodies — are located in the vascular adventitia and are continually perfused with arterial blood. The frequency of nerve impulses transmitted by the afferent pathways (i.e., the sinus nerve which is a branch of the glossopharyngeal nerve, and the aortic nerve which is a branch of the vagus) is very low under normal conditions, but sharply rises when the P_{O_2} decreases or the P_{CO_2} increases in the blood (Biscoe et al., 1970).

The effects of the blood gases on cerebral blood flow have been investigated in careful experiments by Ponte and Purves (1974); they perfused the carotid bodies with blood containing different oxygen and carbon dioxide tensions. The decrease in oxygen or increase in carbon dioxide content in the perfusing blood results in an increase in cerebral blood flow by 63-81%. This effect disappears after dissection of the sinus nerves, i.e., the afferent pathways, as well as the facial nerves which, in all probability, carry some afferents to cerebral blood vessels (see p. 165). However, this effect of carotid chemoreceptors on cerebral blood flow was not corroborated in other studies with dissection of the afferent pathways (Traystman et al., 1978; Traystman and Fitzgerald, 1981). The discrepancy of experimental results can be explained either by the variance in the experimental techniques applied, or by the fact that there are specific chemoreceptors in other parts of the cerebral vasculature that can substitute for the carotid chemoreceptors' function.

Many neural structures, morphologically similar to sensory endings, are distributed in the walls of both cerebral arteries and veins (Kuprianov and Zhitza, 1975). In all probability, they represent functional chemoreceptors (and baroreceptors as well). But in view of the fact that these receptor structures have so far been inaccessible for experimentation with the usual physiological approaches (dissection and stimulation of afferent pathways, electrophysiological studies of their responses, etc.), their

function has not as yet been adequately investigated. One can only speculate that these receptors can respond to changes in oxygen and carbon dioxide levels in the blood and cause, by neurogenic control, respective
changes in cerebral blood flow even under conditions when the carotid and
aortic afferent pathways have been cut.

The neuronal association areas, which play the role of coordinating
centers of cerebral blood flow responses to blood gas changes, have not yet
been localized. It has been shown that different lesions of the brain stem,
hypothalamus, and midbrain (local cooling, destruction or dissection), considerably reduce cerebral vasodilatation in response to hypercapnia and
hypoxia (Molnár and Szántó, 1964; Shalit et al., 1967; Meyer et al., 1969;
Fenske et al., 1975; Capon, 1975; Scremin et al., 1977). However, the
existing physiological data are insufficient to ascertain where the central
neural structures involved in the blood gases' effects are localized and
how they function under normal conditions.

The efferent vasodilator pathways may be included in the facial and
greater superficial petrosal nerves and spread to the nervous plexuses of
the major and pial arteries (see pp. 74–76 and pp. 161–164). However, cerebral vasodilatation in response to hypercapnia, in all probability, occurs
through other pathways located outside these nerves, since the vascular
responses were preserved after dissection of these nerves (Hoff et al.,
1975). The localization of the afferent pathways remains unknown.

Involvement of neural pathways in the responsiveness of the blood vessels feeding the cerebral cortex to carbon dioxide has been shown in
chronic experiments after dissection of pathways connecting the cerebral
cortex with the hypothalamus and other subcortical structures (the method
developed by Khananashvili). The vascular responses to carbon dioxide are
significantly reduced compared to the control hemispheres (Demchenko,
1979). After this operation the functional state of the pial arteries remains unchanged, since their responses to increased cortical activity in
the neuronally isolated cerebral cortex remains intact (Baramidze et al.,
1980).

The possibility that the carbon dioxide effect occurs through a local
neurogenic mechanism cannot be excluded. This conclusion can be drawn
from experiments where an increase in hemispheric blood flow is observed
during perfusion of the carotid system with hypercapnic blood in humans
(Skinhoj and Paulson, 1969). Another possibility cannot be excluded —
namely that carbon dioxide might primarily affect the neuronal activity of
the cortex — which might then influence the local blood flow, to which it
is closely coupled.

Consequently, current data prove that neurogenic dilatation of cerebral blood vessels might be involved in the vascular responses to both increases in carbon dioxide and decreases in oxygen levels in blood. However, many details of the physiological mechanisms accomplishing neurogenic vasodilatation are still unclear and in need of further study. Dis-
crepant results have been obtained in many studies (e.g., Eidelman et al.,
1975; Linton et al., 1975; Heistad et al., 1976). This may be explained
in the following way (Purves, 1979a): first, there may be important draw-
backs in the methods applied for measurement of the cerebral blood flow,
or the experimental conditions are faulty, although the technique is good.
Second, it may be that the techniques are valid, but in fact they do not
measure the required parameters of cerebral blood flow. Third, there may
also be differences among species which may be related to variations in
smooth muscle receptor differences, etc.

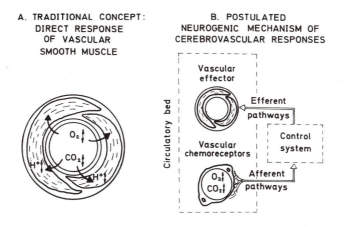

Fig. 4.65.   Feedbacks regulating cerebral blood gas
             levels. (A) The traditional humoral con-
             cept, according to which carbon dioxide
             and oxygen affect the vascular smooth
             muscle directly (or by changing the metab-
             olite contents in the surrounding tissue),
             and (B) the postulated neurogenic mecha-
             nism, according to which the vasomotor re-
             sponses of the specific feeding arteries
             are brought about by neurogenic pathways.

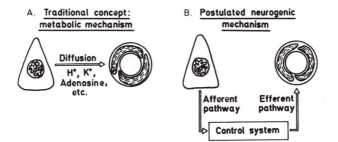

Fig. 4.66.   Feedbacks regulating the adequate blood
             supply to cerebral tissue. (A) The tra-
             ditional humoral concept, according to
             which the metabolic vasoactive substances
             affect the feeding arteries by diffusion
             from the tissue, and (B) the postulated
             neurogenic mechanism, according to which
             the arteries respond to feedback signals
             carried along efferent vasomotor pathways.

The two basic concepts of oxygen and carbon dioxide effects on cerebral blood vessel walls, i.e., the humoral and neurogenic concepts, are summarized in a schematic diagram in Fig. 4.65.

Physiological Evidence for the Involvement of a Neurogenic Mechanism
in the Coupling of Metabolism and Local Blood Flow. The possibility of a

neurogenic mechanism responsible for this type of cerebral blood flow regulation has so far usually been denied. Furthermore, it is still widely believed that only vasoactive substances of metabolic origin directly affect the cerebral vessel walls and thus couple metabolism and blood flow in the brain (see pp. 154-159). However, experimental data have gradually accumulated raising doubts regarding the role of the humoral mechanism in the control of adequate blood supply to brain tissue. In addition, evidence is gradually accumulating that the neurogenic control does participate in this type of cerebral blood flow regulation. The two successive concepts of control mechanisms of cerebral blood flow are schematically presented in Fig. 4.66.

A strong argument for the neurogenic mechanism of the cerebrovascular responses is the very short latent period of local vasodilatation coupled with deficient blood supply of tissue. This latent period was shown long ago in experiments with primary shortages in blood supply to small areas of cerebral cortex. Meyer (1958) found that the latent period of activation of the collateral blood supply is 1-4 seconds, which is much shorter than the minutes required for appreciable changes in metabolite levels in cerebral tissue. Further, the accumulation of metabolites would most likely exert maximum effects inside the ischemic focus while the dilatation of vessels is actually most pronounced at its periphery and beyond. It is hence difficult to imagine that the metabolites accumulated in the ischemic focus could diffuse within a few seconds to vessels located relatively far away. Other evidence for the neurogenic (versus myogenic and metabolic) mechanism of the pial arterial dilatation to the periphery of vascular occlusion was obtained with the micromanipulation technique by this author and his associate (Mchedlishvili and Devdariani, 1964; see also Mchedlishvili, 1972, pp. 96-97).

Additional evidence for the neurogenic mechanism of vascular response has been obtained in experiments with unanesthetized cats, where periodic variations in local blood flow (and oxygen tension) in the cerebral cortex were related to desynchronization of the electrocorticogram. The latent period between these two events lasts about 1 second, but it increases to 10 seconds when the animals have been subjected to general anesthesia. The short latent period in the unanesthetized animals probably results from activation of the neurogenic mechanism in the cerebral cortex (Moskalenko et al., 1980). A very short latent period of vascular response has also been shown during the functional hyperemia caused by rhythmic photoelectric stimulation in cats. The blood vessels dilate and cause an increased blood flow in the visual cortex with a latent period of up to 1 second (Mayorova et al., 1974; Moskalenko et al., 1975). During increased metabolic demand in the cerebral cortex in rabbits the latent period of pial vasodilatation is very short (a few seconds) and of variable duration in different parts of the pial arterial bed. The precortical arteries and the sphincters of pial arterial offshoots respond significantly faster than the adjacent small arterial branches; the longest latent period occurred in the largest pial arteries (Baramidze et al., 1983). This heterogeneity of pial vascular response cannot be due to a direct effect of chemical substances which diffuse from cerebral tissue. This can only be brought about by a neural mechanism. This is particularly likely since the precortical arteries and the sphincters are the most densely innervated (see p. 162).

Additional evidence for the involvement of neural pathways in the responses of the pial arteries was obtained in rabbits by microdissection of the nerves directly connecting the vessel walls with the cortex. Figures 4.67 and 4.68 show that this operation led to an inhibition of the func-

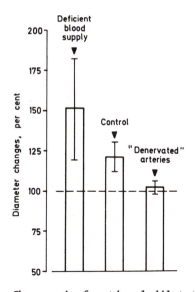

Fig. 4.67. Changes in functional dilatation of pial
            arteries following dissection of the nerves
            connecting the cerebral cortex to the ves-
            sel walls. Pial arteries (100-200 μm in
            diameter) dilate in response to increased
            activity of the cortex after local applica-
            tion of strychnine (control) in rabbits.
            During a deficient blood supply to the ce-
            rebral cortex (resulting from obstruction of
            the precortical arteries by microdiathermo-
            coagulation), the dilatation increases sig-
            nificantly (deficient blood supply) in the
            same animals (0.02 < P < 0.05). But follow-
            ing microdissection of the nerves directly
            connecting the pial arteries with the ce-
            rebral cortex, the dilatation actually dis-
            appears (denervated arteries); the differ-
            ence is significant (P < 0.001). (Modified
            from Mchedlishvili and Nikolaishvili, 1964,
            1967.)

tional vasodilatation in response to increased cortical activity (caused by
strychnine application to the brain surface), as well as inhibition of postischemic vasodilatation (Mchedlishvili and Nikolaishvili, 1964, 1967).
Further, the dilatation of the pial arteries in response to a reduced blood
supply to the cerebral cortex (resulting from drops in systemic arterial
pressure from about 96 down to 32 mm Hg) has been found to be inhibited by
atropine and other specific acetylcholine blockers (Fig. 4.69), thus indicating that the vascular response is caused by cholinergic activation
(Mchedlishvili and Nikolaishvili, 1970). Scopolamine eliminates cerebral
vasodilatation related to the early shift from high- to low-voltage states
in the EEG in rabbits, suggesting that the vascular response involves a
cholinergic mechanism (Pearce et al., 1981). The accumulation of acetylcholinesterase in brain regions subjected to ischemia also seems to point
to neurogenic control of cerebral blood vessel responses (Ott et al., 1975).

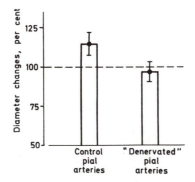

Fig. 4.68.   Changes in postischemic dilatation of pial
             arteries following dissection of the
             nerves connecting the cerebral cortex to
             the vessel walls. Pial arteries (100 μm
             in diameter) in rabbits regularly dilate
             in the postischemic period (after a 1-2
             minute stoppage of cerebral blood flow
             due to a drop in systemic arterial pres-
             sure). But after dissection of nerves
             directly connecting the pial arteries with
             the cerebral cortex (in the same hemi-
             sphere), the postischemic vasodilatation
             disappears. (Modified from Mchedlishvili
             and Nikolaishvili, 1964, 1967.)

     The involvement of sympathetic nerves in the pial vasomotor response
is still difficult to interpret. Cervical sympathetic stimulation, for
example, results in a relatively slight decrease in pial arterial diameter,
significantly less pronounced than that seen in the extracerebral blood
vessels (Marcus and Heistad, 1979; Busija et al., 1982). Furthermore,
there is an "escape" of the vasoconstrictor effect during sympathetic stimulation (Serscombe et al., 1979). The sympathetic vasoconstriction is considerably greater in the larger pial arteries (over 150 μm in diameter)
than in smaller ones (Auer and Johansson, 1981). But the smaller pial
arteries are more active in the regulation of an adequate blood supply to
cerebral tissue. The relatively insignificant effect of sympathetic stimulation on pial arteries, observed since the 1930s, has been considered as
evidence that the cerebral blood vessel responses occur without neural control (Schmidt, 1950). But an alternative explanation is that the experimental approach was inadequate, since the normal behavior of the blood vessels, i.e., the primary dependence of the pial arterial responses on metabolic demands from the cerebral cortex and the characteristic vasodilatation response in the smaller pial arteries (see above), could not be taken
into account (Mchedlishvili, 1972). Chronic sympathectomy in rabbits results in specific disturbances in the responses of active microvascular
segments in the minor pial arterial branches (sphincters at offshoots,
precortical arteries) that regulate adequate blood supply to the cerebral
cortex (Baramidze et al., 1982a). Thus, the sympathetic nerves, which are
vasoconstrictors in nature, are somehow involved in the specific behavior
of minor pial arteries regulating adequate microcirculation in cerebral
tissue.

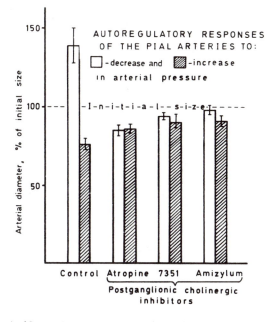

Fig. 4.69.   Disappearance of pial arterial dilatation following postganglionic cholinergic inhibition. The dilatation of rabbit pial arteries due to a decrease in
systemic arterial pressure from ≈90 to 31
mm Hg, which is pronounced in control experiments (white columns), disappears
following i.v. administration of post-
ganglionic cholinergic inhibitors. However, the vasoconstrictor effect due to
an increase in arterial pressure from
≈33 to 85 mm Hg does not change significantly (shaded columns). (Reproduced
from Mchedlishvili and Nikolaishvili,
1970.)

    The dilatation of pial arteries associated with a deficiency in blood
supply to the cerebral cortex is local in nature and always restricted by
the region where metabolic needs are increased (Mchedlishvili and Nikolaishvili, 1966). It is hard to imagine that these vascular responses in any
region of the brain could be controlled from a single neural center. Control by neurons located somewhere inside, or near, the area where the metabolic needs have become increased is more likely. Evidence for this assumption has been obtained in rabbits with chronically dissected pathways
that connect the cerebral cortex with all hypothalamic and other subcortical structures (the method developed by Khananashvili): the functional
dilatation of pial arteries caused by increased cortical activity is not
different from that in the contralateral hemisphere with intact neural
pathways (Baramidze et al., 1980). The nervous pathways directly connecting the pial arteries with the superficial layers of the cerebral cortex
(see p. 164) may be involved in vasodilatation, since it disappears after
nerve dissection as mentioned above.

    The neural receptors in the cerebral tissue near activated neurons are
not yet understood. Bicher (1974) argues about the existence of specific
oxygen sensors in cerebral tissue, since he found that phenoxybenzamine, an
alpha-adrenergic blocker, affects the electroencephalographic changes during hypoxia. Cervós-Navarro (1977) found structures representing nonmyelinated axons, which, according to morphological characteristics, are similar
to afferent receptors in cerebral tissue, and are located relatively far
from the arterioles and capillaries. These receptors can carry afferent
information about metabolic changes in cerebral tissue to neurogenic control centers regulating the diameter of respective arteries, but further
studies of this problem are needed.

    Consequently, experimental evidence is gradually accumulating in favor
of the participation of a neurogenic control mechanism of adequate blood
supply to cerebral tissue; this is gradually being accepted by researchers.
However, the mechanism of this control is still far from being clarified.
If the information required for this control mechanism originates from the
tissue itself, then the presence of specific receptors which would respond
to metabolic changes in the tissue are necessary. But very little is known
about such receptors, and this problem remains open for future research.
Furthermore, almost nothing is known about the pathways and the coordinating centers of this control, although such centers are presumed to exist.
According to the author's opinion, the vasomotor centers of the brain stem,
the hypothalamus, the midbrain, etc., are not likely to participate in this
local blood flow control. Presumably the function of the nervous "centers"
for adequate local blood flow might be carried out by neural structures
located in the cortex itself, near the vascular effectors. Thus, much is
still unclear about the neurogenic control system of adequate blood supply
to small areas of the cerebral cortex.

    Concluding Remarks on the Control of Cerebral Microcirculation by the
Minor Pial and Intracerebral Arterial Branches. The majority of studies
concerning the physiological control of cerebral microcirculation have been
carried out on the pial arteries, but so far no direct evidence exists for
humoral and neural control of the smallest intracerebral arteries and
arterioles. Since the pial arteries can be easily approached, they have
been proved to be the main effectors of the control of cerebral microcirculation. Currently no experimental data exist concerning the *in vivo* functional behavior of and the physiological effects on the intracerebral arterial branches. We are still uncertain of the effect of well-known humoral
factors of metabolic origin (H^+, K^+, adenosine, and others) on the cortical
and other intracerebral arteries, and no data are available regarding neural effects on their walls. It does not seem justifiable to assume that the
physiological effects are similar in the pial and cortical arterial branches since, in addition to differences in their anatomy and chemical environment, their physiological responses are dissimilar. The sources of innervation of the intracerebral arteries are still controversial: the nerves may
originate from the same neurons as those in the pial arteries or nerve
fibers of intracerebral arteries; they may also originate from specific
central neurons. There is also evidence that the innervation of the small
intracerebral arteries is specific and related to blood-brain-barrier function rather than to the vasomotor control of brain vessels (see p. 108).
Thus, the role of the intracerebral arterial ramifications in the control
of cerebral microcirculation, and especially the physiological mechanisms
of vasomotor responses, are still unknown and need further investigation.

4.5. SUMMARY

    The following types of cerebral blood flow regulation are considered
in this chapter: first, the coupling of blood supply to small tissue areas

with the level of neuronal activity and associated metabolic rate; and, second, constant oxygen and carbon dioxide content in the cerebral blood (and tissue) adjusted for by requisite changes in cerebral blood flow. The vascular effectors of these types of cerebral blood flow regulation are chiefly the small pial arteries distributed on the cerebral surface, although constant blood gas content is also maintained by larger vessel responses. The anatomy of the pial arteries provides opportunity for their diameter to change (as is also the case with the major brain arteries) without mechanically affecting cerebral tissue. Significantly, the pial arterial branches represent a very specific microvascular system in which abundant vascular interconnections are present. Thus, in the evolutionary process multiple arterial microcircles have formed and gradually increased in number on the cerebral surface, from which radial arteries originate and feed into small cortical areas. This arrangement, and the specific behavior of the pial microvascular bed, provide fast redistribution of blood to meet the metabolic demands of particular tissue areas without disturbing the blood supply to adjacent regions. In spite of the fact that pure humoral feedback by the blood gases and metabolic substances directly affecting the cerebral vessel walls has always been considered the chief physiological mechanism controlling both adequate blood supply and constant blood gas content, strong evidence is gradually accumulating indicating that the neurogenic control of cerebral blood flow should also play an important role as the feedback and the feedforward mechanisms of these types of regulation of brain circulation. However, many specific problems of these mechanisms are still unsolved and require further investigation.

Chapter 5. Pathological Arterial Behavior:

Vasospasm and Vasoparalysis

Pathological behavior of cerebral arteries usually implies inadequate vasoconstriction or dilatation. Such vascular behavior is especially dangerous for the brain, which requires a particularly well-regulated blood supply. The metabolic rate and the related blood flow rates are very high in cerebral tissue not only during brain activity, but also during rest and sleep. Furthermore, no stores of carbohydrates or other energy reserves, including oxygen, are present within the brain; cerebral metabolism is therefore completely dependent upon the continual transport of substances from the blood to brain tissue. Disturbances in blood supply to the brain immediately result in functional disorders in neurons, which are the most sensitive cells in the body to oxygen deficiency. Derangements occur within seconds of arrest of microcirculation, and if the stoppage of blood supply continues for a few minutes, irreversible changes and even death of neurons can occur. Finally, the regulatory system of cerebral blood flow is known to be highly vulnerable to the action of various pathogenic factors. The foregoing considerations explain why disturbances in cerebral blood flow are the most frequent causes of various disorders in normal brain function and result in neurological disorders.

Pathological vasoconstriction can cause a deficiency in blood flow in various areas of the brain, as well as interfere with the collateral blood supply. This disturbance in cerebral blood flow was not thought to be due to vasospasm by the majority of neurologists prior to the 1960s, since it was impossible to identify vasospasm in patients because of the lack of appropriate diagnostic means. In addition, it was impossible to identify and investigate cerebral vasospasm in post-mortem pathomorphological sections in patients who suffered from neurological disorders prior to death. Since thrombosis and stenosis of cerebral arteries are seldom detected during brain infarcts (Koltover et al., 1975), the latter might be caused in other cases by vasospasms, which could not be identified after death (Kreindler, 1975).

Interest in cerebral vasospasm has considerably increased since the 1960s due to the growing knowledge of the functional behavior of the cerebral arteries under different physiological and pathological conditions and progress in angiographical, neurosurgical, and tomographical techniques, which allowed for direct observation of cerebral vasospasm in large brain

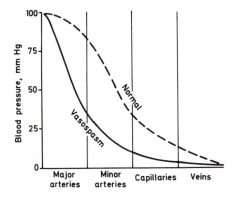

Fig. 5.1. Pressure gradient in a peripheral vascu-
           lar bed during vasospasm of the major
           arteries, which inevitably results in a
           considerable decrease in the microcircu-
           lation rate.

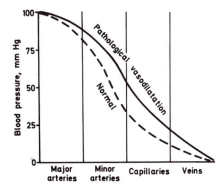

Fig. 5.2. Pressure gradient in a peripheral vascu-
           lar bed during pathological vasodilatation,
           or vasoparalysis, of the feeding arteries,
           which inevitably results in a considerable
           rise in blood pressure and flow in the
           microvascular bed.

arteries. Cerebral vasospasm observed in patients is most commonly associated with perivascular hematomas following head trauma and with the subarachnoid hemorrhage related to arterial aneurysms (Symon, 1973). Neurosurgeons are interested in this type of vasospasm and have contributed to
extensive experimental work concerned with the vasospasm of large cerebral
arteries caused by damage of their walls and perivascular hematomas (we
shall often cite their experimental results in the forthcoming sections of
this chapter). However, cerebral vasospasm can develop due to other
causes.

    Vasospasm creates a considerable resistance to blood flow in the af-
fected arteries and, if the collateral blood supply is insufficient, results in a drop in blood pressure in the microvessels (Fig. 5.1) and in a

reduction in flow velocity in the microcirculation. Thus the blood supply
to cerebral tissue significantly decreases, causing ischemic changes.

Pathological vasodilatation, in contrast to vasospasm, does not interfere considerably with blood flow in arteries and therefore does not lead
to cerebral blood flow insufficiency. The pressure gradient decreases
along the feeding arteries (Fig. 5.2) and the flow rate in the microvascular bed is increased. The rise of intravascular pressure can cause additional disturbances, for example rupture of arterial walls, provided that
they were damaged by sclerotic processes, aneurysm, etc. The increased
blood pressure inside the capillaries can result in a bulk flow of water
across their walls with ensuing brain edema. In addition, pathologically
dilated cerebral arteries lose their ability to regulate cerebral blood
flow adequately and can therefore cause various cerebrovascular disorders.
Below we shall consider pathological vasodilatation in the brain as having
an opposite nature to cerebral vasospasm.

5.1. VASOSPASM RELATIVE TO THE NORMAL BEHAVIOR OF CEREBRAL ARTERIES

Physiological and Pathological Vasoconstriction. By definition, vasospasm is a sharp and often persistent contraction of the blood vessel, reducing its caliber and blood flow (Webster, 1981). Therefore, whether
vasospasm could be a normal physiological phenomenon is questionable, since
a sharp and persistent vasoconstriction would inevitably disturb the normal blood supply to the tissue. The endeavor to definitively differentiate
physiological vasoconstriction and pathological vasoconstriction from
the viewpoint of the actual events in the circulation (Mchedlishvili, 1974,
1977a, 1981) has led to the following conclusion. Physiological vasoconstriction may be related only to normal regulation of blood flow under
physiological conditions, for instance when the constriction occurs following functional hyperemia, and results in the recovery of the normal rate of
microcirculation. On the other hand, physiological vasoconstriction might
be a manifestation of compensation for pathological disturbances. An
example of this is the constriction of the major brain arteries in response
to a sharp elevation in systemic arterial pressure or to an accumulation
of excess blood volume in the cerebral vasculature (see Chapter 3). Another example of vasoconstriction which compensates for pathological events
is a sharp constriction of damaged peripheral arteries, thereby preventing
bleeding. Pathological vasoconstriction, or vasospasm, is, on the contrary, a type of arterial behavior that neither leads to reestablishment
of physiological homeostasis (including coupling of blood flow and metabolic rates), nor is it directed to compensate for some pathological condition. Pathological vasoconstriction results in an inappropriate increase
in vascular resistance, entailing a considerable reduction in arterial
blood flow rate; this causes ischemic changes resulting from a deficient
blood supply to cerebral tissue. These two types of arterial constriction
are schematically presented in Fig. 5.3.

Vasospasm is a vasoconstriction brought about by active contraction
of vascular smooth muscle, requiring a considerable consumption of energy
generated by the cell metabolism. An artery that was in a state of spasm
during life loses its wall contractility after death because of the arrest
of metabolic processes in muscle cells. This explains why arterial spasm
is not usually detected post-mortem even when ischemic changes in the related brain tissue areas are evident.

Characteristics and Identification of Vasospasm. Vasospasm is an inappropriate vasoconstriction resulting in an increase in vascular resis-

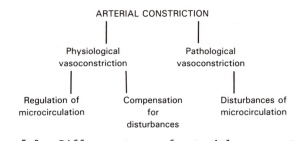

Fig. 5.3. Different types of arterial vasoconstric-
           tion and their significance.

tance, which is physiologically useless and is even harmful for the tissue
elements and for the organ's function. If the collateral blood supply is
insufficient, this leads to ischemic tissue changes.

Vasospasm, or pathological vasoconstriction, can occur naturally only
in the vessels whose anatomy and function are adjusted to active changes
in vascular lumina, i.e., in muscular arteries (see Chapter 1). In the
largest arteries in the body, such as the aorta and its branches, whose
walls contain many elastic fibers but a comparatively thin muscular layer,
spasm is not typical. The capillaries are deprived of specific contractile elements and are not apt to undergo spasm development. Nor is it characteristic of veins, particularly in the brain, where the vessel walls do
not contain a continuous muscular layer.

Because of the great ability of the peripheral vasculature to compensate for disturbances in blood flow in individual vessels, it is impossible
to identify vasospasm from the quantitative characteristics of vasoconstriction. The degree of vessel contraction during vasospasm can be quite
different; it can be a comparatively slight contraction to practically complete obstruction of the arterial lumina. Therefore, vasospasm cannot be
identified only on the basis of the degree of vascular constriction.

The duration of vasospasm can also be highly variable: it can last
for minutes, hours, and even days. From the viewpoint of the pathogenic
significance of vasospasm duration with respect to blood supply disturbances in tissue, the sensitivity of the affected tissue structure to a deficiency in blood supply is very important. Ischemic changes appear in a
tissue only in those cases when the microcirculation is inadequate for a
long period relative to tissue resistance, but if the tissue elements are
already necrotized, the duration of the vasospasm is no longer significant.

Vasospasm along the arterial branchings can develop in various ways:
it can range from a few millimeters to many centimeters in length. The
absolute length of the vasospasm along the arteries is not as important as
the value of the actual rise in resistance in the vessels, since the blood
supply deficiency is determined only by this rise in resistance.

Vasospasm and physiological vasoconstriction are difficult to differentiate by quantitative characteristics of arterial constriction. Thus,
identification of vasospasm in individual cases, both in animal experiments
and in medical practice, is sometimes difficult due to the absence of general quantitative criteria for distinguishing physiological from pathological vasoconstriction (Mchedlishvili, 1977a; Mchedlishvili, Purves, et
al., 1979). A deficiency in blood flow to tissue is likewise not an essen-

tial criterion of vasospasm because normal microcirculation can be maintained through collateral pathways even though arteriograms of the feeding
artery demonstrate spasm.

The differentiation of physiological and pathological vasoconstriction
is also complicated because vasoconstriction can have a dual significance,
i.e., compensation for one disturbance might simultaneously cause another
disorder. For instance, pronounced development of brain edema is compensated for by constriction of the major and pial arteries of the brain (Mchedlishvili and Akhobadze, 1961). Vasoconstriction can result in a deficient
blood supply to brain tissue, and a compensatory decrease in systemic arterial pressure level can be observed during the same period (Mchedlishvili,
1968; Mchedlishvili, Kapuściński, et al., 1976). Another example of the
dual significance of vasoconstriction is the response of the major brain
arteries following a temporary arrest in cerebral blood flow: vasoconstriction compensates for the development of postischemic brain edema, but augments the deficiency of blood supply to cerebral tissue (Mchedlishvili,
1968, 1972). It follows that identification of vasospasm is difficult in
particular cases (i.e., its differentiation from physiological vasoconstriction) and requires further theoretical and practical consideration.

Vasospasm of Brain Arteries in Relation to Leading Physiological Concepts of Cerebral Blood Flow Regulation. An assumption that vasospasm
could appear in the cerebral vasculature was probably made when arterial
vasomotor responses became generally known to physiologists. However, this
assumption contradicted the leading physiological concepts of cerebral
blood flow regulation for a long time.

As mentioned earlier (p. 17), the basic physiological concept of the
19th century concerning cerebral circulation was the "Monro-Kellie doctrine." Its authors speculated that the cerebral vascular diameter, and
hence cerebral blood flow, were always invariable since there were three
incompressible substances inside the rigid skull: blood, cerebrospinal
fluid, and brain tissue (Hill, 1896). This implied that, unlike other
peripheral arteries in the body, neither vasomotor responses nor vasospasm
could occur in the cerebral arteries. This view did not change for decades.
Cerebral blood flow was then believed to be changed only by variations in
systemic arterial or venous pressures. Thus, vasospasm was not thought to
appear in the cerebral vasculature.

In the 1920s and 1930s investigations of the pial arteries by Forbes
and his associates (summarized, in particular, in Forbes, 1940) proved that
active cerebrovascular responses might occur during changes in systemic
arterial pressure, etc. However, the natural constrictor responses of the
pial arteries were found to be relatively small, and no convincing evidence
was then available that spasm could develop in the cerebral arteries under
natural conditions. In the 1940s and 1950s, considerable progress in cerebral blood flow investigations in both animals and humans was made due to
the development of new techniques (Schmidt, 1950; Kety, 1960). However,
the data obtained then were still inadequate to result in a change in the
concept of cerebral vasospasm, which was still not considered to be an important cause of cerebrovascular disturbances. Accordingly, transient cerebrovascular insufficiencies were thought to appear only from a temporary drop
in systemic arterial pressure (Corday et al., 1953).

Accumulation of experimental evidence concerning cerebral vasospasm
was rapid in the 1960s when the functional behavior of specific cerebral
arteries, mainly large ones, was investigated in detail during regulation
of cerebral blood flow and development of spasm (Mchedlishvili, 1964).
Neurosurgical and angiographic techniques advanced during this period and

CONCEPTIONS OF CEREBRAL   CEREBRAL
BLOOD FLOW CONTROL: VASOSPASM:

19th century:

CBF = constant .... rejected

Prior to 1930s:

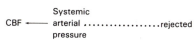

Systemic
CBF ⟵—— arterial .... rejected
pressure

1940s-1950s:

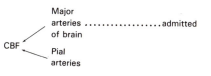

Systemic
arterial
pressure
CBF

Cerebrovascular
resistance .... rejected
(arterioles only).

1960s-1970s:

Major
arteries .... admitted
of brain
CBF

Pial
arteries

Fig. 5.4. Views on cerebral vasospasm as related to
concepts of cerebral blood flow regulation in various historical eras. See explanation in text.

provided direct observations of spasm in large cerebral arteries in humans
(Raynor and Ross, 1960). Cerebral vasospasm then became widely accepted
as a probable and frequent cause of cerebrovascular disturbances.

Figure 5.4 shows schematically how vasospasm in cerebral vasculature is
related to the leading physiological concepts of cerebral blood flow regulation.

Typical Localization of Vasospasm in Cerebral Vasculature Relative to
the Physiological Behavior of Cerebral Arteries. Both physiological and
pathological vasoconstriction result from contraction of vascular smooth
muscle; they are thus consequences of the coupling of specific stimuli and
contractile events in muscle cells. The development of spasm of any type
of cerebral artery may be related to its characteristic physiological behavior. If so, cerebral vasospasm should then occur most easily in vessels which constrict to the greatest extent in the course of cerebral blood
flow regulation. In support of this hypothesis, a parallel can be drawn
between the degree of vasoconstrictor behavior of specific cerebral arteries during regulation of cerebral blood flow and the typical distribution
of vasospasm in the cerebral arterial bed (Mchedlishvili, 1972, 1977a).

As mentioned earlier (see previous chapters), over a period of many
decades many physiologists thought that the principal resistance vessels
in the circulatory bed, in the brain in particular, are the smallest precapillary arteries, i.e., the arterioles (Kety, 1960). However, systematic investigations carried out during the 1960s resulted in accumulation

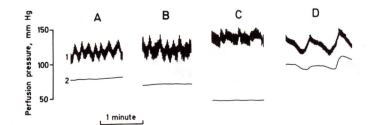

Fig. 5.5. Spasm development in the major arteries of the brain.
Simultaneous recording of arterial pressures in the
aorta (record 1) and the circle of Willis (record 2)
in dogs demonstrated an increasing rise in the pressure gradient along the major arteries of the brain
(internal carotid and vertebral arteries) indicating their progressive constriction in the course of
one hour during spasm development (records A-C), but
in record D the arteries spontaneously dilated and
the gradient respectively decreased. (Reproduced
from Mchedlishvili, 1964.)

of a large body of evidence indicating that it is not the cerebral precapillary arterioles, but principally the much larger cerebral arteries, that
are actively involved in the regulation of cerebral circulation. The most
active portions of the cerebral arterial bed were then found to be the
major brain arteries and the pial arteries (especially the smallest pial
arteries).

     According to the data considered in Chapter 3, the major arteries of
the brain, including the internal carotid and the vertebrals, as well as
other large cerebral arteries, are primarily involved in regulation of cerebral blood pressure and flow against changes in systemic arterial pressure. They undergo constriction, entailing a respective increase in cerebrovascular resistance during rising arterial pressure, thus providing
for the maintenance of a constant cerebral blood flow and pressure (see
pp. 49-56). Constriction of the major arteries has also been demonstrated during excess blood volume accumulation within the brain vessels
caused either by obstructed venous outflow or excessive arterial inflow.
This constriction is recruited to eliminate blood accumulation by restricting blood inflow to cerebral vasculature (see pp. 60-69). The degree of
constriction of the major arteries of the brain is normally adjusted to
the needs of cerebral blood flow regulation, but can be considerably more
pronounced, up to a complete closure of the vascular lumina, under certain
experimental conditions (Mchedlishvili, 1977a). The dilatation of major
arteries is usually less pronounced, since their resistance is approximately 15-20% of the total cerebrovascular resistance during rest and hence
cannot be decreased much further. No appreciable dilatation of the major
arteries has been detected even when the cerebral tissue suffered from
great deficiencies in blood supply either locally or within larger cerebral territories (Mchedlishvili,1972). Thus, there are sufficient grounds
for the conclusion that the major brain arteries do not appreciably compensate for the deficient blood supply to cerebral tissue, the more so since their
most typical response is constriction (see Chapter 3). A progressive
constriction of all major arteries (internal carotid and vertebral arteries), leading to a deficient blood supply in the brain, has been observed

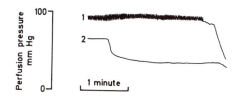

Fig. 5.6.   Spasm development in the major arteries of
            the brain. Simultaneous recording of ar-
            terial pressures in the aorta (record 1)
            and the circle of Willis (record 2) in rab-
            bit chest-head preparation (Mchedlishvili,
            1962) showed a case where the pressure
            gradient suddenly increased, indicating
            that vasoconstriction of the whole set of
            major arteries of the brain occurred. Sud-
            den death of the animal ensued; the cardiac
            contractions stopped and the systemic ar-
            terial pressure dropped immediately. (Re-
            produced from Mchedlishvili, 1964.)

in experiments with dogs and rabbits during estimation of the pressure
gradient in these vessels (Fig. 5.5).   Vasoconstriction occurs sometimes
suddenly and results in the animal's death (Fig. 5.6).

    Pathological constriction of the major brain arteries has been shown
both in patients and animals exposed to harmful factors and under certain
pathological conditions. This has been observed, in particular, in humans
following surgical stripping of the carotid canal (Pool, 1957), or administration of X-ray contrast media into the internal carotid arteries
(Raynor and Ross, 1960; Wackenheim et al., 1972), as well as in animals
during traumatic shock (Vasadze, 1960), during X-ray radiation (Nadareishvili, 1963), or prolonged posthemorrhagic arterial hypotension (Amashukeli,
1969). This indicates that vasospasm might readily develop in the major
and adjacent larger arteries of the brain.

    The functional behavior of the pial arteries is different from that
of the major cerebral arteries (see Chapter 4). The responses of the pial
arteries are directed mainly toward adjusting blood supply to cerebral tissue to meet its metabolic needs. The pial arteries, especially the smallest vessels, generally dilate in response to increased cerebral metabolic
rates and to primary deficiencies in blood supply to cerebral tissue. The
most typical response of the pial arteries, with respect to all kinds of
cerebral blood flow regulation, is dilatation (see pp. 141-143). The constrictor responses of the pial arteries to direct application of physiologically active substances are usually small. In earlier studies by
Forbes and his associates, adrenaline caused insignificant vasoconstriction that did not exceed 30% of the initial diameter in arteries larger
than 50 μm (Forbes and Wolff, 1928; Fog, 1939). Corresponding data were
obtained later (Wahl et al., 1971-1972). An insignificant and transient
constrictor effect has also been found following direct application of
serotonin to the pial arterial walls in cats, baboons, and rabbits (Raynor
and McMurtry, 1963; Symon, 1967; Ormotsadze et al., 1969). Accordingly,
pial arterial spasm does not develop easily under natural conditions.
Spasm-like constriction in pial vessels has been observed only during artificial (mechanical and electrical) stimulation of their walls (Schultz,
1866; Florey, 1925; Echlin, 1942; Lende, 1960).

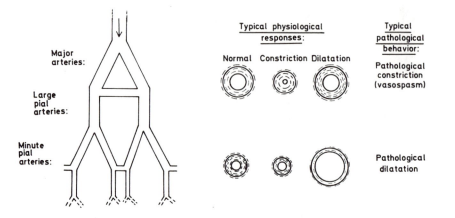

Fig. 5.7.   Relationship between pathological vascular responses and the
            typical physiological behavior of cerebral arteries. The major
            arteries of the brain, whose typical physiological response
            (during regulation of cerebral blood flow) is to constrict rath-
            er than dilate, are more apt to develop pathological constric-
            tion (vasospasm) rather than pathological vasodilatation. In
            contrast, the minute pial arteries, which are more liable to
            dilate than to constrict under physiological conditions (i.e.,
            while regulating cerebral blood flow), accordingly are more apt
            to pathologically dilate than to develop vasospasm.

     Thus, it may be concluded that the development of spasm of cerebral
arteries is closely related to their specific physiological behavior during regulation of cerebral blood flow. Figure 5.7 shows schematically how
the typical localization of vasospasm in the cerebral vasculature is related to the normal functional behavior of the cerebral arterial bed.

5.2.   PATHOLOGICAL VASODILATATION RELATIVE TO THE NORMAL
       BEHAVIOR OF CEREBRAL ARTERIES

     Physiological and pathological vasodilatations are often difficult to
differentiate not only in medical practice but also in animal experiments
(Fig. 5.8). Consideration of this problem is especially urgent because of
the scarcity of data on pathological vasodilatation, as a pathophysiological problem, in the scientific literature. Only recently has pathological
vasodilatation been specially considered at a session of the Fourth Tbilisi
Symposium on Cerebral Circulation (Gannushkina, 1979).

     It is well known that physiological vasodilatation is usually seen in
the regulation of the peripheral circulation, including that of the brain.
Previous chapters in this book contain examples of vasodilatation of physiological significance. Physiological dilatation of cerebral arteries maintains the constancy of cerebral blood flow despite a decrease in the systemic
arterial pressure level (see Chapter 3), or it serves to maintain constant
levels of oxygen and carbon dioxide in cerebral blood and tissue (see Chapter 4). Physiological vasodilatation is especially important in adjusting
the microcirculation rate to the metabolic needs of cerebral tissue (see
Chapter 4), which is required either when the tissue metabolic rate becomes
primarily increased or the blood supply to the tissue becomes restricted.
In addition, physiological vasodilatation compensates for various distur-

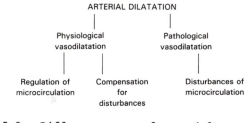

Fig. 5.8. Different types of arterial vasodilatation
and their physiological significance.

bances in cerebral circulation. A typical example of such vasodilatation
is postischemic, or reactive, hypermia; another example is the dilatation
of particular cerebral arteries related to the collateral blood supply to
cerebral tissue that occurs following obstruction of some feeding brain
arteries.

Pathological vasodilatation, distinct from physiological vasodilatation, results in disturbances of the normal blood supply to tissue leading
to an excessively high blood pressure and perfusion rate in the microcirculation in respective brain regions.

Pathological vasodilatation, like vasospasm, takes place principally
in muscular peripheral arteries, although pathological expansion of the
vascular lumina can also occur in capillaries and veins. However, both
the capillaries and veins are deprived of the vasomotor activity characteristic of the arteries of muscular type. In addition, the luminal expansion
of the capillaries and veins affects blood flow in the peripheral circulation in a different manner than that caused by the arterial dilatation.
Proceeding from this, while considering pathological vasodilatation we
shall imply only dilatation of the cerebral arteries.

Pathological vasodilatation is the *functional expansion* of arteries,
but not necessarily a distension of their walls — like that seen in arterial aneurysms. Some specific structural changes in the vascular walls may
appear either preceding pathological dilatation of arteries or secondarily
(see p. 194). The essential characteristic of pathological vasodilatation
is that it is in principle a functional event and therefore can become reversible, if its duration is restricted to a definite time interval, e.g.,
no more than 20-30 minutes under certain experimental circumstances
(Strandgaard et al., 1976; MacKenzie et al., 1977).

From a functional point of view, the principal feature of pathological vasodilatation is that it does not regulate cerebral blood flow. Thus
it can neither actively maintain constancy of circulatory parameters nor
actively adjust the regional cerebral blood flow to the metabolic needs of
cerebral tissue. This feature of pathological dilatation is related to
the fact that the vessel walls have lost their ability to change their
lumina in response to natural regulatory stimuli. Therefore, the blood
flow and blood volume in the vessels cannot be actively regulated or significantly restricted anymore. Hence, pathological dilatation of cerebral
arteries leads to disturbances in cerebral blood flow in the areas supplied
by the dilated vessels.

It is often difficult to define whether vasodilatation is pathological or physiological, since this vascular response can play a dual role.
Vasodilatation may, on the one hand, be a compensatory mechanism (i.e., a
pure physiological phenomenon) contributing to an adequate blood supply to

cerebral tissue and, on the other hand, it can simultaneously be a pathological phenomenon, provoking disturbances in microcirculation. This dual
response is usually observed following a 1-2 minute arrest of cerebral
blood flow in experimental animals when a sharp dilatation of the pial arteries contributes to an increase in blood supply to cerebral tissue (postischemic hyperemia), while also augmenting excess blood accumulation in the
cerebral vasculature (see p. 66-67 in Chapter 3) and even brain edema development. Comparable vasodilatation, having a dual significance, occurs in an
ischemic focus (e.g., following occlusion of the middle cerebral artery).
It is certainly a physiological dilatation directed toward recovery of flow
to ischemic areas through collateral canals and elimination of the consequences of ischemia. But, its occurrence is also related to ischemic damage to vessel walls which then cannot increase in vascular tone in response to vasoconstrictor stimuli, so that extensive hyperemia and even
local edema develops. Such vasodilatation cannot be definitely classified
as a physiological or a pathological event. Very often vasodilatation and
the ensuing hyperemia appear to be harmful rather than beneficial when they
occur shortly after the onset of ischemia or in previously ischemic brain
areas (Heiss et al., 1976; Morawetz et al., 1978). The dual significance
of vasodilatation may be even more pronounced than vasoconstriction, which
can also have a dual significance.

Pathological vasodilatation can be accompanied by compensatory events
in the cerebrovascular bed. When a pronounced pial vasodilatation occurs
in the whole brain following a 1-2 minute stoppage of cerebral blood flow,
the major arteries become uniformly constricted (see p. 66 in Chapter 3).
This is certainly a compensatory event to protect the brain from the effect of considerable pial arterial dilatation, i.e., the ensuing circulatory disorder. A compensatory event protecting the arteries against pathological dilatation includes hypertrophy of the vascular media occurring in
the arterial walls of experimental animals subjected to chronic arterial
hypertension (Johansson and Nordborg, 1978). Similarly, stenosis and occlusion of the carotid arteries protect the pial arteries against pathological dilatation during arterial hypertension (Johansson, 1976).

Criteria for pathological vasodilatation cannot be easily defined because it is difficult, even impossible, to differentiate between physiological and pathological vasodilatation by only quantitative characteristics of either arterial expansion or an increase in cerebral blood flow.
From a theoretical point of view, pathological vasodilatation is a condition of cerebral arteries that are considerably dilated due to any cause
when dilatation is not required for adequate blood supply to tissue. Further, it occurs when natural vasoconstrictor stimuli to arterial walls do
not result in an adequate response. However, these events can hardly be
clarified in animal experiments and even less so in medical practice.

If the parameters of pathological vasodilatation were quantitatively
distinguishable from the parameters of physiological vasodilatation,
researchers and medical workers would be able to easily differentiate between these two types of vasodilatation. However, in all probability,
such quantitative criteria do not exist in reality. Indeed, a maximal degree of vascular wall expansion can occur in a given artery during both
pathological and physiological vasodilatation. The spread of dilatation
along the arterial branches can likewise be quite variable in both physiological and pathological vasodilatation. There is also uncertainty about
the duration of vasodilatation. Actually, the duration of physiological
arterial dilatation can be restricted in time only if it is matched with
an increase in the functional activity and metabolic rate of cerebral tissue lasting a particular period. However, there are cases of physiologi-

cal vasodilatation, e.g., related to collateral blood supply (following obstruction of an arterial branch), which are of infinite duration.

The following functional test for identifying pathological vasodilatation may be applied: administration of vasoactive agents that constrict
normal arteries, but have no effect on pathologically dilated arteries.
This seems not to be true for the cerebral arteries, since it is well known
that even normally functioning brain arteries do not readily respond to ex-
trinsically administered vasoconstrictor agents, which may easily disturb
normal cerebral blood flow regulation.

The most characteristic feature of pathological vasodilatation is
probably the inadequacy of blood supply to tissue and the occurrence of
pathological events in the microcirculatory bed fed by the dilated arteries.

A suitable criterion for identifying pathological vasodilatation is
the estimation of excessively high blood flow in the cerebral vasculature,
termed "luxury perfusion" (Lassen, 1966). There is a specific symptom,
namely, an increase in oxygen content in the venous blood, which indicates
that the actual cerebral blood flow considerably exceeds the metabolic demands of the tissue, and therefore the tissue is not necessarily consuming
the oxygen transported by the arterial blood to the cerebral vasculature.*
This symptom, called "red venous blood" or "red cerebral veins" (Waltz,
1969, Sundt and Waltz, 1971), has great significance in clinical practice.
"Luxury perfusion" with hyperoxygenation of cerebral venous blood is often
observed in patients having a stroke.

Pathological vasodilatation is further characterized by a considerably
lowered resistance in the arteries which are dilated, and hence by a tangible rise in blood pressure in related microvessels (Fig. 5.2). This is
especially dangerous when systemic arterial pressure is increased simultaneously (the latter may contribute, in turn, to further development of
pathological vasodilatation; see below). The coupling of these two events,
i.e., increased systemic arterial pressure and reduced cerebrovascular resistance, results in an enormous rise in blood pressure in corresponding
microvessels. The latter, in turn, causes dysfunction of the blood-brain
barrier resulting in excessive filtration of water, bulk flow of ions, and
even passage of protein molecules into cerebral tissue. Thus, edema develops either in smaller brain areas or in larger regions of the cerebral
tissue, such as when the feeding vessels are pathologically dilated
(Johansson et al., 1970; Dinsdale et al., 1974; Gannushkina and Shafranova,
1976, 1977).

Typical Localization of Pathological Dilatation in the Cerebral Arterial Bed. Abnormal vasodilatation can occur in various portions of the cerebral arterial bed, including the major, the pial, and the intracerebral
(parenchymal) arterial branches. However, the typical localization of
pathological vasodilatation, similar to vasospasm, is probably related to
the inherent functional behavior of specific cerebral arterial portions.
The most typical locus of pathological vasodilatation in the brain is the
pial arteries, especially the smaller vessels (see Fig. 5.7 and text on
p. 183). This seems to be related to the following facts: (a) pathological vasodilatation has been observed virtually only in pial arteries (Bara-

---

*However, this event can be related, at least partially, to the lowering of
the metabolic rate of oxygen in brain tissue during ischemia (Meyer, 1968).

midze, 1979); (b) normally the most typical response of the pial arteries
is dilatation, which is usually observed when the cerebral blood flow is
regulated (see Fig. 4.45 and the text in Chapter 4); and (c) during dilatation of the pial arteries (under various conditions, e.g., in the postischemic state, asphyxia, during a sharp rise in systemic arterial pressure,
etc.) neither the major arteries nor the intracerebral arteries show marked
dilatation (see Chapters 3 and 4). Almost no evidence, however, exists regarding pathological vasodilatation of the intracerebral (parenchymal)
arteries. This is probably at least partially related to the absence of
appropriate techniques for *in vivo* investigation.

Pathological vasodilatation often affects only certain segments of the
pial arteries, especially when the vasodilatation is provoked by a sharp increase in intravascular pressure. It most frequently affects those pial
vessels that have a mainly straight course, i.e., those that have no significant bendings and shoot off from the feeding arteries at the most acute
angles (Gannushkina et al., 1977a). According to the findings of this research group, pathological dilatation occurs most frequently in arterial
anastomoses of the boundary zones of the middle, anterior, and posterior
cerebral arteries (see p. 15 in Chapter 1); it is also related to comparatively poor adrenergic nerve supply of the arterial anastomoses.

5.3. THE OBJECTIVES IN SOLVING THE PROBLEM OF MECHANISMS
OF PATHOLOGICAL BEHAVIOR OF CEREBRAL ARTERIES

The problem of understanding the pathophysiological mechanisms involved in the development of cerebral vasospasm (as well as pathological
vasodilatation), like many modern biomedical concerns, is becoming very
complicated. An enormous amount of experimental and clinical data have
gradually accumulated in the world's scientific periodicals. To classify
all the data, to clarify their significance, and to find efficient methods
for further research in this field, a systems analysis of the problem of
pathological behavior of cerebral arteries may be valid. Attempts to carry
out systems analyses of the problem of vasospasm development have been
made in recent years (Mchedlishvili, 1977a, 1981).

The main objectives for obtaining the solution of the problems of
pathological behavior of cerebral arteries have been formulated for the
Fourth Tbilisi Symposium on Cerebral Circulation, which was devoted to the
mechanisms of regulation of cerebral blood flow (Mchedlishvili, Purves, et
al., 1979). These objectives are enumerated below (in slightly altered
form for the present edition). The consideration of these objectives in
relation to the ensuing text of this chapter will give the reader an idea
of the extent of the problem concerning the mechanisms of development of
vasospasm and of pathological vasodilatation in the cerebral arterial bed,
and strategies for solution of this problem.

The objectives related to the study of the mechanism of development
of pathological vasoconstriction (vasospasm) of the cerebral arteries are
as follows:

1. To elucidate the nature and diagnostic criteria of the pathological constriction (vasospasm) from pathophysiological and clinical points of
view;

2. To analyze the involvement of biophysical factors (intravascular
pressure, luminal radius, etc.) in the development of vasospasm;

3.   To determine possible changes in arterial smooth muscle, which can cause the development of vasospasm of cerebral vessels;

4.   To analyze the involvement of various physiologically active substances in the development of cerebral vasospasm;

5.   To consider the involvement of the neurogenic vasomotor mechanism in development of vasospasm;

6.   To consider the principles of vasospasm elimination in the cerebral arterial bed.

Actually similar objectives pertain to the development of pathological vasodilatation (vasoparalysis) in the cerebral arterial bed.

A systems analysis of the problem under consideration (like that of any other scientific problem), such as that outlined in the list of enumerated objectives, cannot be definitive. In fact it can only reflect the present-day experience of researchers. With advances in knowledge and accumulation of new data, the objectives will certainly be in need of additional specifications to reflect the current level of scientific understanding of the problem under consideration.

5.4.   THE ESSENCE OF PATHOLOGICAL ARTERIAL BEHAVIOR FROM THE STANDPOINT OF VASCULAR SMOOTH MUSCLE PHYSIOLOGY

The nature and mechanism of development of cerebral vasospasm had remained basically unclear until the 1970s. This may be explained by several factors. First, because of lack of knowledge about the functional organization of the cerebral arterial bed, the mode of localization of vasospasm in it had not been elucidated; it had been unclear where to investigate to achieve satisfactory results. In early studies of vasospasm (Schultz, 1866; Florey, 1925; Echlin, 1942; Lende, 1960; and some others) the pial arteries were used, probably because they had been the easiest to approach; they were not very informative for the problem's solution. Second, no adequate methods had been developed for a proper experimental analysis of the pathophysiological mechanisms of spasm development in those cerebral arteries where it appears most readily under "natural" conditions. Third, the knowledge of physiology, biochemistry, and biophysics of the vascular smooth muscle responsible for vasospasm development was still insufficient.

But from the 1960s and through the 1970s these limitations were overcome, step by step. The functional peculiarities of different portions of the cerebral arterial bed and the related modes of localization of vasospasm in it have been elucidated. Furthermore, considerable progress has been achieved in the analysis of events inside the vascular smooth muscle cells related to constriction and dilatation (Somlyo and Somlyo, 1968; Bülbring et al., 1970; Orlov et al., 1971; Gurevich and Bernstein, 1972; Johansson and Somlyo, 1980; Jones, 1980; Butler and Davies, 1980; Kramer and Hardman, 1980; Hartshorne and Gorecka, 1980). However, the pathophysiological mechanisms of spasm development have not been considered in any of these scientific contributions. Therefore, the actual difference between physiological and pathological vasoconstriction from the viewpoint of smooth muscle physiology and biomechanics has not been properly considered in these works. Nevertheless, they encouraged detailed investigation into pathophysiological mechanisms of vasospasm development.

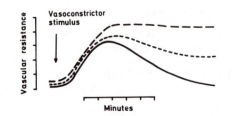

Fig. 5.9. Differences between normal and spasmodic
           contraction-relaxation coupling in vascu-
           lar muscle. The proportional sizes of
           constriction and dilatation are specific
           for normal constrictor responses in vas-
           cular smooth muscle, while a deficiency
           in dilatation is seen during pathologi-
           cal vasoconstriction, or vasospasm, of
           the artery. See text for details. (Re-
           produced from Mchedlishvili, 1981.)

     Investigations of this problem should be carried out primarily in
animal experiments, since the complicated interaction of physiological and
pathological events leading to vasospasm in human patients interferes with
the accumulation of sufficiently informative data. The conditions of vasospasm development should therefore be considerably simplified in order to
exclude the effects of numerous complicating factors that occur under
natural conditions and interfere with elucidation of the mechanisms of
vasospasm development. Such conditions could be achieved in research by
isolating the arteries anatomically and/or functionally by complicated experimental procedures which are impossible to perform in humans. The results of systematic studies of the pathophysiological mechanisms of cerebral vasospasm development in the 1960s and through the 1970s have been summarized by the author in a monograph (Mchedlishvili, 1977a) and several review articles (Mchedlishvili, 1974, 1981).

     The Essence of Vasospasm. Proceeding from knowledge accumulated in
the course of investigations of the development and relief of cerebral
vasospasm under various conditions, the following concept of the essential
difference between normal and pathological constrictor responses of blood
vessels has been proposed (Mchedlishvili, 1973, 1974, 1977a). The normal
constrictor response to comparatively brief stimuli consists of two
coupled processes — contraction and subsequent relaxation of the vascular
smooth muscle, during which the initially increased muscular tone decreases
again to its initial level. Therefore, the inevitable coupling of two
active processes takes place in muscle cells: the contraction and the subsequent relaxation **return the** muscle to the initial resting state. Vasospasm may be a manifestation of the following disturbance of this coupling:
upon stimulation the muscular contraction attains a normal or even increased amplitude, while the subsequent relaxation of the muscle cells is
delayed or more or less inhibited, resulting in a sustained state of contraction of the vascular wall (Fig. 5.9).

     The normal coupling of the two active processes — contraction and re-
laxation — is typical for any smooth muscle, as well as for striated
muscle. Studies of the two processes in isolated internal carotid arteries in dogs (for a description of the method see Mchedlishvili, 1972;

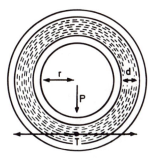

Fig. 5.10. Forces determining the width of arterial
lumen. The intravascular pressure (P),
related to luminal radius (r) and thickness of vessel wall (d), determines the
widening of arteries, while the tangential tension (T) of the vascular wall
determines the luminal contraction. The
relationship between these forces is
$T \approx P \cdot r/d$. See text for details. (Reproduced from Mchedlishvili, 1977a.)

Mchedlishvili and Ormotsadze, 1979; and pp. 62-63 in Chapter 3) show that the
duration of the smooth muscle contraction is usually shorter than that of
relaxation under normal conditions, i.e., when spasm does not develop. In
randomly selected "normal" responses the duration of relaxation is approximately three times longer than that of contraction and the relationship is
actually independent of the size of the vascular response. Thus, a relatively shorter contraction than relaxation in the internal carotid artery
walls under experimental conditions can be considered to be normal (Mchedlishvili, 1977a).

It seems obvious from present knowledge that the size and duration of
vasoconstriction in response to normal stimuli (e.g., during regulation of
blood circulation in an organ) are efficiently determined by a controlling
feedback mechanism. In contrast to the normal situation, the feedback
mechanism associated with relaxation is defective in vasospasm. The delay
in arterial smooth muscle relaxation, indicative of vasospasm, is variable
and may sometimes lead to a complete absence of relaxation, thus resulting
in a sustained state of vascular constriction (Fig. 5.9). It follows that
during changes in vascular smooth muscle which entail increased inclina-
tion to vasospasm (e.g., considerable activation of muscle contraction
processes or inhibition of the processes related to the relaxation), any
normal constrictor stimulus can cause an inappropriate vasoconstriction,
i.e., vasospasm. An insight into the pathophysiological mechanisms of
vasospasm development led to the conclusion that this disturbance in the
contraction-relaxation coupling of the vascular smooth muscle is actually
based on disorders in the same processes occurring during normal vascular
smooth muscle function (Mchedlishvili, 1977a, 1981).

An important role is certainly played in the development of vasospasm by biomechanical factors described in the law of Laplace (Fig. 5.10):
$T \approx Pr/d$, where T is the tangential tension of the vascular wall, P is the
intravascular pressure, r is the radius of the vascular lumen, and d is
the thickness of the vascular wall (Voronin, 1947; Burton, 1951; Rushmer,
1961; Damask, 1978). An unchanged vascular diameter means that the forces

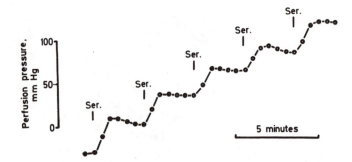

Fig. 5.11. Staircase phenomenon caused by repeated constrictor
            stimuli to an artery prone to vasospasm. During
            disturbances in relaxation processes in vascular
            smooth muscle, the constrictory stimuli repeatedly
            affecting the vascular wall result in the develop-
            ment of a "staircase phenomenon" leading to con-
            siderable vascular spasm. This experiment was per-
            formed in the isolated *in situ* dog's internal carotid
            artery continuously perfused with Ringer-Krebs bi-
            carbonate solution by constant-output pump. The
            arterial tone is expressed in terms of the level of
            perfusion pressure. (Reproduced from Mchedlishvili,
            Kometiani, et al., 1970-1971.)

in the equation are in equilibrium. However, following a constrictor stimulus the vascular muscle tone (T) increases and results in reduction in the
luminal radius (r) as well as in increase in thickness of the vascular wall
(d). Under these conditions the vascular tension (T) overcomes the intravascular pressure more easily and causes a progressive decrease in the vascular radius (r). Therefore vasoconstriction occurs more easily in vessels
with a smaller diameter: Complete closure of the vascular lumen is impossible only because the length of the perimeter of the vascular intima cannot be decreased to zero (or almost zero). Vasoconstriction causes thickening of the vascular intima; the internal elastic membrane becomes sharply
bent. In this situation the endothelial cells, which are normally flat,
become cylindrical in shape, and this leads to a considerable decrease in
the vascular lumen (Hutt and Wick, 1954; Kovalevsky, 1963; Esipova et al.,
1967).

    The prevalence of muscular contraction over relaxation in vascular
smooth muscle predisposed to vasospasm development can lead to the appearance of a "staircase phenomenon," if constrictor stimuli reach the vascular wall repeatedly. This phenomenon, shown in Fig. 5.11, has been observed in the isolated internal carotid artery in dogs during repeated
intraarterial administration of serotonin (Mchedlishvili, Kometiani, et
al., 1970-1971).

    The essence of pathological vasodilatation in some respects resembles
vasospasm, but differs in others. Contraction and relaxation in vascular
smooth muscle are also disturbed, and the disturbance is manifested in
lack of conformity between the length of relaxation and subsequent contraction of muscle cells following specific dilator stimulation. But unlike
vasospasm, it is relaxation that prevails over contraction of the muscle

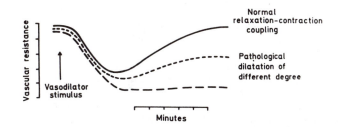

Fig. 5.12.   Differences between relaxation-contraction coupling
in normal and pathologically dilated vessels. The
proportional sizes of dilatation and subsequent constriction are specific for the normal dilator response of vascular smooth muscle to a single dilator
stimulus, while a deficiency in contraction leads to
pathological dilatation of the artery. See text for
details.

during pathological vasodilatation. Normally smooth muscle responds to
vasodilator stimuli by relaxation and subsequent contraction of equal amp-
litudes and, therefore, the muscle tone completely recovers following the
dilatator response. In case of a "vasoparalysis," however, the constriction seems to be deficient, so that following the relaxation-contraction
cycle the vascular smooth muscle remains dilated (Fig. 5.12).

When the arterial diameter is steadily regulated under normal conditions, vasodilator responses, i.e., the vascular muscle relaxation and
subsequent contraction leading to recovery of the initial tone, are controlled by specific feedback mechanisms. However, if the intrinsic characteristics in muscle cells related to contraction are deficient, the artery remains dilated for a longer time than necessary, i.e., in a state of
pathological vasodilatation.

Biomechanical factors involved in development of pathological dilatation are, in all probability, considerably more important than those involved in the development of cerebral vasospasm. The biomechanical factors are described above and include: the tangential tension of the vessel wall (T), the intraluminal pressure (P), the luminal radius (r), as
well as the thickness of the vascular wall (d). These factors are schematically presented in Fig. 5.10 with respect to the following relationship:
$T \approx Pr/d$.

The contribution of these factors to pathological vasodilatation is
very important, especially the intraluminal pressure (P), which contributes
to stretching of the arterial wall. A sharp increase in intravascular
pressure, which provokes pathological vasodilatation, can be dependent on
both an increase in systemic arterial pressure and a reduction in vascular
resistance along the path between the aorta and a given artery. A rise in
intravascular pressure in cerebral arteries following a sharp increase in
systemic arterial pressure during arterial hypertension (provided that constriction of the major arteries of the brain does not compensate for the
pressure increase, see Chapter 3) promotes pathological dilatation of pial
arteries. When this occurs, it results in an enormous increase in blood
pressure within corresponding microvessels, resulting in disturbances in
the microcirculation.

An increase in the radius of the vascular lumen (r) contributes, in turn, to subsequent stretching of the arterial walls if dilatation has already been initiated (even when the dilatation is originally of a physiological nature) and can also promote a progressive increase in dilatation. The concomitantly occurring decrease in thickness of the arterial wall (d) contributes to further vasodilatation and interferes with the recovery of the initial size of the vascular lumen. These forces can be counteracted only by the tangential tension of the vascular wall (T), which is primarily dependent on the active contraction of vascular smooth muscle. However, a primary disturbance in the contractile process determining the vascular tone may contribute significantly to pathological vasodilatation. Disturbances may occur in different links in the process (considered below) and may hence contribute to the development of pathological vasodilatation. Extensive further study of pathological vasodilatation is needed, since almost no experimental data concerning this important problem is available thus far.

When pathological vasodilatation has already occurred, i.e., the cerebral arteries remain in the state of an inappropriate dilatation for a long time, certain morphological changes might appear in the considerably expanded vascular walls. The internal elastic membrane is straightened and appears to be covered with flat muscle cells with thin, elongated nuclei. There is an increased permeability of plasma proteins into the walls of chronically dilated arteries (Gannushkina and Shafranova, 1975, 1977). Fibrinous deposits in the arterial media may be caused by the penetration of blood plasma that squeezes and damages smooth muscle cells (Goldby and Beilin, 1972). These changes in the vascular muscle cells might lead either to their necrosis or to their hypertrophy.

Basic processes in vascular smooth muscle causing vasospasm and vasoparalysis are, in all probability, the same as those determining muscle contraction and relaxation under normal conditions. Experimental evidence shows that the intrinsic processes determining pathological vascular responses, particularly vasospasm, actually consist of similar links outside and inside the smooth muscle cells to those found in normal physiological vascular behavior (Mchedlishvili, 1977a, 1981).

The inappropriate constriction and dilatation of cerebral arteries can be produced by different mechanisms. Although any kind of schematization of these mechanisms would inevitably possess some limitations, their classifications nevertheless seem to assist in understanding the essence of development of pathological constriction and dilatation of cerebral arteries. In all probability, a classification emphasizing the basic pathogenic points in the mechanisms of development of both vasospasm and vasoparalysis could be most helpful. These points are as follows: first there may be a prolonged action of specific endogenous vasoactive substances resulting in a sustained state of vasoconstriction or vasodilatation, which is actually aimless from the point of view of regulation of cerebral circulation. Second, a change in the reactivity of vascular smooth muscle produced, for instance, by some physiologically active substance, results in a sustained state of constriction or dilatation in response to even normal stimuli regulating cerebral circulation. Third, primary disturbances in the normal functioning of the plasma membrane, as well as intracellular membranes, in smooth muscle cells may render them incapable of recovering the normal resting state of the vascular tone and hence produce a sustained state of constriction or relaxation. Fourth, the primary disturbances in the intracellular processes may be related to contraction and relaxation of vascular muscle cells, especially the calcium ion carrier mechanisms. Fifth, primary disorders in the contractile

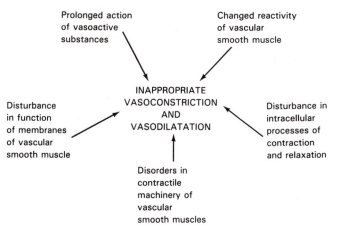

Fig. 5.13.   Factors provoking pathological vascular
behavior.

machinery of vascular smooth muscle cells can result in a sustained state
of contraction or relaxation, i.e., vasospasm or vasoparalysis. The putative pathogenic factors provoking pathological arterial behavior are schematically presented in Fig. 5.13.

It is quite probable that under normal conditions these points in
muscle cell contraction and relaxation do not function independently. For
instance, even when vasospasm is produced by prolonged action of an un-
usual and quantitatively excessive stimulus, it always eventually affects
the membrane and intracellular processes, which have been undisturbed initially. On the other hand, disturbances in the membrane and/or intracellular processes of vascular smooth muscle may produce vasospasm, as well as
pathological vasodilatation, even when vasoactive substances or vasomotor
nerve impulses normally involved in the regulation of cerebral blood flow
are still at normal levels. The classification of factors involved in the
development of pathological cerebral vascular responses is aimed at stress-
ing the main link disturbed in the contraction-relaxation cycle of vascular
smooth muscle cells. This is necessary not only for a better understanding
of the mechanisms of vasospasm and vasodilatation, but also for their appropriate diagnosis and treatment in patients.

5.5.   EXTRINSIC EFFECTS ON VASCULAR SMOOTH MUSCLE THAT MAY BE
       INVOLVED IN THE DEVELOPMENT OF CEREBRAL VASOSPASM

The pathophysiological mechanism of vasospasm development proceeds
from a series of interconnected events which finally lead to formation of
pathological vasoconstriction. The initial links of this mechanism may be
some physiological or pathological events which may or may not be related
to the regulation of cerebral blood flow. Individual links of the mechanism are in a cause-effect relationship, so that the initial changes may
finally result in a disturbance in the normal contraction-relaxation cycle
of vascular smooth muscle typical of vasospasm (see above, p. 190).

Pathological vasoconstriction, like any physiological reaction of the
arterial walls, appears most often in response to some extrinsic physiological stimuli affecting vascular muscle. The constrictor stimuli can
vary: (a) myogenic effects of muscle in response to various degrees of

stretch; (b) direct effects of some metabolic products originating in the
surrounding tissue and reaching the vascular walls by diffusion; (c) neurogenic vasomotor effects reaching the vascular smooth muscles via the efferent nerve fiber neurotransmitters; and, (d) effects of vasoactive substances originating in or from the vascular walls, or from the circulation.

Under normal conditions the above-mentioned physiological stimuli may
be involved in the regulation of blood circulation or other physiological
processes, and thus they can affect vascular smooth muscle secondarily.
To induce vasospasm the stimuli should: (i) cause contraction of vascular
smooth muscle cells, and/or (ii) change the contractile process of the vascular smooth muscles in a specific direction, i.e., increase and contract,
and/or (iii) cause specific disturbances in the process of relaxation of
vascular smooth muscle cells, thus resulting in a sustained and inappropriate state of vasoconstriction.

Physiological stimuli directly affecting the vascular wall may include
the myogenic response to arterial wall stretch of varying degrees and the
effects of metabolic products originating in the surrounding tissue that
diffuse to the vascular walls. The effects of specific vasoconstrictor
substances of endogenous origin which might affect the vascular wall will
be considered below (pp. 197-207).

The myogenic contractile response of vascular smooth muscle to stretch
has been well known for many years (see pp. 83-84). The effect is manifested both in mechanical and electrical responses of vascular smooth
muscles to stretch (Johnson, 1980). However, the net myogenic contractile
response is relatively small in contrast to the sharp constriction of arteries characteristic of vasospasm. In addition, the net myogenic response
usually has a relatively short duration, while vasospasm typically is a
sustained vasoconstriction. Thus, the net myogenic response of normal vascular smooth muscle is probably not involved in the development of cerebral vasospasm. However, if the contractile and relaxation processes in
vascular smooth muscle have been specifically disturbed (see pp. 216-220
and 223-227), a sudden distension of the vascular walls caused by a sharp
rise in intravascular pressure may become a stimulus resulting in a sustained vasoconstriction of vasospasm type.

The metabolic products originating in the tissue surrounding the vessel walls that directly affect vascular smooth muscle are probably not involved in the development of vasospasm. Such a regulatory mechanism can
work only on the smallest precapillary arteries inside the cerebral tissue,
while vasospasm predominantly affects the larger cerebral arteries, which
are inaccessible to the metabolic substances diffusing through cerebral
tissue. Furthermore, all of the presently considered metabolic vasoactive
products, like carbon dioxide, hydrogen and potassium ions, and adenosine,
are dilator substances in physiological concentrations and therefore cannot be involved in the development of cerebral vasospasm.

However, any physiological stimulus causing vasoconstriction, in
spite of its myogenic or metabolic (as well as neurogenic) origin, might be
involved in the production of vasospasm. But this would happen only under
special conditions when the contractile and, more importantly, the relaxation processes in the arterial smooth muscle have been changed. This
event is schematically presented in Fig. 5.14.

Involvement of Specific Vasoactive Substances in the Development of
Cerebral Vasospasm. Various vasoconstrictor substances of endogenous
origin, like serotonin, catecholamines, various prostaglandins, etc., can

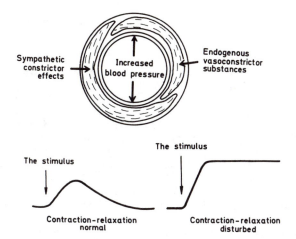

Fig. 5.14. Vasospasm occurring in response to
            physiological vasoconstrictor stimuli.
            Even normal vasoconstrictor stimuli in-
            volved in cerebral blood flow regula-
            tion can cause a spasmodic contraction
            of cerebral vascular smooth muscle if
            the latter is predisposed to enhanced
            contraction and the relaxation mecha-
            nism is impaired.

be involved in development of vasospasm. Such substances can affect vascular smooth muscle while they are circulating in blood, or released inside
the vascular wall or in its vicinity. Thus, such substances can specifically affect vascular muscle cells and cause physiological or pathological
vasoconstriction. Abundant experimental results concerning the vasoconstrictor effects of such substances have been summarized elsewhere (Sokoloff, 1959; Carpi, 1972; von Essen, 1973; Olesen, 1974; Edvinsson and
MacKenzie, 1977; Mchedlishvili, 1977a; Kuschinsky and Wahl, 1978; Bevan et
al., 1980; Burnstock, 1980; Needleman and Isakson, 1980).

   Many endogenous vasoactive substances participate in the regulation of
cerebral blood flow. In some instances they transmit neurogenic efferent
impulses related to cerebral blood flow regulation to vascular smooth
muscle. However, under certain conditions they might also play a role in
disturbances of this regulation and, in particular, in the development of
vasospasm. The significance of such substances in pathological vasoconstriction has been largely attributed to the development of vasospasm in
the close vicinity of hemorrhage and blood clotting. It has been suggested
that this vasospasm develops as a result of blood platelet aggregation and
subsequent liberation of vasoconstrictor substances like serotonin (Zervas
et al., 1973; Watts, 1977; Linder and Alksne, 1978) or liberation of fib-
rinolytic products (Arutiunov et al., 1975).

   Serotonin (5-hydroxytryptamine), produced by the mast cells throughout
the body, can circulate in blood in relatively large amounts (Zervas et
al., 1973). Serotonin can also originate from blood platelets during blood
clotting either inside the vascular lumen during the formation of a parietal thrombus or adjacent to the vascular wall following bleeding, e.g., from

a damaged aneurysm (Raynor et al., 1961; Arutiunov et al., 1970; Symon, 1971). In addition, serotonin might be produced inside the arterial wall in response to some specific stimuli. Evidence for the production of serotonin in the wall of the internal carotid artery isolated *in situ* has been obtained in experiments with dogs under the conditions of shock produced by the intravenous administration of heterogeneous blood (Mchedlishvili, Garfunkel, et al., 1972).

The constrictor effect of serotonin on brain vessels is greater than that of catecholamines, and blood vessels in the majority of peripheral organs outside the brain (mesentery, kidney, extremities) show a smaller constrictor response to serotonin than the cerebral arteries (Bohr and Elliott, 1963; Daugherty et al., 1968). But even in the brain vasculature, the effect of serotonin is not identical for different cerebral arteries: the vasoconstriction is comparatively strong in the internal carotid artery, but is significantly smaller in the pial arteries (Ormotsadze et al., 1969), as shown in Fig. 5.15. The constrictor effect of serotonin on the isolated internal carotid artery of dogs (the principle of the technique is on pp. 62-63) is easily seen when the serotonin concentration inside the vascular lumen is on the order of 0.01 µg per ml of perfusion fluid. This concentration is much less than that in the blood of the same species [where serotonin concentration has been found by Zervas et al. (1973) to be up to 0.37 µg/ml] as well as in other animals and man (Kursky and Baksheev, 1974). Hence it may be concluded that serotonin exerts a specific constrictor effect on the major brain arteries.

The constrictor effect of serotonin on cerebral arteries is related to the presence of serotonin-specific receptors in the plasma membranes of smooth muscle cells. This has been proved by inhibition of serotonin effects on the internal carotid artery by a specific blocker, Deseril (methysergide, Sandoz) given either before or following the administration of serotonin in the artery (Mchedlishvili, Ormotsadze, et al., 1971). Figure 5.16 demonstrates the constrictor effect of serotonin on the internal carotid artery, which is inhibited by Deseril. The serotonin receptors are located, in all probability, on the surface of muscle cell plasma membrane, since serotonin is not soluble in lipids and therefore penetrates plasma membranes slowly (Born, 1970). The constrictor effect of serotonin on the internal carotid artery inversely correlates with the resting tone of the vessel wall (Fig. 5.17).

From the viewpoint of vasospasm development, it is essential that no habituation (tachyphylaxis) be observed during repeated or prolonged action of serotonin on cerebral vessel walls (Mchedlishvili, Kometiani, et al., 1970-1971; von Essen, 1973). Therefore serotonin can cause cerebral vasospasm in cases when it is continuously affecting the arterial wall (Fig. 5.16). This might occur because of a process comparable to the "accumulation" of serotonin in the vascular walls. This has been proved in experiments with reserpine, which is known to cause liberation of serotonin from its stores (Carpi, 1972). Figure 5.18 demonstrates that following intraarterial administration of reserpine the tone of the internal carotid artery increases with a subsequent decrease below original levels. This occurs, in all probability, due to liberation and then depletion of serotonin from the stores inside the vascular wall. However, after blockade of the serotonin receptors by Deseril the constrictor phase disappears, thus proving that the vascular tone was determined by the prolonged action of the serotonin intrinsic to the vascular wall. This is evidence that serotonin might be responsible for a steady state of constriction of the internal carotid artery during vasospasm. A continued effect of serotonin

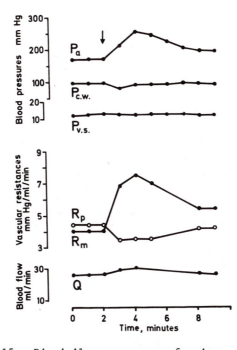

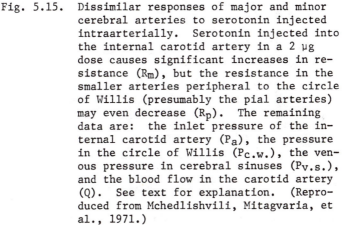

Fig. 5.15.   Dissimilar responses of major and minor
             cerebral arteries to serotonin injected
             intraarterially. Serotonin injected into
             the internal carotid artery in a 2 µg
             dose causes significant increases in re-
             sistance (R_m), but the resistance in the
             smaller arteries peripheral to the circle
             of Willis (presumably the pial arteries)
             may even decrease (R_p). The remaining
             data are: the inlet pressure of the in-
             ternal carotid artery (P_a), the pressure
             in the circle of Willis ($P_{c.w.}$), the ven-
             ous pressure in cerebral sinuses ($P_{v.s.}$),
             and the blood flow in the carotid artery
             (Q). See text for explanation. (Repro-
             duced from Mchedlishvili, Mitagvaria, et
             al., 1971.)

might also appear when its destruction inside the vascular wall has been
inhibited. If the enzyme monoamine oxidase, which is responsible for serotonin catalysis, is inhibited by Iproniazid, Niamide, or Nardil, the serotonin effect on the internal carotid artery becomes significantly increased and prolonged (Mchedlishvili, Kometiani, et al., 1970-1971), as is
demonstrated in Fig. 5.19.

    Therefore, elimination of vasospasm, caused by a prolonged effect of
serotonin on cerebral arteries, can be accomplished by the application of
specific blockers to serotonin receptors (e.g., by Deseril), or by reserpine, which eliminates the binding of serotonin with the vascular smooth
muscle cells.

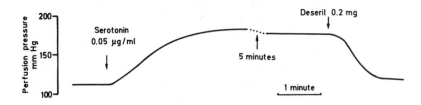

Fig. 5.16.   The continuous constrictor effect of serotonin on the internal
              carotid artery and its inhibition by Deseril. The constrictor
              effect of serotonin, added to the perfusion fluid of the iso-
              lated (*in situ*) internal carotid artery of a dog, can be con-
              stant for several minutes, but disappears as soon as a specific
              blocker of the serotonin receptors in smooth muscle cells, Des-
              eril (methysergide, Sandoz), is added to the fluid.   (Repro-
              duced from Mchedlishvili, 1977a.)

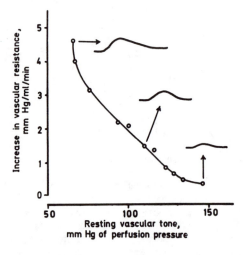

Fig. 5.17.   Dependence of the serotonin constrictor
              on the resting tone of the internal ca-
              rotid artery. The constrictor effect of
              serotonin (0.4 µg) is greater in vessels
              with lower resting vascular tone (ex-
              pressed in terms of the perfusion pres-
              sure). The data are obtained from ex-
              periments with an isolated internal ca-
              rotid artery (of a dog) continuously per-
              fused with Ringer–Krebs bicarbonate
              solution by a constant-output pump.
              (Reproduced from Mchedlishvili, Ormot-
              sadze, et al., 1971.)

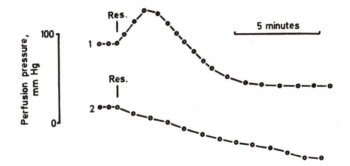

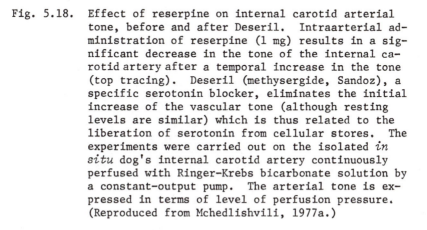

Fig. 5.18. Effect of reserpine on internal carotid arterial
            tone, before and after Deseril. Intraarterial ad-
            ministration of reserpine (1 mg) results in a sig-
            nificant decrease in the tone of the internal ca-
            rotid artery after a temporal increase in the tone
            (top tracing). Deseril (methysergide, Sandoz), a
            specific serotonin blocker, eliminates the initial
            increase of the vascular tone (although resting
            levels are similar) which is thus related to the
            liberation of serotonin from cellular stores. The
            experiments were carried out on the isolated *in
            situ* dog's internal carotid artery continuously
            perfused with Ringer-Krebs bicarbonate solution by
            a constant-output pump. The arterial tone is ex-
            pressed in terms of level of perfusion pressure.
            (Reproduced from Mchedlishvili, 1977a.)

The alpha-adrenomimetic substances — *the catecholamines* (adrenaline,
noradrenaline, and dopamine) — might arise from sources within arterial
walls: they can be liberated from the adrenergic nerve terminals close to
the smooth muscle cells (Gershon, 1970; Bevan et al., 1980) and they can
circulate through the vascular lumen. The amount of catecholamines in the
blood might be significantly increased under different physiological and
pathological conditions (Carpi, 1972). The catecholamines are probably the
most widespread vasoconstrictor substances of endogenous origin in the body
that directly affect vascular smooth muscle. In addition, they have been
found to change the responsiveness of vascular smooth muscle in the direction
characteristic of vasospasm (see below).

It is known that the constrictor effect of the catecholamines is determined by the function of specific alpha-adrenergic receptors, which are
numerous in the arterial smooth muscles. Therefore, the effects of the
vasoactive amines are abolished following blockade of these receptors by
specific agents like dihydroergotoxin, phentolamine, phenoxybenzamine,
etc. (Bevan et al., 1980).

The characteristic constrictor effect of alpha-adrenergic substances
on the cerebral arteries is considerably smaller than that of serotonin
(Bohr and Elliott, 1963; Ormotsadze et al., 1969; Toda and Fujita, 1973;
Edvinsson and Owman, 1975). This agrees with recent data indicating that
the walls of large cerebral arteries (namely the basilar artery) contain a
limited number of alpha-like adrenoreceptors (Bevan, 1981). The adrenergic effects on the cerebral arteries probably have a certain physiological significance. It is well known that an increase in adrenaline content

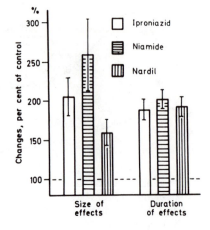

Fig. 5.19.   The effect of monoamine oxidase inhibition on the constrictor effect of serotonin on the internal carotid artery.
Following inhibition of monoamide oxidase in the wall of the internal carotid
artery by Iproniazid, Niamide or Nardil,
the constrictor effects of serotonin become significantly increased and prolonged. A delay in serotonin destruction in the arterial wall contributes to
a sustained state of contraction in vascular smooth muscle, characteristic of
vasospasm. The experiments were carried
out on the isolated *in situ* dog's internal carotid artery continuously perfused with Ringer-Krebs bicarbonate solution by a constant-output pump. The
change in arterial tone is expressed in
terms of level of perfusion pressure.
(Reproduced from Mchedlishvili, 1977a.)

in the blood is an important physiological mechanism responsible for maintaining and increasing the level of the systemic arterial pressure in the
body. This effect is dependent on the constrictor response of the majority
of the body's arteries to the direct effect of adrenaline. However, because of the comparatively slight constrictor response of the cerebral arteries, they do not constrict significantly under these circumstances and,
therefore, do not reduce the blood supply to the brain tissue when it is
unnecessary.

From the viewpoint of vasospasm development, it is very important
that the catecholamines induce specific alterations in the genuine constrictor response of the cerebral blood vessels to physiological stimuli.
This has been demonstrated in experiments with isolated internal carotid
arteries in dogs (Mchedlishvili, Borodulya, et' al., 1972). Following
catecholamine administration, the size and duration of arterial constrictor
responses to other constrictor stimuli (e.g., serotonin) increased significantly (Fig. 5.20). Furthermore, following the action of catecholamines
a greater response to the serotonin vasoconstrictor effect was observed in
the majority of cases (almost 90%). This specific effect of catecholamines

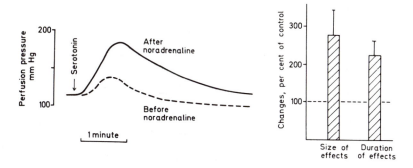

Fig. 5.20.   The effect of noradrenaline, a catecholamine, on the constrictor response of the internal carotid artery caused by serotonin.
The successive administration to the perfusate of the dog's
artery isolated *in situ* of 0.2 µg serotonin, 5 µg noradrenaline, and again 0.2 µg serotonin revealed that the constrictor
effect of serotonin has specifically changed; its size and
duration are significantly increased.   The lower tracing is
the control effect of serotonin and the upper tracing is the
serotonin effect after the administration of noradrenaline. On
the right the mean increase in constrictor effect (M ± SE) is
demonstrated (the size of constrictor response is expressed as
a rise in perfusion pressure).   The experiments were carried
out on the isolated *in situ* dog's internal carotid artery perfused with Ringer–Krebs bicarbonate solution by a constant-
output pump.   The arterial tone is expressed in terms of the
level of perfusion pressure.   (Reproduced from Mchedlishvili,
Borodulya, et al., 1972.)

might be explained by their stimulatory action on metabolic processes in
the vascular smooth muscle cells (Somlyo and Somlyo, 1968).

    Thus, catecholamines might be involved in development of vasospasm in
spite of the fact that the number of alpha-adrenergic receptors in the cerebral arterial walls is relatively small.

    Prostaglandins, as vasoactive substances, have attracted the atten-
tion of researchers since the 1960s.   These substances are produced in
various tissues throughout the body (Christ and Van Dorp, 1972) including
arterial walls.   The synthesis and the destruction of prostaglandins occur
in a relatively short period, and hence their effect is assumed to be predominantly local.   They are therefore considered to be "local hormones."
The majority of prostaglandins are vasoactive substances that directly affect vascular smooth muscle (Needleman and Isakson, 1980).   It is believed
that there are specific prostaglandin receptors on the plasma membranes of
vascular smooth muscle cells.   In cases when prostaglandins cause a constrictor effect on the arteries, depolarization of the muscle cell occurs
with a subsequent flux of Ca^{++} into the cytoplasm (Strong and Bohr, 1967).

    Numerous studies have demonstrated that prostaglandins A_1, B_1, E_2, and $F_2\alpha$
cause constriction of cerebral arteries (Morgan et al., 1972; Yamamoto et
al., 1972; Pickard, 1973; Allen et al., 1974; White et al., 1975; Kapp et
al., 1976; Needleman and Isakson, 1980) and, therefore, they might participate in the genesis of cerebral vasospasm.   From the point of view of spasm

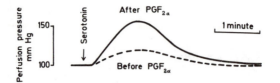

Fig. 5.21. Alteration of the constrictor response
of serotonin by prostaglandin $F_{2\alpha}$ on the
internal carotid artery of a dog. The
lower tracing is the serotonin control
effect (0.8 µg) and the upper tracing
is the serotonin effect (0.8 µg)
after prostaglandin administration (1
µg). The tracings represent the perfusion pressure changes in the isolated
internal carotid artery continuously perfused with Ringer-Krebs bicarbonate solution by a constant-output pump. (From
the experiments of Mchedlishvili and
Ormotsadze.)

development, the effects of prostaglandins on the cerebral vessels have
been characterized (as demonstrated in the isolated internal carotid artery; see Mchedlishvili and Ormotsadze, 1979). First, repeated intraarterial administration of vasoconstrictor prostaglandins (A_1, B_1, E_2, and $F_{2\alpha}$)
does not cause any decrease in their effects, i.e., no tachyphylaxis is
evident (tachyphylaxis has been observed only in the repeated vasodilator
effects of prostaglandin E_1). Second, the vasoconstrictor prostaglandins
considerably potentiate the constrictor arterial responses of serotonin
(Fig. 5.21). Third, the residual contraction of vascular smooth muscle
seen following the vasoconstrictor effects of prostaglandins provides evidence that the relaxation process of the muscle becomes disturbed.

    Vasopressin (antidiuretic hormone), after being produced in the posterior
pituitary, is taken by its vein directly into the cavernous sinus. Therefore
its concentration in the blood surrounding the walls of internal carotid
arteries can sometimes be considerably increased, which may affect the
arteries under natural conditions. The vasopressin vasoconstrictor effect on the internal carotid arteries of dogs has been found to have a significantly long duration. It also specifically changes the reactivity of
the vascular smooth muscle with respect to the effects of other vasoconstrictor stimuli; this is especially essential for spasm development
(Mchedlishvili, 1977a). For example, the vasoconstrictor effect of serotonin becomes considerably increased in size and duration if the vessel
wall has been previously treated with vasopressin (Fig. 5.22).

    The comparative significance of the endogenous vasoconstrictor sub-
stances in the development of vasospasm may be elucidated when their effects are compared under similar experimental conditions. Such results
have been obtained in isolated internal carotid arteries of dogs. This
technique (see p.62-63) enables one to carry out experiments on the cerebral artery, which especially tends to develop spasms and is a site where
the effects of vasoconstrictor substances can be properly analyzed (Mchedlishvili and Ormotsadze, 1979). The vasoconstrictor substances administered intraarterially cause effects of different sizes on the vascular
smooth muscle. Serotonin causes the greatest constrictor effect on arterial walls in the smallest doses. A similar, but somewhat smaller, effect

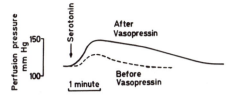

Fig. 5.22. Alteration of the constrictor response
of serotonin by vasopressin on the internal carotid artery of a dog. The
tracings represent the perfusion pressure of the artery continuously perfused by a constant-output pump with
Ringer-Krebs bicarbonate solution. The
lower tracing is the control effect of
serotonin (0.1 µg) and the upper tracing is the serotonin effect (0.1 µg)
after vasopressin administration (0.01
IU). (Reproduced from Mchedlishvili,
1977a.)

is obtained after injection of hypertensin. As for noradrenaline and the
prostaglandins, the amplitude of their effects is comparatively variable
in different experiments: effects of similar size might be obtained with
various doses. The dose-response relationship of the vasoconstrictor substances studied on the internal carotid artery is shown in Fig. 5.23.

The following differences between the effects of serotonin and hypertensin on the internal carotid artery have been found under conditions
when they were administered repeatedly: the constrictor effect of serotonin never decreases (at the beginning of the experiments it even increases). But tachyphylaxis of the effect of hypertensin (i.e., the rapid
development of tolerance) has been regularly observed: the effect steadily decreases during repeated action. For instance, during the second administration of hypertensin, the vascular response decreases on the average by 44%, and during the third, by 68%, from the initial size. When other
vasoconstrictor substances, i.e., noradrenaline, prostaglandins, and vasopressin, are administered repeatedly into the perfusion fluid of the artery,
no tachyphylaxis has been observed.

The duration of vasoconstrictor responses of the internal carotid artery caused by different agents varies significantly. To compare the duration of the effects obtained in all cases, irrespective of differences in
the size of smooth muscle contractions, the comparative duration of vascular responses, i.e., related to 1 mm Hg of the size of the responses, were
calculated. Figure 5.24 shows the comparative duration of vasoconstrictor
effects, including contraction and relaxation of vascular smooth muscle
responses to different vasoconstrictor substances. The data show that the
shortest vasoconstrictor response was caused by serotonin and the longest
by vasopressin, the latter being almost ten times longer than the former. The effect of other investigated vasoconstrictor substances is intermediate in duration between these two substances: serotonin < prostaglandin A_1 < hypertensin and prostaglandin E_2 < prostaglandin B_1 and noradrenaline < vasopressin.

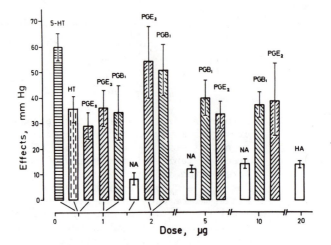

Fig. 5.23. Dose-response relationship between various vasoconstrictor substances on the internal carotid artery.
The sizes of the constrictor responses are related
to the doses of substances administered into the
perfusion fluid (bicarbonate Ringer-Krebs solution)
pumped into the isolated internal carotid artery of
dogs under standardized conditions. 5-HT, serotonin; HT, hypertensin; PGE_2, PGB_1, and PGA_1, prostaglandins E_2, B_1, and A_1, respectively; NA, noradrenaline. The constrictor effects manifest themselves as an increase in vascular smooth muscle
tone, expressed as increase in perfusion pressure.
(Reproduced from Mchedlishvili and Ormotsadze,
1979.)

     The relaxation time of smooth muscle following contraction also varies
in response to different vasoconstrictor substances. Randomly selected
"normal" responses of arterial smooth muscle to intraarterial administration of 0.1-0.4 µg of serotonin show that the duration of relaxation is
about 295 ± 20.8% of the duration of contraction. This relationship, called
the relaxation index, compares the duration of smooth muscle relaxation in
percent to the duration of contraction, taken as 100%. Figure 5.25 shows
that the most rapid relaxation of the vascular smooth muscle in response to
different vasoconstrictor substances follows serotonin administration.
During vasoconstrictor responses to the other substances under investigation, the relaxation index gradually increases in the following sequence:
serotonin < prostaglandin E_2 < hypertensin < prostaglandin B_1 < noradrenaline < prostaglandin A_1 < vasopressin. The differences in effect between
some of these substances are not always statistically significant.

     Following the vasoconstrictor effects of the studied substances, a re-
sidual contraction of the vascular smooth muscle has been observed in some
cases. In randomly selected responses such residually increased vascular
tone has been observed after serotonin effects in 13.2% of responses observed, after prostaglandin A_1 in 12.1%, after noradrenaline in 32.3%,
after prostaglandin B_1 in 42.5%, after prostaglandin E_2 in 58%, and after
vasopressin in 83.3% of responses.

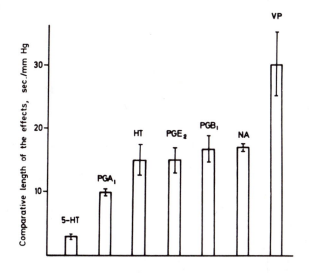

Fig. 5.24. Comparative duration of vasoconstrictor effects of
various vasoactive substances on the internal carotid artery of dogs. 5-HT, serotonin; HT, hypertensin;
PGE_2, PGB_1, and PGA_1, prostaglandins E_2, B_1, and A_1;
NA, noradrenaline; and VP, vasopressin were administered into the perfusion fluid of the artery under
standardized conditions. (Reproduced from Mchedlishvili and Ormotsadze, 1979.)

In addition to their own vasoconstrictor activities, some substances
change the effects of other vasoconstrictor substances. Since the internal cartoid artery uniformly responds to the action of serotonin, the effects of other vasoconstrictor substances on serotonin responses have been
studied under conditions in which the substances are administered subsequently: serotonin, then the studied substance, and then serotonin again.
Hypertensin does not affect the constrictor response of serotonin, but noradrenaline, prostaglandins, and vasopressin increase it significantly.
Figure 5.26 shows the extent of potentiation of the serotonin effect following the administration of these vasoconstrictor agents.

As mentioned above (pp. 190-191), pathological vasoconstriction is a
consequence of disturbances in the normal constriction-relaxation cycle of
vascular muscle. Vasospasm typically appears during derangements in the
relaxation of vascular muscle; this often occurs simultaneously with an increase in muscle contraction. Therefore each specific vasoconstrictor affecting the internal carotid artery can be considered from the point of
view of having a possible role in the development of arterial spasms:

(a) Vasoactive substances play an important role in the development
of arterial spasms, especially those having potent constrictor effects.
Among the mentioned vasoconstrictors, serotonin and hypertensin cause the
greatest effects, noradrenaline has the least, and the prostaglandins have
intermediate effects. Differences in the effect of vasoactive substances
on the artery may be dependent on the quantity of specific receptors on
smooth muscle cell plasma membranes. On the other hand, differences in effect might be caused also by permeability differences. The vasoconstrictor
substances studied affected the vascular walls of the internal carotid ar-

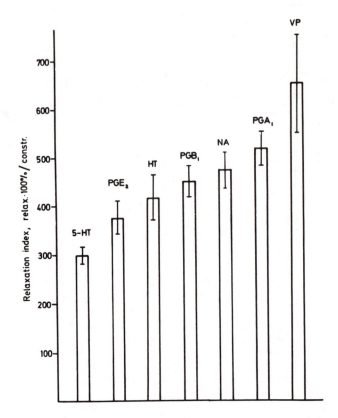

Fig. 5.25. Duration of relaxation of internal carotid artery
            walls following contractile responses to various
            vasoconstrictor substances. The relaxation index
            of arterial smooth muscle, i.e., the duration of
            relaxation in percent relative to the duration of
            contraction, was measured following the intra-
            arterial administration (under standardized condi-
            tions) of different vasoconstrictor substances:
            5-HT, serotonin; PGE_2, PGB_1, and PGA_1, prosta-
            glandins E_2, B_1, and A_1; HT, hypertensin; NA, nor-
            adrenaline; and VP, vasopressin. (Reproduced from
            Mchedlishvili and Ormotsadze, 1979.)

tery from the inside (since they were administered intraarterially). This
type of experimentation does not take into account differences in their
permeability through the internal layers of the blood vessel walls, i.e.,
between arterial lumen and smooth muscle cells. Therefore it is possible
that the relationship of constrictor effects would be different, depending
on whether the substances were produced inside the vascular wall or would
affect it from outside, but this particular problem is in need of special
study.

    (b) Vasoactive substances might play an important role in the develop-
ment of arterial spasm if the vascular wall does not show any habituation
during repeated (or prolonged) action. Among the investigated vasoconstrictor substances, only hypertensin has been found to develop tolerance.

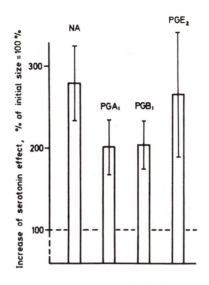

Fig. 5.26. Increase of the serotonin vasoconstrictor
effect on internal carotid artery of dogs
following the action of noradrenaline and
prostaglandins A_1, B_1, and E_2. In all
cases the initial effects of serotonin
calculated as 100%; legend as to Fig. 5.25.
(Reproduced from Mchedlishvili and Ormotsadze, 1979.)

Nevertheless, this does not completely exclude it from participating in the
development of vasospasm, especially if there are corresponding changes in
the vascular smooth muscle plasma membranes or intracellular processes.
These changes could result in a sustained state of contraction of the arterial wall even during physiological vasoconstrictor stimuli that regulate
the vascular lumina (see pp. 216-220 and 223-227). Under such conditions
even the short-time action of angiotensin would augment the development of
an internal carotid artery spasm.

(c) Vasoactive substances may play an important role in the development of arterial spasm if the relaxation of vascular smooth muscle following contraction is considerably delayed. From this standpoint, the most
prolonged relaxation of the internal carotid artery followed the action of
vasopressin. Significantly shorter relaxation of smooth muscle has been
observed after prostaglandins and hypertensin administration, and the
shortest relaxation has followed the action of serotonin. In addition,
some vasoconstrictor substances can cause a residual contraction after the
normal vasoconstrictor response, including the contraction and relaxation
of vascular smooth muscle, is complete. Among the vasoconstrictor substances studied, the prostaglandins B_1 and E_2 and vasopressin are thought
to cause such an effect.

(d) Vasoactive substances can play an important role in the development
of arterial spasm if they change the reactivity of the vascular smooth
muscle by potentiating its response to other vasoconstrictor stimuli and
thus, the relaxation of the smooth muscle tends to be delayed. Among the
vasoconstrictor substances investigated, the most significant ones that

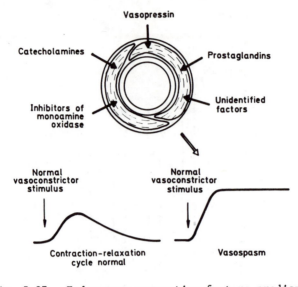

Fig. 5.27. Endogenous vasoactive factors predispos-
           ing cerebral vascular smooth muscle to
           spasmodic contraction. See text for de-
           tails.

appear to cause such an effect are noradrenaline and the prostaglandins.
If a substance possesses the capacity to change vascular smooth muscle reactivity, then even normal vasoconstrictor stimuli reaching the vascular
wall, e.g., during regulation of cerebral circulation, may cause a sustained state of constriction of the artery resulting in disturbances of the
blood flow therein. Additionally, if the collateral blood flow is insufficient, a deficiency of blood supply to some regions of the brain may occur. This
effect is schematically demonstrated in Fig. 5.27.

     Thus, all of the investigated vasoactive substances might contribute
to the development of arterial spasms under certain circumstances. Of the
endogenous vasoconstrictor substances thought to be involved in production
of cerebral vasospasm, an essential role might be attributable to those
which cause the most potent constrictor effects without tachyphylaxis, or
those which result in specific changes in smooth muscle reactivity (increased contraction, impaired relaxation) to subsequent vasoconstrictor
stimuli.

     The Neurogenic Mechanism Provoking Cerebral Vasospasm. The adren-
ergic nerve control of cerebral arteries, which can be involved in any type
of cerebral blood flow regulation, has been considered in Chapters 3 and 4
of this book. There is no doubt about the effect of vasoconstrictor nerves
on the cerebral vascular tone. It also seems quite probable that neurogenic vasoconstrictor effects on cerebral arteries can be involved in the
development of cerebral vasospasm. However, evidence for the influence of
vasomotor nerves in the occurrence of pathological vasoconstriction in the
brain is still quite poor.

     The involvement of the neurogenic mechanism in the development of ce-
rebral vasospasm has been studied repeatedly in recent years. The animal
model of experimental vasospasm usually applied for this purpose is developed by administering blood or its constituents into the subarachnoid

space surrounding the large cerebral arteries in chronic experiments. When vasospasm appears in these cases and is identified by angiographic techniques, alpha-adrenergic blockade by phenoxybenzamine (White et al., 1979) or 6-hydroxydopamine (Simeone et al., 1979) does not attenuate or potentiate the vasospasm. These results provide evidence that this type of vasospasm can develop independently of neurogenic vasoconstriction of the cerebral arteries. But, on the other hand, chronic bilateral sympathectomy results in some decrease in pathological vasoconstriction of the large cerebral arteries directly caused by subarachnoid hemorrhage (Mabe, 1978; Endo and Suzuki, 1979).

Electron microscopy has repeatedly revealed significant alterations in nerves surrounding the cerebral arteries subjected to spasm development from subarachnoid hemorrhage (Dobrovolsky, 1975). A striking loss of noradrenaline fluorescence in the cerebral arterial walls under the same conditions has been observed even in vascular regions outside the hemorrhage (Peerless and Kendall, 1975). The small cored vesicles in arterial wall terminals change and even disappear during spasm of the basilar artery (Endo and Suzuki, 1979). However, it is difficult to conclude definitively at present whether this is due to a primary change in the course of development of vasospasm or whether the terminals change secondarily when the spasm has been already developed due to direct (humoral) effects of circulating constituents or the products of the extravasated blood on the cerebral vessel walls. Yet no convincing evidence indicates that pathological constriction of cerebral arteries results from efferent nerve impulses of any frequency, unless some specific effect (see above) on the arteries and/or the primary specific changes of the contraction-relaxation cycle of the vascular muscle cells are present.

Typical vasospasm can readily develop in the isolated internal carotid arteries of dogs, continuously perfused with Ringer-Krebs bicarbonate solution, after deprivation of an efferent neurogenic control to the artery hours after the death of the animal. In addition, vasospasm seen during life does not disappear and changes considerably if the artery is later deprived of neural control in the same way. Further, in accordance with the results of other studies, spasm of the internal carotid artery is not affected by the administration of adrenergic blockers, but readily disappears after intraarterial administration of myogenic spasmolytic drugs, such as papaverine, methylxanthines, and apovincaminate derivatives (Mchedlishvili, 1977a; Mchedlishvili and Ormotsadze, 1981).

The experimental conditions used to investigate the neurogenic mechanism of vasospasm development may be insufficient for forming definitive conclusions about this problem. In particular, as far as we know, nobody has applied chronic stimulation to the neural pathways affecting the major brain arteries. Clinically, chronic excitation of periarterial plexuses resulting in neurological symptoms including pathological constriction of vertebral arteries is seen during osteochondrosis of neck vertebrae in humans.

The neurogenic mechanism may, however, be involved in the development of cerebral vasospasm under specific circumstances. For instance, some changes in arterial muscle cell function cause them to respond to normal vasoconstrictor stimuli, such as those occurring during blood flow regulation, with a pathological spasmodic contraction. This disturbance in vascular smooth muscle function may be related to specific changes in the excitation of plasma membranes, to specific disturbances in intracellular processes, or to disorders in the function of contractile proteins (see below in this chapter). The vessel contraction then becomes considerably more pronounced than necessary for blood flow regulation, and the relaxation of the arterial wall becomes insufficient. Thus, a sustained state of vasoconstriction, typical of vasospasm, would be seen.

"Neurogenic vasospasm" probably appears most frequently in the arteries of the brain which are most often subjected to vasoconstriction under physiological conditions and which possess the most abundant vasoconstrictor nerve supply. Such vessels include the major brain arteries (internal carotids and vertebrals) and their largest branches located at the base of the brain (see Chapter 3).

Furthermore, as mentioned earlier (pp. 202-203), catecholamines (and noradrenaline in particular) can change the reactivity of vascular smooth muscle when a predisposition of the arterial wall to spasm development becomes evident. Therefore, the neurogenic control mechanism affecting the arterial walls by regulating the catecholamine content of the vascular smooth muscle might be directly involved in the development of vascular spasm.

Consequently, neurogenic effects might be the cause of pathological arterial behavior in the brain in the following ways. First, if vascular smooth muscle is specifically impaired, then even normal neurogenic stimuli might cause development of vasospasm. Second, neurogenic stimuli induce accumulation of vasoactive substances in the vascular muscle cells, and hence specifically change their reactivity, so that even normal vasoconstrictor stimuli regulating the cerebral blood flow could immediately cause vasospasm. Third, we can also speculate (since no evidence exists thus far) that pathological activity (in the form of convulsive activity), which originates in neurons related to cerebral arteries, can cause severe spasmodic contraction of blood vessels.

5.6. FACTORS INDUCING PATHOLOGICAL VASODILATATION IN CEREBRAL ARTERIES

The mechanisms of pathological vasodilatation have not been adequately considered so far in scientific literature. Experimental data are also scarce. Therefore, more speculation than firm experimental evidence exists concerning the development of pathological vasodilatation of cerebral arteries.

Various physical and chemical factors affecting the cerebral arteries might be involved in the development of pathological vasodilatation. Their affects are often comparable to normal physiological effects on arterial walls. But usually pathological vasodilatation develops when the affecting factors are abnormal either in size or in duration. In general, pathological vasodilatation might be induced by stimuli which cause mechanical expansion of vascular lumina and/or induce excessive relaxation of vascular smooth muscle and/or result in specific disturbances in the contraction process of vascular smooth muscle leading to a sustained and inappropriate state of vasodilatation. Pathological dilatation of arteries may occur following physiological stimuli that do not actually differ from those which regulate cerebral blood flow under normal conditions.

A hemodynamic factor which can induce, or contribute to, inappropriate vasodilatation is a sharp increase in intravascular pressure. As earlier mentioned (pp. 193-194), this factor is considerably more important in the development of pathological dilatation than the lowering of intravascular pressure is for the development of vasospasm. The intravascular pressure in any peripheral, including a cerebral, artery can certainly never rise above the aortic pressure; it is always lower. The difference between these pressure levels is determined by the vascular resistance along the arterial branches from the aorta to the given peripheral arteries. On this basis the intraarterial pressure can rise considerably in a cerebral artery only if the systemic arterial pressure level sharply increases and the cerebrovascular resistance has not increased proportionately. It is well known that under normal conditions the blood pressure level is regulated in the cerebral vasculature by active changes in resistance along the cerebral arteries, especially the major brain arteries (see Chapter 3). Naturally, this regulatory mechanism can maintain constant blood pressure in cerebral vessels only within certain limits. If the systemic arterial pressure becomes excessively high, regulation by the major arteries might become insufficient; then the intravascular pressure correspondingly increases in the pial arteries. This can provoke the development of pathological dilatation in the pial arteries.

In addition, the mode of branching and the anatomical character of individual pial arteries are also significant with respect to the development of pathological dilatation. Gannushkina and her associates (Gannushkina and Shafranova, 1976, 1977; Gannushkina et al., 1977a) have shown that during a sharp rise in systemic arterial pressure in rabbits the extent of vascular expansion is most pronounced in those pial arteries which follow a straight path and whose angles of offshoot from the feeding vessels are rather oblique (as compared to those vessels with obtuse branching angles). Therefore, the rise in intravascular pressure leading to the passive expansion of pial arteries in response to a sharp increase in systemic arterial pressure is considerably more pronounced in those parts of pial arterial branches where the hydraulic resistance associated with the vascular geometry is the least. Such arteries dilate more readily when the intravascular pressure increases.

Furthermore, the predisposition to such a dilatation also depends on the resting diameter of the pial arteries. The extent of vascular expansion is inversely proportional to the initial vascular caliber. Thus, the smaller pial arteries expand considerably more than the larger vessels during increased systemic arterial pressure (Gannushkina et al., 1977b; Auer and Johansson, 1980). This is shown in Fig. 5.28. Hence evidence has shown that the ability of the pial arteries to passively expand during increases in intravascular pressure is actually the same as that seen during active dilatation that occurs during the regulation of cerebral blood flow. active dilatation occurs in response to a deficient blood supply to cerebral tissue or to changes in the carbon dioxide level in cerebral blood and tissue (see pp. 104-106 and 119 in Chapter 4). Thus, the smaller the resting caliber of the pial arteries, the greater their predisposition to pathological dilatation.

Extrinsic effects on cerebral arterial walls, similar to those which cause their dilatation under natural conditions, can be involved in the development of pathological vasodilatation. Since the pial arteries are most apt to undergo pathological dilatation and a deficiency of blood supply to cerebral tissue causes dilatation of the pial arteries under natural conditions, we should consider those factors which can affect the pial arterial walls during ischemia and thus contribute to pathological vasodilatation. In this case, vasodilator products of tissue origin can be involved in the development of pathological vasodilatation, but only under the following specific conditions: (a) when they have accumulated in considerable amounts over a long period of time in close proximity to vascular walls and (b) when their accumulation is small and of short duration, but the re-

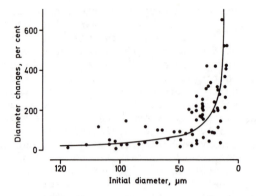

Fig. 5.28. Dilatation of pial arteries of various
            resting diameter during rises in sys-
            temic arterial pressure, which exceed
            the limits of regulation of constant
            cerebral blood pressure and flow (see
            Chapter 5). The pial arteries of cats
            of smaller resting diameter dilate more
            significantly than the larger vessels.
            (Reproduced with permission from Auer
            and Johansson, 1980.)

sponsiveness of the vascular smooth muscle has been specifically altered
so that the relaxation process becomes considerably enhanced and the contractile process is markedly impaired. Thus the relaxed vascular walls
cannot recover their initial tone and hence cannot properly control the
vascular resistance and blood flow to the appropriate microvascular beds.

Vasodilator metabolites can appear in large amounts in brain tissue
due to a decrease in oxidative processes and the development of lactacidosis (Sjesjo, 1978). These metabolites accumulate in brain tissue and the
cerebrospinal fluid, diffuse through cerebral vessel walls, and thus might
directly affect vascular smooth muscle, promoting the continued relaxation
which is typical of pathological vasodilatation.

Hydrogen ions regularly appear as by-products during hypoxic
changes of cerebral metabolism and are known to induce dilatation of the
pial arteries when directly applied to their walls (see pp. 154-155 in
Chapter 4). Hydrogen ions that accumulate in brain tissue and cerebrospinal fluid during ischemia (Hossmann and Kleihues, 1973; Lundgren et al.,
1974; Mchedlishvili, Antia, et al., 1974; Astrup et al., 1977; Nemoto and
Frinak, 1981) can probably participate in the development of postischemic
vasodilatation and hyperemia. In this case the vasodilatation might become pathological if the pial arteries are inadequately dilated and cannot
return to their initial state when the compensatory increase in blood
supply is no longer needed. Thus, hyperoxygenation of the cerebral venous
blood is often found in patients with intracerebral hemorrhage who are deep-
ly comatose at the time of investigation. This indicates the presence of
"luxury perfusion" related to pathological dilatation of the cerebral ar-
eries. This phenomenon has been found to coincide with the presence of a
marked noncompensated lactic acidosis (mean value = 7.74 mEq/liter) in
cerebrospinal fluid. Furthermore, a close correlation (r = 0.7) has been
revealed between an increase in cerebral venous P_{O_2} and the cerebrospinal
fluid lactate concentration in these patients (Kaasik, 1979b).

Although no strict correlation between an accumulation of hydrogen ions in cerebral tissue and vasodilatation has been revealed during ischemia and the postischemic period (Mchedlishvili, Antia, et al., 1974), the prolonged acidosis may nevertheless be important for the development of pathological vasodilatation in the brain. Metabolic disturbances that cause acidosis in brain tissue and cerebral vascular walls may disturb the normally operating regulation mechanisms of cerebral blood flow (especially neurogenic control) resulting in an inability to control the cerebral arterial width. Thus, cerebral vessels would respond to hydrogen ion accumulation in the tissue by marked dilatation, which would not be further regulated. In addition, the normal function of vascular smooth muscle might also become disturbed by the deprivation of adequate energy supply due to breakdown of adenine nucleotides under these conditions.

As mentioned in Chapter 4 (p. 155), potassium ions may also play a role in the appearance of vasodilatation following increased activity of cerebral tissue. Concerning their contribution to development of pathological vasodilatation, one can speculate that during a marked deficiency in blood supply to the cerebral tissue the active transport of potassium ions in the cellular plasma membranes may be disturbed, thus contributing to accumulation of the ions in extracellular spaces (Hossmann et al., 1977). However, the dilator effects of potassium ions are evident only in cases in which an increase in potassium concentration does not exceed 10-12 mM. Higher concentrations cause, on the contrary, a constrictor effect on arteries (Mchedlishvili, 1977a) and therefore would not be involved in the pathological vasodilatation. In addition, the vasodilator effect of potassium ions on cerebral arteries is relatively short and therefore cannot contribute significantly to occurrence of pathological vasodilatation in the brain (see p. 156).

It has also been suggested that the immediate cause of pathological dilatation of pial arteries might be a disturbance in the myogenic response of vascular smooth muscle to stretch (Gannushkina, 1979). The decisive role of vascular tone in the development of pathological dilatation (especially if the intravascular pressure is primarily increased) is beyond any doubt. However, it is another question as to whether it is the myogenic response of vascular smooth muscle to stretching that is decisive in maintaining normal vascular tone or the tone is actually related to humoral or neurogenic stimuli continuously affecting the arterial walls. This problem has not yet been solved. The questionable role of direct myogenic responses in the maintenance of constant cerebral blood pressure and flow despite changes in systemic arterial pressure has already been considered in Chapter 3. The net myogenic response of vascular smooth muscle probably does not play a role in the occurrence of pathological vasodilatation either, since this vasodilation frequently occurs following a primary increase in the intravascular pressure when no primary disturbances in the myogenic response can be found. Primary disturbances in myogenic responses as a causal factor in the development of pathological vasodilatation could be proved experimentally if all other factors remained constant, but this has not been shown so far.

It is well known that cerebrovascular smooth muscle cells contain a considerable number of specific receptors for cholinergic and beta-adrenergic substances (Saratikov et al., 1979; Burnstock, 1980; Bevan et al., 1980). Thus, cerebral arteries respond by dilatation if these substances of endogenous origin reach the vessel wall. In addition, the cerebral arteries respond by dilatation to other specific endogenous vasodilator substances, i.e., histamine, vasoactive intestinal polypeptide, etc. (Saratikov et al., 1979; Sparks, 1980; Burnstock, 1980; Needleman and Isakson, 1980). However, nobody has yet analyzed the effects of these substances

on specific cerebral arteries from the point of view of the development of
pathological vasodilatation, as has been done with the vasoconstrictor substances related to the development of cerebral vasospasm (see pp. 196-210).
Therefore, it is still difficult to say conclusively whether all these
natural vasodilator effects could be involved in occurrence of pathological
vasodilatation in the brain and if they are, to what extent.

We can speculate that when other factors causing expansion of pial
arterial walls, particularly increased intravascular pressure, are present,
or if there are disturbances in the contractile process of vascular smooth
muscle, then the vasodilator effects of the aforementioned substances might
provoke pathological vasodilatation. However, this problem is in need of
further detailed experimentation.

5.7. DISTURBANCES IN SMOOTH MUSCLE CELLS THAT PROVOKE ARTERIAL PATHOLOGICAL RESPONSES

Although pathological vasoconstriction and vasodilatation can be induced by different stimuli affecting the arterial walls, the specific
changes in the contraction and relaxation processes which are characteristic of vasospasm and vasoparalysis ultimately occur in the vascular
smooth muscle. Pathological responses of smooth muscle are undoubtedly
determined by the same physiological factors at the cellular and subcellu-
lar levels affecting both physiological activation and contraction-relaxation processes of vascular smooth muscles. Pathological changes in activation and in contraction-relaxation of vascular muscle can be dependent on
processes related to muscle cell function: events in their plasma membranes, intracellular ionic mechanisms that couple extrinsic stimuli with
the contractile machinery of cells, and the functioning of the latter.
The forthcoming section deals with just those functional events in vascular smooth muscle cells which may be responsible for the pathological behavior of cerebral arteries.

The cellular processes related to vascular smooth muscle function are
too complex to be a subject of this book, but they have been reviewed in
a series of publications in detail (Somlyo and Somlyo, 1968; Bülbring et
al., 1970; Orlov et al., 1971; Gurevitch and Bernstein, 1972; Bohr et al.,
1980; Adelstein, 1980). Only those processes which contribute to a better
understanding of how they can determine the appearance of pathological
constriction (vasospasm) and pathological dilatation (vasoparalysis) of
cerebral arteries will be described below.

Involvement of Plasma Membranes in Excitation-Contraction Coupling.
The plasma membranes of smooth muscle cells are responsible for cell activation
and determine the effect of extrinsic factors on vascular smooth muscle
contraction. The plasma membrane actively transports ions to provide a
distinct ionic composition in the inside medium and the outside medium
of the smooth muscle cell and hence an ionic gradient across the membrane.
Determinants of this gradient include the univalent ions, characterized
by their great mobility, i.e., potassium, sodium, and chloride ions. Differences in their concentration and mobility results in plasma membrane
polarization; the outside is positively charged compared to the inside.

Activation of vascular smooth muscle cells, leading to contraction,
starts with depolarization of their plasma membranes. This provides
transmission of messages at rates that greatly surpass those achieved by
diffusion of molecules or by physiological bulk flow of fluid (Johansson
and Somlyo, 1980). For a better understanding of the role of vascular

smooth muscle cell plasma membranes in the development of vasospasm and pathological vasodilatation it is necessary to consider their normal function in some detail.

It is well known that potassium ions are predominantly distributed inside the cell, while sodium ions are primarily concentrated in the extracellular medium. Inside muscle cells the concentration of sodium ions is about 50 mM and that of potassium ions 98 mM per liter of intracellular water (Somlyo and Somlyo, 1968); in the extracellular fluid the concentration of sodium ions is much higher, about 150 mM per liter, and that of potassium is lower, about 4-5.5 mM. These values can vary considerably in different blood vessels in various species (Jones, 1980). Overall, the concentration gradient for K^+ across the muscle cell plasma membranes is considerably greater than that for Na^+. The transport mechanism responsible for active ion movement across the plasma membrane against their concentration gradient is rather complex. This transport requires a continual and considerable expenditure of energy which is provided by the cellular metabolism — mainly the oxidation of adenosine triphosphate and other high-energy compounds.

The unequal distribution and mobility of the univalent and larger ions across the plasma membrane of vascular smooth muscle cells is closely related to the transmembrane electrical potential (Johansson and Somlyo, 1980). This potential is thought to be mainly determined by the permeabilities and distribution of K^+ and Cl^-, whereas Na^+ seems to be of little importance. The permeability of the plasma membrane to K^+ and Cl^- is considerably higher than that for Na^+ under resting conditions, although the latter ions also contribute to the transmembrane potential. Therefore, the exit of K^+ from the cell and the opposite movement of Cl^- into it makes the intracellular space negatively charged in comparison to the extracellular fluid under resting conditions. The resting transmembrane potential measured with intracellular microelectrodes in smooth muscle in various segments of the vascular tree of different species range between —25 mV and —65 mV in physiological saline (Johansson and Somlyo, 1980). Recent estimates in the larger brain arteries (the basilar and the middle cerebral arteries) show the transmembrane potential to be equal to —50 to —55 mV (Fujiwara et al., 1981). Following the presentation of activating stimuli, e.g., noradrenaline (acetylcholine in other smooth muscle), the transmembrane potential in the vascular smooth muscle decreases. This is related to the depolarization of the plasma membrane and results in a decrease in the membrane potential to about half of the resting level (Somlyo et al., 1971; Wahlström, 1973). In this case, depolarization is thought to be dependent on the redistribution of univalent ions according to their concentration gradient across the plasma membrane.

Under normal conditions, depolarization is very short and then the active transport of ions against their concentration gradient across the plasma membranes leads to cell repolarization. A change in electrical potential in the walls of arteries can be recorded during this period lasting usually no more than half a second. This potential is called the action potential because it is followed by activation and contraction of vascular muscle, although there are cases when an action potential does not precede muscle contraction (Johansson and Somlyo, 1980). The ionic currents responsible for action potentials in vascular smooth muscle are not yet definitely known, and it is assumed that the ionic gradients differ in different vessels. The activation of vascular smooth muscle cells in response to depolarization of their plasma membranes triggers the contractile process of muscle. It seems probable that the activation of vas-

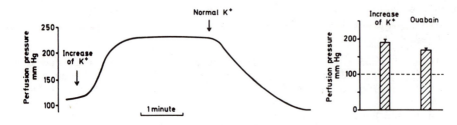

Fig. 5.29.   Spasmodic vasoconstriction of internal carotid artery caused
             by sustained depolarization of vascular smooth muscle plasma
             membranes. A graph (on the left) and a histogram (on the
             right) demonstrate the effect of sustained depolarization of
             vascular smooth muscle cell plasma membranes on the vascular
             tone of dog's isolated (*in situ*) internal carotid artery that
             was continuously perfused by a constant-output pump with
             Ringer-Krebs bicarbonate solution. The vascular tone changes
             are expressed in terms of the perfusion pressure changes in
             the artery. In the left-hand tracing the K^+ concentrations
             have been increased from 5.9 to 29.5 mM. The bars on the
             right represent the mean effects (M ± SE) of a 4- to 5-fold
             increase in K^+ levels and a 1 mg increase in ouabain (admin-
             istered intraarterially) on the artery. Explanation in the
             text. (Modified from Mchedlishvili, Kometiani, et al., 1972.)

cular smooth muscle plasma membranes also plays an important role in pathological constriction and dilatation of cerebral arteries.

     Coupling of activation (related to depolarization) to the contraction
of smooth muscle cells is accomplished by calcium ions, which function as
messengers from the plasma membrane to the contractile machinery of the
muscle cell (Somlyo and Somlyo, 1968). This coupling is considered to
occur simultaneously with the depolarization of plasma membranes, since
the membrane permeability for Ca^{++} increases considerably. Because the
concentration of Ca^{++} is considerably higher in the extracellular fluid and
the plasma membrane than in the cytoplasm, the ions begin to flux, according to
their concentration gradient. This flux of Ca^{++} into the cytoplasm of
muscle cells has been proven to be the principal trigger of contraction.
The subsequent relaxation of muscle cells occurs when Ca^{++} is again removed
from the cytoplasm. However, if the depolarization of muscle cell plasma
membranes becomes sustained, the active uphill transport of Ca^{++} from
muscle cell cytoplasm following their contraction will be hindered. Furthermore, the high concentration of Ca^{++} remaining in the site of muscle
cell filaments would inevitably result in a sustained state of contraction
of vascular smooth muscle; this results in vasospasm and its corresponding
changes in blood flow in the arteries.

     Vasospasm Due to Disturbances in Plasma Membrane Function. To eluci-
date the role of plasma membranes in the development of vasospasm, experiments were based on the well-established fact that depolarization of the
plasma membrane of smooth muscle cells could be produced either by increased potassium ion concentration in their outside medium or by inhibition of the Na-K-ATPase pump which provides the energy for active ion
transport in plasma membranes, e.g., by ouabain (Friedman and Friedman,
1963; Somlyo and Somlyo, 1968). In experiments with isolated internal
carotid arteries of dogs (the principle of this method has been discussed
on pp. 62-63 and described in detail in Mchedlishvili, 1972, and Mchedlish-

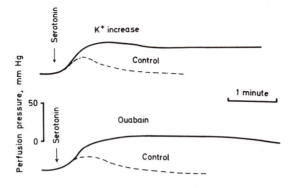

Fig. 5.30. Changes in the serotonin constrictor response of internal carotid artery evoked by disturbances in the
repolarization of vascular muscle cell plasma membranes. The serotonin effect (0.1 μg) on an isolated
(*in situ*) internal carotid artery of the dog is
changed by sustained depolarization induced by increased K$^+$ levels (up to 11.8 mM) in the perfusion
fluid and by intraarterial administration of ouabain
(0.3 mg). The tracings represent the perfusion pressure in the artery continuously perfused by a constant-output pump with Ringer-Krebs bicarbonate solution. The lower tracings denote the control effect
of serotonin and the upper tracings denote serotonin
effect in the same dose following partial depolarization of the plasma membranes. (Reproduced from
Mchedlishvili, Kometiani, et al., 1971-1972.)

vili and Ormotsadze, 1970, 1979), it has been shown that a 3- to 5-fold
increase in the K$^+$ concentration in the perfusion fluid of the artery,
i.e., to 18-30 mM (at the expense of Na$^+$) causes sustained vasoconstriction comparable to vasospasm, during which the resistance in the artery
increased by more than 70% of the resting level. This lasts as long as
the potassium content in the perfusion fluid remains high, but the vessel
wall readily relaxes as soon as the level of potassium becomes normal
(Fig. 5.29).

A similar effect has been obtained after intraarterial administration
of ouabain (Reanal) in a dose of 1 mg: the resistance in the artery increased by about 50% of the resting level. If ouabain is administered to
the artery when its walls have already been contracted by an increased
potassium concentration in the perfusion fluid, an additional increase in
the vascular resistance is seen (Mchedlishvili, Kometiani, et al., 1970-
1971, 1972; Mchedlishvili, 1977a). Thus, sustained depolarization of vascular smooth muscle plasma membranes independently results in a sustained
constriction of the artery similar to vasospasm (Fig. 5.29).

When an increase in the potassium ion concentration in the arterial
perfusion fluid or the dose of ouabain are relatively small, the contraction of the arterial wall is also small or even absent. But the intraarterial administration of a bolus of serotonin (which causes a comparatively short vasoconstriction) under these circumstances results in a
strong, sustained contraction of the vascular smooth muscle with a considerably delayed onset of relaxation (Fig. 5.30).

The constrictive effects of increased concentrations of potassium ions and ouabain remain even after blockade of serotonin and alpha-adrenergic receptors in the vascular smooth muscle by specific blockers (by Deseril and DH-ergotoxin, respectively). This proves that the mechanism of the pathological arterial response may be independent of these physiological vasoconstrictor stimuli on the vascular muscle. But, on the other hand, after the elimination of Ca^{++} from the vascular wall by continuous perfusion of the artery with a fluid containing EDTA or EGTA but no Ca^{++}, the constrictor effect of potassium ions and ouabain are abolished. This proves that coupling between the plasma membrane depolarization and a spasm-like contraction of the vascular smooth muscle is accomplished by Ca^{++}, which is also the messenger for other constrictor effects on vascular smooth muscle.

Thus, we may conclude that disturbances in the normal function of vascular smooth muscle plasma membranes, which result in a tendency to a sustained state of their depolarization, may become a cause of vasospasm. Under natural conditions such disturbances may be related to disorders in the structure of membranes, as well as in the metabolism of proteins and lipids, from which the membranes are built. Disturbances in the intracellular metabolism that provides energy for the ions' active transport across the membranes can also affect plasma membrane function.

Disorders in the vascular smooth muscle cell membrane function might contribute to the development of pathological vasoconstriction in old age, when the ability of cellular membranes to repolarize can readily be disturbed (Frolkis, 1970). This probably explains the appearance of vasospasm associated with certain cerebrovascular disorders in the elderly.

Another membrane mechanism involved in the development of vasospasm has been suggested by Orlov and his associates (1975), who have observed spontaneous contractions of smooth muscle, with a frequency of 5-6 per minute, in *in vitro* isolated internal carotid arteries of dogs and humans (taken from the curvature and the cavernous portion of the vessels). The spontaneously active smooth muscle cells were found to be highly sensitive to an increase in potassium ions in the surrounding medium; even insignificant increases in potassium or the addition of serotonin to the medium immediately resulted in a sustained state of contraction of the vascular muscle lasting up to 30 minutes. From these findings, the authors suggested that spasm of the internal carotid artery can develop following the activation of the vascular smooth muscle by spontaneously active muscle cells. Extrinsic stimuli of either a neural or humoral nature can activate this pacemaker mechanism and cause a sustained state of vasoconstriction in the form of vasospasm.

Consequently, alterations in the vascular smooth muscle cell plasma membrane function can become a cause of vasospasm, if these alterations occur primarily due to any pathological cause. Under such circumstances, even normal vasoconstrictor stimuli, which regulate the cerebral blood flow, would result in vasoconstriction in the form of vasospasm.

Pathological vasodilatation due to a disturbance in plasma membrane function has not yet been considered in the scientific literature. However, specific disturbances of vascular smooth muscle cell membrane function may play an important role in the occurrence of pathological vasodilatation. Orlov (1979b) has assumed that when the vessel walls are stretched by increase intravascular pressure, the muscle cell plasma membrane permeability might change. A reduction in transmembrane active transport of ions results in a decrease in vascular tone and vasodilatation. As mentioned above (p. 193), the essence of pathological vasodilatation consists

of a disturbance in the relaxation-contraction cycle of vascular smooth
muscle when the contraction is deficient. Therefore, if the contraction
of the vascular muscles is disturbed by structural or functional disorders
in plasma membranes, the arteries will lose their tone regardless of constrictor stimuli reaching the vascular walls. Under these conditions, the
vascular smooth muscle cells, which remain relaxed in response to any
physiological or pathological stimuli, cannot reestablish their resting
vascular tone. This mechanism of pathological vasodilatation might operate in the ischemic focus where a deficiency of oxygen and energy supply
to vascular smooth muscle plasma membranes might result in a state of sustained vasodilatation having a pathological character. However, these
considerations are as yet only speculation and are in need of special
further study.

The Intracellular Processes in Vascular Muscle Related to Vasospasm
and Vasoparalysis. As we have mentioned above, the activation of vascular
smooth muscle cells initiated by a depolarization of the plasma membrane
results in a flux of Ca^{++} into the cytoplasm (Somlyo, 1979; Jones, 1980).
These ions are thought to trigger the contractile process of muscle performed by the myofilaments. Under resting conditions, the muscle cell
cytoplasm has a free Ca^{++} concentration of about 10^{-7} M; it rises to 10^{-5} M
to initiate muscle contraction. The low concentration of Ca^{++} inhibits
the ATPase activity in smooth muscle. This inhibition is reversed by
phosphorylation of myosin light chains which is regulated by Ca^{++} binding
protein, calmodulin, and by the cyclic AMP-dependent protein kinase (Adelstein, 1980). After the myofilaments contract, Ca^{++} is subsequently eliminated from the cytoplasm, which induces relaxation of vascular smooth
muscle. It is reasonable to suppose that all these intrinsic processes
in muscle cells may also be affected by the specific disturbances in the
contraction-relaxation cycle seen during pathology of the cerebral arteries.

Two types of disturbances in the intrinsic function of arterial smooth
muscle may result in the development of vasospasm and pathological vasodilatation. The first of them is a disturbance in Ca^{++} transport and the
second one, a disturbance in the contractile machinery of the vascular
muscle cell. Both of these processes can probably result in such changes
in the intracellular processes that even normal vasoconstrictor stimuli
result in a sustained state of muscular contraction characteristic of vasospasm. On the other hand, the intracellular processes can probably be
changed so that normal vasodilator stimuli initiate a sustained state of
relaxation of the vessel wall characteristic of pathological vasodilatation.
However, there is still very little experimental evidence directly demonstrating the involvement of these processes in the development of vasospasm
and vasoparalysis.

At rest vascular smooth muscle contains stores of calcium ions located mainly in the extracellular medium, the pinocytotic vesicles of the
plasma membranes, and in the endoplasmic reticulum as well as in mito-
chondria inside cells. The estimation of free Ca^{++} concentration in the
extracellular and intracellular water showed a concentration gradient of
10^4 (Blaustein, 1977). The concentration of Ca^{++} in the cytoplasm, i.e.,
in the environment of myofilaments, is very low, and hence the cells remain
in a relaxed state. The actual concentration of Ca^{++} in the vascular
muscle cell cytoplasm determines the tone of vessel walls. Therefore, the
sustained state of vascular wall contraction, which is characteristic of
vasospasm, might be induced by the maintenance of high concentrations of
Ca^{++} inside the vascular muscle cell cytoplasm.

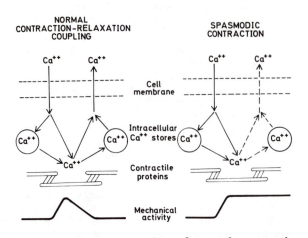

Fig. 5.31.   Spasmodic contraction of vascular smooth muscle
caused by the retention of calcium ions in the cell
cytoplasm. Normal contraction-relaxation coupling
due to Ca^{++} fluxes are shown on the left and spasmodic contraction of the vascular walls due to specific changes in Ca^{++} fluxes in muscle cell plasma
membranes are shown on the right. See text for
explanation.

In response to vasoconstrictor stimuli, the diffusion of Ca^{++} across
the muscle cell plasma membranes increases considerably. Hence, Ca^{++} ions
start to flux according to their concentration gradient into the cytoplasm,
surround the contractile myofilaments where the Ca^{++} concentration increases, and induce contraction of muscle cells (Seidel and Bohr, 1971).
Subsequent relaxation of muscle cells occurs as soon as the Ca^{++} ions are
removed from the environment of the contractile myofilaments and then out
of the cytoplasm, leading to a decrease in the concentration of Ca^{++} to the
resting level. This process of Ca^{++} flux against its concentration gradient out of the cytoplasm is, certainly, an active process, which needs a
considerable expense of energy in the form of adenosine triphosphate.
Thus, calcium ions are transported into the cisternae and vesicles of the
endoplasmic reticulum, into the plasma membranes, and then into the extracellular spaces. Accordingly, at least two types of "calcium pumps" probably exist in smooth muscle cells. One of them operates with the assistance of Ca-ATPase and maintains the intracellular homeostasis by pumping
excess calcium through the plasma membrane to the outside, and the other
provides absorption of Ca^{++} by the sarcoplasmic reticulum. The energy required for Ca^{++} transport against the gradient is provided by the breakdown of adenosine triphosphate. These "calcium pumps" thus provide, first,
an active flux of Ca^{++} from the contractile proteins of the myofilaments
and, second, the absorption of Ca^{++} by the sarcoplasmic reticulum (Rasmussen and Tenenhouse, 1968; Jones, 1980). The relationship between Ca^{++}
transport and the mechanical activity of vascular muscle cells during the
normal contraction-relaxation cycle is schematically presented in Fig.
5.31 (left side). It can be assumed that if Ca^{++} removal out of the cytoplasm
is delayed, relaxation of the muscle would be disturbed and would result
in a sustained state of muscular contraction which is characteristic of
vasospasm. This is schematically shown in Fig. 5.31 (right side).

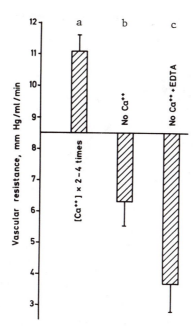

Fig. 5.32.   The effect of calcium ions on the rest-
             ing tone of the internal carotid artery.
             The effects of changes in the Ca^{++} levels
             on vascular wall resting tension (ex-
             pressed in terms of resistance changes)
             were studied in experiments with a dog's
             isolated *in situ* internal carotid artery
             continuously perfused by a constant-out-
             put pump with Ringer-Krebs bicarbonate
             solution, (a) during increased calcium
             ion concentration in the perfusion fluid;
             (b) during deprivation of Ca^{++} from the
             perfusion fluid; and (c) the same as "b"
             with the addition of EDTA (ethylenediamine-
             tetraacetate, 400 mg/liter). See text
             for explanation. (Data from Mchedlish-
             vili, 1977a.)

Evidence for "Calcium Pump" Disturbances Involved in the Development
of Vasospasm. The existing evidence that a delay in the removal of calcium ions from the vascular muscle cell cytoplasm can be the cause of a
sustained state of contraction, i.e., vasospasm, is still very poor. The
evidence obtained from dogs in isolated internal carotid arteries continuously perfused with Ringer-Krebs bicarbonate solution is primarily indirect. Calcium ions have been shown to play a significant role in the
maintenance of the resting vascular tone of the artery (Mchedlishvili,
Kometiani, et al., 1971); following the elimination of Ca^{++} from the vascular walls (by a 15- to 20-minute-long perfusion of the artery with Ca-
free EDTA, or EGTA, containing Ringer-Krebs solution) the tone of the
arterial wall decreases significantly (Fig. 5.32). In addition, the
elimination of Ca^{++} from the arterial wall results in a considerable reduction (by an average of 89%) in the constrictor responses of the artery
to serotonin and other vasoconstrictor substances (noradrenaline, hyper-

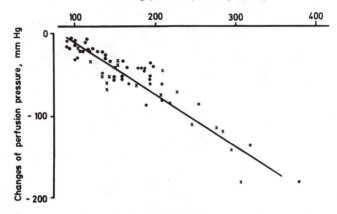

Fig. 5.33. Dependence of vasodilatatory responses of internal
            carotid artery on resting vascular tone. The
            vasodilatatory effects of theophylline (black
            circles) and papaverine (crosses) are proportional
            to the resting vascular tone of the internal ca-
            rotid artery of dogs, expressed in terms of the
            perfusion pressure in the isolated (*in situ*) in-
            ternal carotid artery continuously perfused by a
            constant-output pump with Ringer-Krebs bicarbonate
            solution. The vasodilator effect is expressed in
            terms of the changes in perfusion pressure. (Re-
            produced from Mchedlishvili, 1977a.)

tensin, and vasoconstrictor prostaglandins). The constrictor responses of
the artery to a sustained depolarization of vascular smooth muscle induced
by an increase in K^+ in the perfusion fluid or by intraarterial administration of ouabain are also decreased in this experimental model (Mchedlishvili, Kometiani, et al., 1970-1971, 1972).

    Evidence for the involvement of Ca^{++} retention in the muscle cell
cytoplasm in the production of a sustained state of vascular wall contraction has been provided by the author's experiments with the well-known
spasmolytic pharmacological agents, theophylline and papaverine (Carpi and
Giardini, 1972). Their action is presumably dependent on facilitating the
active removal of Ca^{++} from the muscle cell cytoplasm (Ferrari and Carpenado, 1968). The conclusion that the retention of Ca^{++} in muscle cells is
actually involved in a sustained state of contraction would be proved if
the vasodilator effect of the drugs could be shown to be dependent on the
removal of Ca^{++} from the cells. In experiments carried out with the isolated *in situ* internal carotid artery of dogs, the intraarterial administration of theophylline (5-10 mg) or papaverine (1-2 mg) causes a significant
decrease in the vascular tone. This dilatory effect inversely correlates
to the resting vascular tone (Fig. 5.33). The effect is independent of
whether the innervation of the artery is intact (in experiments carried out
under superficial anesthesia) or removed (more than 30 minutes after the
death of the animal with continuous perfusion of the vessel). Therefore,
the vasodilator effect is myogenic, i.e., fulfilled by the direct effect
of the drugs on vascular smooth muscle. Additional experiments were carried out under conditions of artificially increased vascular tone by different causes: either by serotonin (added to the perfusion fluid in doses

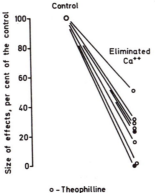

Fig. 5.34. Significant decrease in the dilatatory
response of the internal carotid artery
to theophylline and papaverine is observed during elimination of Ca^{++} from
the vascular wall. This effect was
studied in the isolated (*in situ*) carotid arteries of dogs continuously perfused by a constant-output pump with
Ringer-Krebs bicarbonate solution. The
resistance changes in the arteries are
expressed in terms of the perfusion
pressure changes. To eliminate the
Ca^{++} from the vascular walls, the arteries were continuously perfused with
Ca-free EDTA-containing solution. See
text for explanation. (Data from
Mchedlishvili, Kometiani, et al., 1972.)

of 0.01-0.1 µg/ml or when it has been synthesized in the vessel wall under
the influence of heterogeneous blood; see Mchedlishvili, Garfunkel, et al.,
1972), or by depolarization of the vascular muscle cells (because of a
high content of K^+ in perfusion fluid, or following the action of ouabain).
Under these conditions the following evidence for the dependence of the
relaxing effects of the drugs on vascular muscle on Ca^{++} removal from the
muscle cell cytoplasm has been obtained: first, under conditions of comparable vessel tone, the dilator effects of theophylline and papaverine are
considerably smaller when calcium ions have been removed from the vessel
walls (Fig. 5.34). Second, during continuous perfusion of the artery with
Ca-free EDTA (or EGTA) containing Ringer-Krebs bicarbonate solution, which
causes elimination of Ca^{++} primarily from the extracellular spaces of the
vessel walls, the repeated administration of theophylline or papaverine in
the perfusion fluid caused gradual decreases in the dilator responses (Fig.
5.35). This effect can be explained as follows: during each relaxation
of the vascular muscle, a portion of Ca^{++} was removed into the extracellular space and immediately chelated by EDTA, or EGTA. Therefore, the intracellular Ca^{++} concentration gradually decreases and, thus, the effects of the
drugs (normally accomplished by Ca^{++} removal from the cytoplasm) steadily
weakens. If the relaxation of the vascular wall in a sustained state of
contraction is actually dependent on the removal of Ca^{++} from the muscle
cell cytoplasm, then we may conclude that the retention of Ca^{++} should, on

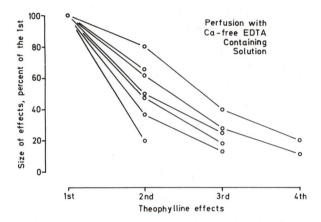

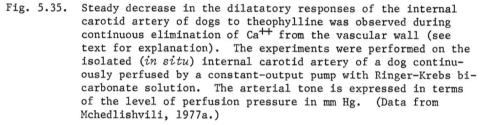

Fig. 5.35. Steady decrease in the dilatatory responses of the internal
            carotid artery of dogs to theophylline was observed during
            continuous elimination of Ca^{++} from the vascular wall (see
            text for explanation). The experiments were performed on the
            isolated (*in situ*) internal carotid artery of a dog continu-
            ously perfused by a constant-output pump with Ringer-Krebs bi-
            carbonate solution. The arterial tone is expressed in terms
            of the level of perfusion pressure in mm Hg. (Data from
            Mchedlishvili, 1977a.)

the contrary, result in a spasmodic constriction of arteries. However,
further studies are required to obtain more convincing evidence concerning
the existence of this mechanism of vasospasm development.

      The active fluxes of calcium ions in the vascular smooth muscle cell
compartments during relaxation are dependent on the metabolism of high-
energy compounds such as adenine nucleotides (Butler and Davies, 1980).
Cyclic AMP (adenosine 3',5'-monophosphate), which is formed from ATP by
the reaction catalyzed by adenylate cyclase in muscle cell plasma membranes,
may play an important role in muscular relaxation (and possibly in constriction as well) (Kramer and Hardman, 1980). The presence of cyclic AMP
has a noticeable effect on the tone of cerebral arteries, since activation
of adenylate cyclase (which is responsible for the production of cyclic
AMP) and inhibition of phosphodiesterase (which is responsible for the
hydrolysis of cyclic AMP) in the wall of dogs' internal carotid arteries
resulted in a significant decrease in the constrictor effect of prostaglandin E_2. Conversely, the inhibition of adenylate cyclase and the activation of phosphodiesterase, which leads to a decrease in the amount of
cyclic AMP, cause a significant potentiation of vasoconstriction of the
internal carotid artery brought about by the prostaglandin E_2 (Mchedlishvili and Ormotsadze, 1980). Consequently, the metabolic processes in the
cerebral vascular muscle cells resulting in the production or degradation
of the cyclic AMP can have a considerable influence on the active Ca^{++}
fluxes. Disturbances of these processes might result in a decrease in
Ca^{++} removal from the muscle cell cytoplasm and, thus, lead to a sustained
state of vascular smooth muscle cell contraction, i.e., to vasospasm.

      Contractile Protein Machinery Changes Responsible for the Development
of Vasospasm and Vasoparalysis. There is no experimental evidence so far
which proves that primary changes in the contractile proteins of arterial
smooth muscles result in a sustained state of contraction characteristic

of vasospasm. We can only suggest the possibility of such pathological events in the vascular muscle cells (proceeding from the presently available knowledge of the processes during normal conditions).

It is presently established (Somlyo, 1979; Hartshorne and Gorecka, 1980; Adelstein, 1980) that the contraction of smooth muscle, like that of striated muscle, is determined by a specific interaction between the main contractile muscle proteins, actin and myosin. Contraction centers around the attachment and detachment of a globular portion of the myosin molecule to the actin filament. This results in sliding of the filaments past each other. The energy for the actin-myosin interaction is supplied by adenosine triphosphate. The actin-myosin interaction is regulated by the concentration of free calcium ions in the cytoplasm (see above). One can speculate that some conformational changes in the contractile proteins or the depletion of high-energy phosphate compounds within the smooth muscle cells may be involved as immediate causes in the development of the vasospasm. Such vasospasm could develop when all the preceding links of contractile or relaxing processes remain normal and the physiological stimuli regulating the arterial behavior reach the vascular walls. Thus, some primary changes in the machinery of contractile proteins might be involved in the mechanism of vasospasm development, although this remains speculation at present.

Some evidence for such a mechanism in the development of vasospasm has been obtained in experiments with isolated internal carotid arteries in dogs (Mchedlishvili, 1977a). The vasospasm which may be dependent on such a mechanism has been observed during 1968-1978 in experiments following the repeated action of vasoconstrictor substances, e.g., serotonin, or following long plasma membrane depolarization by a drastic increase in K^+ content in the perfusion fluid, or by administration of ouabain into the artery. The continued perfusion of the artery by a Ca-free EDTA-containing Ringer-Krebs solution also seemed to promote occurrence of such a vasospasm in some cases. Evidence that the vasospasm was related only to a disturbance in the contractile machinery of the muscle cell was seen — the spasm could not be eliminated by theophylline and papaverine, whose relaxing effect on the arterial muscle under normal conditions is, in all probability, related to the removal of Ca^{++} from the cytoplasm. Sometimes, however, these drugs evoked an opposite effect, causing a more potent contraction of the vessel wall. However, the molecular processes in the contractile proteins of the vascular muscle cells which were actually involved in the development of the vasospasm remained unclear, and the problem is in need of further detailed study.

On the other hand, it cannot be excluded that some disturbances in the vascular smooth muscle machinery could be involved in disorders of the contractile process and result in a sustained state of relaxation, i.e., pathological vasodilatation. However, no evidence for these kinds of disturbances has been obtained at present, and the problem is in need of special investigation.

5.8. COMPENSATORY EVENTS ACCOMPANYING PATHOLOGICAL ARTERIAL RESPONSES

Both pathological constriction and dilatation of the cerebral arteries are harmful for the blood supply to tissues which are fed by the vessels. Therefore circulatory disturbances tend to be compensated for in the brain vasculature. Since vasospasm and vasoparalysis are in a sense opposite to each other, the related compensatory events in the cerebrovascular bed are also different and hence are considered separately.

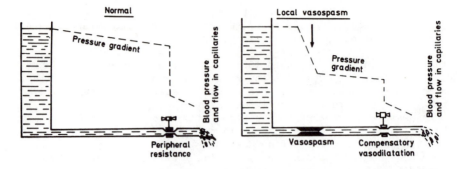

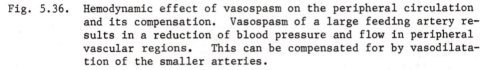

Fig. 5.36. Hemodynamic effect of vasospasm on the peripheral circulation
            and its compensation. Vasospasm of a large feeding artery re-
            sults in a reduction of blood pressure and flow in peripheral
            vascular regions. This can be compensated for by vasodilata-
            tion of the smaller arteries.

Compensatory events in cerebral vasculature accompanying vasospasm
are directed toward elimination of the effect of inappropriate vasoconstriction, which causes an increased resistance and a reduced blood flow
in the affected arteries. To this end, a compensatory decrease in resistance should occur along the route of blood flowing to the brain areas that
have been previously fed by the spasmodic arteries. The decreased resistance usually occurs in the periphery of the arterial obstruction as well
as in the neighboring arterial branches through which collateral blood inflow to the microvascular regions exposed to deficient blood supply can be
thereby accomplished.

If the degree of arterial luminal contraction during vasospasm is not
pronounced, the vasodilatation along the adjacent vascular portions might
completely compensate for the increased resistance in the spasmodic arteries. Since vasospasm develops most frequently in the major brain arteries
(see pp. 181-184), vasodilatation often occurs in the peripheral arterial
branches. This vasodilatation might compensate for the increased resistance in the spasmodic vessels so that the microcirculation remains normal,
and is schematically presented in Fig. 5.36.

Gannushkina (1973) has thoroughly investigated the circulatory phenomena during the development of collateral circulation in the brain. It
has been shown that following arterial obstruction a diffuse dilatation
occurs first in the pial arteries, but later on the vasodilatation becomes
restricted to the particular arterial pathways which supply the tissue
areas exposed to deficient circulation (caused by arterial obstruction).
In the subsequent period, specific morphological changes occur in the walls
of arteries whose diameter has continuously increased. Hence, structural
changes may be detected in the arterial walls, either hyperplasia and
hypertrophy: the volume and the number of nuclei in vascular smooth muscle
cells increase, the amount of nucleic acids increases, and the RNA and DNA
stain more intensively.

Three factors determine the collateral blood flow during arterial obstruction: (a) anatomical, (b) hemodynamic, and (c) physiological (Mchedlishvili, 1977a).

(a) The anatomical factor includes the preexistence of collateral arterial pathways which can supply the territory normally fed by the obstructed arteries. The cerebral arterial bed provides an especially large availability of collateral pathways at various levels of arterial branching: at the circle of Willis, the larger pial arteries (macroanastomoses in the boundary zones of the anterior, middle, and posterior cerebral arteries), and the minor pial arterial ramifications (microanastomoses), described in Chapters 3 and 4. However, in individual cases the extent of development of these collateral pathways may vary and there might be developmental anomalies, especially at the circle of Willis (Riggs and Griffiths, 1938).

(b) The hemodynamic factor of collateral blood flow is represented by the increase in the pressure gradient along the collateral arterial pathways in cases of arterial obstruction (due to vasospasm or some other cause). As soon as obstruction appears in an artery, the blood pressure peripheral to it drops immediately. On the other hand, the blood pressure in the larger arteries proximal to the site of obstruction have a tendency to rise (although the regulation of systemic arterial pressure interferes with the pressure increase in the large arterial branches). Since the collateral arterial pathways are located parallel to the obstructed vessels, the pressure gradient along the collateral pathways increases, thus contributing to blood inflow to the tissue areas exposed to deficient blood supply. The maintenance of a normal level of systemic arterial pressure in this case is of significant importance for keeping up the pressure gradient in the collateral arterial pathways. If the arterial pressure level decreases, a restriction of collateral blood inflow to the ischemic area can result (Kosmarskaya and Kapustina, 1953).

(c) The physiological factor facilitating the collateral blood supply to the tissue areas exposed to deficient blood flow is the active dilatation of smaller arterial branches beyond the obstructed vessel (i.e., exposed to vasospasm or any other type of vascular obstruction). This dilatation is probably the manifestation of an adequate blood supply regulation to cerebral tissue (see Chapter 4), and results in a decrease in the resistance in the arterial pathways feeding the tissue which suffers from ischemic changes.

During vasospasm (as well as other kinds of arterial obstruction), the efficiency of collateral blood supply to respective portions of tissue may differ. First, the congenital collateral arterial pathways are developed to different degrees and do not function identically (at different levels of phylogeny). Second, even in the same organism the physiological mechanisms providing collateral blood supply may operate differently (as for all kinds of regulation in the body). In particular, regulation might be easily disturbed under the influence of harmful factors. Further, when the arterial walls undergo sclerotic processes, their ability to dilate is restricted, which interferes with the collateral blood inflow. Third, the increased use of a collateral blood supply might have a dual effect; simultaneous compensation for one kind of circulatory disorder may cause another. For instance, the recovery of blood supply to ischemic tissue results in postischemic hyperemia (Mchedlishvili, 1960c; Sundt and Waltz, 1971; Gannushkina, 1973; Mchedlishvili, Nikolaishvili, et al., 1974). The rate of microcirculation in this case can overcome actual metabolic needs and appear as "luxury perfusion" (see p. 187). Postischemic hyperemia, with an increased blood supply to the tissue and a considerably higher intravascular pressure, can contribute to the development of postischemic brain edema (Mchedlishvili, Kapuściński, et al., 1976).

    Compensatory events in cerebral vasculature accompanying pathological vasodilatation are directed toward eliminating the decreased peripheral resistance and the ensuing rise in blood pressure and flow in the micro-vasculature of the respective cerebral areas, which are harmful for the tissue. Compensatory increases in the resistance in the other portions of arterial branches located either proximally or distally to the site of pathological vasodilatation are the main way of eliminating disturbances.

    Since pathological vasodilatation usually occurs mainly in the branch-es of the smaller pial arteries, constriction of the major brain arteries usually compensates for this pathological event. This has been observed under various experimental conditions when a significant pial arterial dilatation has occurred during asphyxia, the postischemic state, and even widespread functional cerebral hyperemia (see pp. 65-67 in Chapter 3).

    It has already been mentioned (pp. 212-213) that pathological vasodilata-tion is especially dangerous when it is related to an increase in systemic arterial pressure (for instance, during hypertension of any kind). In this case, a general narrowing of cerebral arterial branches and even a decrease in the number of capillaries can be observed in the brain (Sokolova et al., 1981).

5.9. SUMMARY

    This chapter deals with the pathological behavior of cerebral arter-ies, namely pathological vasoconstriction (vasospasm) and pathological vasodilatation ("vasoparalysis" or "vasoparesis"). Knowledge of these vascular responses has increased considerably in the last decade due to in-vestigations of the physiological behavior of the brain arteries during the regulation of cerebral blood flow and the physiology of the contrac-tion and relaxation of the smooth muscle cells. Pathological vascular re-sponses characteristically occur in the cerebral and other peripheral ar-teries of the muscular type. The localization of pathological vascular re-sponses seems to be closely related to the inherent behavior of these cerebral arteries when they are regulating cerebral blood flow: vasospasm most commonly affects the major brain arteries, while pathological dilata-tion usually occurs in the smallest pial arteries. The differentiation be-tween pathological and physiological arterial responses is often difficult, first, because of the absence of distinctive quantitative criteria and, sec-ond, because of the dual effect of the vascular compensation, i.e., they might compensate for some while causing other circulatory disturbances in the brain. The essence of vasospasm consists of a disturbance in the normal contraction-relaxation cycle where due to vasoconstrictor stimuli the con-traction of vascular smooth muscle is enhanced while the relaxation is defi-cient. In contrast, pathological vasodilatation develops when vascular muscle contraction is deficient, especially during sharp increases in intra-vascular pressure. The development of pathological arterial responses is related to the inherent functional events in vascular smooth muscle cells, which are responsible for the normal arterial behavior, but have been changed specifically. The specific events at the cellular and subcellular levels which are responsible for development of vasospasm and vasoparalysis are considered in this chapter. However, much is still unknown about the mechanisms of these pathological vascular responses. The elucidation of the pathophysiological mechanisms of the development and release of cere-bral vasospasm and vasoparalysis is necessary for a better understanding of the cerebrovascular events which are most important for effective treat-ment of many neurological and neurosurgical patients.

Chapter 6. Transport of Blood and Oxygen to Brain Tissue

This chapter deals with the blood flow phenomena that occur in the microcirculation as a result of the arterial behavior which was analyzed in previous chapters. Oxygen transport to cerebral tissue is considered here only from the perspective of red cell transportation in the peripheral circulation. This transportation occurs, to a certain degree, independent of plasma flow in the blood stream, since the red cell:plasma ratio undergoes considerable changes in the flowing blood under various conditions; this, in turn, modifies the oxygen supply to tissues. The problems discussed in this chapter will be restricted to those already mentioned. We will not consider the exchange of substances transported by flowing blood to and from the environment of microvessels. Thus, neither the diffusion of oxygen into the blood from lung alveoli and from blood to tissue, nor the chemical aspects of oxygen binding with hemoglobin, will be considered in this book. In this chapter, we shall only consider the variety of circulatory phenomena in microvessels related to whole blood and its principal constituents — the red cells and plasma — which are determined chiefly by the functional behavior of feeding arteries.

6.1. FUNDAMENTALS DETERMINING THE RATE OF MICROCIRCULATION

Principal Physiological Parameters Characterizing Microcirculation. There are numerous parameters which are characteristic of circulatory phenomena in microvessels. These parameters include the velocity of blood flow, the red cell:plasma ratio (the concentration of red blood cells, or hematocrit), the transmural pressure, the pressure gradient, the viscosity of blood, the resistance to blood flow, the proportion of active and closed capillaries, etc. Each of these parameters is important from some physiological point of view. However, for a better consideration of microcirculation both in the research field and in medical practice, it is necessary to single out its principal parameters. The main purpose of the peripheral circulation, for simplification's sake, is to supply tissue with all essential substances and to remove waste products from the tissue. Proceeding from this viewpoint, the following three parameters of microcirculation can be singled out and specified as the principal ones: (a) the

PRINCIPAL PARAMETERS OF MICROCIRCULATION

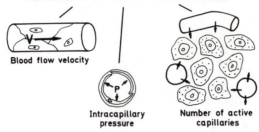

Fig. 6.1.   Parameters identified according to the
            main functions of microcirculation, i.e.,
            (a) transportation of blood gases and
            various other substances to and from the
            tissue, and (b) their exchange between
            blood and tissue.

blood pressure in the capillaries, (b) the blood flow velocity in individual capillaries, and (c) the number of active capillaries in a given capillary bed (Fig. 6.1).

    (a) The blood pressure in the capillaries is an important parameter
since it must overcome the frictional force resisting blood flow. Then,
the pressure across the vessel walls (the transmural pressure) provides
energy for distending the vascular lumen by counteracting the smooth muscle
and connective tissue tension of the vessel wall as well as of the surrounding tissue structures. Thus, the transmural pressure determines, to a degree, the luminal diameter of the microvessels. In addition, the intravascular blood pressure determines to a great extent the water exchange between blood and the surrounding tissue, as well as the passive transport
of various substances (those transported in a dissolved form along with
water) from blood to tissue and vice versa. The blood pressure in capillaries is closely related to central arterial and venous pressures, as
well as to resistances in both arterial and venous routes of blood that
connect the given capillaries with the central circulation.

    (b) The blood flow velocity in the capillaries is important because
it determines how much oxygen and other essential substances are transported by the blood to the given microareas of tissue in a given time, and
how much carbon dioxide and other metabolic products are removed. The
blood flow velocity in individual capillaries is closely related to the
distribution of blood in the whole capillary network, since the majority
of individual capillaries do not originate directly from arteriolar microvessels and do not terminate in venular microvessels, but are connected at
their origin and terminals with the other capillaries. Therefore, the
blood flow mechanics in the branching capillary network is of major importance. Capillary blood flow velocity is directly dependent on parameters
such as the pressure gradient in the microvessels and the blood fluidity
(versus viscosity) in them.

    (c) The number of active capillaries is very significant for deter-
mining the rate of microcirculation by changing the cross-sectional area
of the capillary bed. For instance, increases in cross-sectional area result in enhancement of the volumetric blood flow rate without a significant increase in the linear velocity of flow in capillaries. Thus, in the

case of an increased number of active capillaries, the rate of microcirculation increases without a considerable expense of energy to overcome the concomitant increase in resistance because of a higher linear velocity of flow. Furthermore, the active capillaries actually provide the supply of oxygen and other essential substances to the tissue and remove its metabolic products. The number of active capillaries determines, first, the distance substances must diffuse between the blood and tissue elements and, second, the area of capillary walls, i.e., the blood-tissue barrier, through which substances are transported (both passively and actively) from blood to microvascular environment, and vice versa. The changeable number of the active capillaries is characteristic of microvessels rather than small arteries and veins. The number of active capillaries is closely related to various phenomena in the microvascular bed, in particular to the red cell:plasma ratio and flow velocities in different capillaries, to the intravascular pressure, to the "contractility" of the capillary walls, etc. (see pp. 271-273).

Factors Determining Blood Flow Rate in Microvessels. The blood flow in capillaries is usually devoid of pulsatile fluctuations such as those in heart palpitation and respiration, which are normally damped along the feeding arteries before the blood reaches the capillaries. The blood flow velocity in capillaries is usually determined in the same manner as the velocity of red cell flow along the microvessels. Under normal conditions, the average flow velocity in capillaries of amphibians (e.g., frogs) is 0.3-0.6 mm/sec and in mammals, 0.5-1.0 mm/sec. However, in the capillaries of the cerebral cortex in cats, the blood flow velocity has been recently found to be very high: mean 1.5 mm/sec, varying approximately from 1 to 3 mm/sec (Pawlik et al., 1981). Even under resting conditions, the flow velocity can be quite different in the neighboring capillaries of a microvascular network. The variations may increase considerably under different physiological and, especially, pathological conditions.

The average blood flow velocity in capillaries is related to the blood volume flowing through the microvascular bed and its total cross-sectional area which is, in turn, dependent on the number of active capillaries and their diameter. This dependence is expressed by the equation $Q = vS$ or $v = Q \div S$, where Q is the volume of flowing blood, v is its mean velocity in microvessels, and S is the total cross-sectional area of the microvascular bed. When the feeding arteries undergo dilatation (arterial hyperemia), the volume of blood flowing in the microvascular bed (Q) becomes increased; this results in an increase in the flow velocity in capillaries (v), although the total cross-sectional area of the microvascular bed is increased because of a rise in the number of active capillaries (since v increases more than S). Conversely, following constriction or partial obstruction of the feeding arteries, the blood volume flowing in the microvascular bed (Q) decreases (ischemia), and this results in a reduction in the blood flow velocity in capillaries (v), in spite of the fact that the total cross-sectional area of the microvascular bed (S) decreases due to a reduction in the number of active capillaries (since v decreases more than S). During venous blood stagnation caused by the obstruction of draining veins, in spite of an increase in the total cross-sectional area of the microvascular bed (S), the volume of blood flowing in the tissue (Q) decreases, since the velocity of blood flow in capillaries (v) decreases more significantly. However, in an area of acute inflammation the cross-sectional area of the microvascular bed (S) increases to such an extent (due to a sharp increase in number of active capillaries and a very significant increase in their luminal diameter) that the velocity of blood flow (v) in the capillaries decreases significantly in spite of the increase in blood volume (Q) flowing through the microvascular bed (Mchedlishvili, 1952).

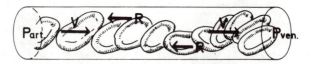

Fig. 6.2.   Main factors which determine blood flow velocity (v)
            in the microvessels, according to the principal law
            of flow. The flow is determined by the pressure
            gradient ($P_{art} - P_{ven}$) that drives the flow, and the
            resistance (R) that counteracts the flow of red
            cells and plasma in microvessels.

The blood flow in individual microvessels is determined by the principal
law of flow already mentioned (pp. 6, 44, and 103):

$$Q = \Delta P/R,$$

where Q is the blood flow, ΔP is the pressure gradient along the blood vessel, and R is the resistance to flow in the vessel. This relationship
means that the blood flow velocity is directly proportional to the pressure
gradient and inversely proportional to the resistance in the microvessel.
The relationship between these parameters is schematically presented in
Fig. 6.2.

The driving force of blood flow in microvessels is the pressure gradient along a vessel or a group of vessels, since a certain pressure energy
is necessary to overcome the frictional forces associated with blood flow.

Numerous attempts have been made to directly measure the blood pressure in small blood vessels. The results obtained were highly variable.
This is probably related to the fact that the pressure in a given microvessel is a function of various factors pertaining to both the central and
peripheral circulation.

The blood pressure in any point of a microvascular bed is greatly dependent on the central arterial pressure (in the aorta and its branches),
since from a physical point of view the foremost source of energy, and
hence of pressure, in the circulatory system is the heart work. Accordingly, the blood pressure in the arterial and capillary microvessels is
primarily dependent on the central arterial pressure, but is considerably
lower because of the expenditure of its major part in overcoming the frictional forces resisting blood flow along its route to the microvessels.

Proceeding from the principal law of flow, the blood flow in microvessels is directly correlated to the pressure gradient (ΔP) in the vessel. ΔP actually means ($P_a - P_v$) where P_a is the input pressure, i.e., the
pressure at the arterial end or the entrance of the vessel, and the P_v is
the output pressure, i.e., the pressure at the venous end or the exit of
the vessel. Accordingly, when the pressure gradient in a microvessel is
greater, the P_a is higher and the P_v is lower.

The input pressure of a microvessel, P_a, can be expressed as the central arterial pressure (in the aorta and its branches) minus the energy
expended along the route of blood from the aorta via all afferent branches
to the microvessels under consideration (Fig. 6.3). Since the expended
pressure is proportional to the resistance in the afferent, or feeding,

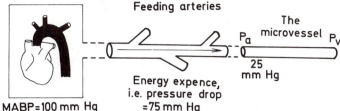

Fig. 6.3.   Input pressure of a microvessel (P_a) amounts
to the difference between the mean arterial
blood pressure (MABP) in the aorta and its
branches, and the pressure expended on overcoming the resistance in feeding arterial
branches (100 − 75 = 25 mm Hg in this example).

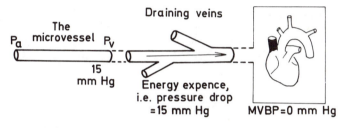

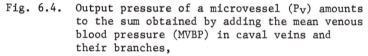

Fig. 6.4.   Output pressure of a microvessel (P_v) amounts
to the sum obtained by adding the mean venous
blood pressure (MVBP) in caval veins and
their branches,

vessels, it decreases during their constriction, and vice versa. On the
other hand, the output pressure in the venous end of a microvessel, P_v, is
to a great extent dependent on the venous outflow from the vessel and the
level of the central venous pressure, i.e., in the caval veins and their
main branches. The P_v in a microvessel can be expressed as the level of
systemic venous pressure plus the blood pressure expended along the veins
carrying blood from the microvessel to the right ventricle (Fig. 6.4).
Accordingly, if the resistance to blood flow in the efferent veins increases (for instance, because of compression of the veins from the outside or the appearance of a thrombus in their lumina), the P_v would increase in the microvessels, leading to a decrease in blood velocity in
them.

A significant rise in venous pressure due to obstruction of venous
outflow results in a venous blood stagnation in the microvascular bed.
This may cause several blood flow anomalies in the capillary network.
First, pulsatile flow of blood is seen — with each systole of the heart
and concomitant systolic rise in arterial pressure, the blood starts to
move in an orthograde direction, i.e., to the veins, but during the diastolic decrease in arterial pressure the movement of red cells slows down
or stops completely in the capillaries. In the case of a more severe venous blood stagnation, a "pendulum movement" of blood can be observed in
the capillaries — the orthograde flow appears only in the systolic rises
in arterial pressure, while the retrograde flow of blood takes place during the diastolic periods. The extent of orthograde and retrograde blood
movements depend on the degree of venous blood stagnation: the more this
stagnation is pronounced, the greater is the retrograde movement and the

smaller is the orthograde movement. But the retrograde movement can never
be greater than the orthograde movement. Both of these blood flow anomalies are related to the sharp rise in blood pressure in the capillaries
(due to venous blood stagnation). When the capillary blood pressure
reaches the level of diastolic pressure in the feeding arterial vessels,
a pulsatile movement of blood appears. Thus, an orthograde arteriovenous
pressure difference appears only during cardiac systoles, bringing about
the orthograde blood flow to the veins. But when venous blood stagnation
is even more expressed, the capillary pressure becomes higher than diastolic pressure in the feeding arteries; then the arteriovenous pressure difference reverses in the capillaries in diastolic periods (i.e., the pressure close to the arteries becomes lower than that close to the veins).
Hence, retrograde flow occurs — the blood moves in one direction and then
in another in a pattern called "pendulum flow." The reverse movement of
blood can occur in this case because of the elasticity of arterial walls
and the tissue surrounding capillaries close to the arteries as well.

    Resistance to blood flow in microvessels is usually estimated from
the law of flow mentioned above (pp. 6, 44, 103, and 234), as the pressure gradient (mm Hg) divided by the volume velocity of blood (ml/sec).
The resistance is dependent on several circulatory parameters in the microvessels.

    Various factors involved in the blood flow resistance in microvessels
are presented in Poiseuille's equation, or law:

$$\Delta P = \frac{8L\eta}{\pi r^4} Q,$$

where ΔP is the pressure gradient reflecting the resistance to flow in
microvessels, L is the length of the vessels, η is the viscosity, r is vessel radius, and Q is the flow rate. Thus, the resistance is directly proportional to the velocity of blood and the viscosity of blood, and inversely proportional to the fourth power of the microvessels' radius (the vessel length remains constant).

    However, considerable difficulties have always been faced in attempts
to estimate the resistance in microvessels quantitatively from Poiseuille's
equation. It is impossible at the present level of technology to evaluate
the blood viscosity in microvessels, since it is a very changeable parameter (see below).

    From the perspective of active regulation of microvascular blood flow
and its pathological changes, it is necessary to consider in more detail
factors which might affect the resistance in the microvascular bed. Two
parameters need not be considered in this discussion: the length of the
microvessels, which remains constant under any condition, and the blood
flow velocity, which is the parameter to be regulated in the microvascular
bed, and therefore should not be considered here. Thus, there are two remaining parameters which are important for changes in microvascular resistance, namely the vessel radius and the blood viscosity.

    Under physiological conditions the microvascular radius is of major
importance for the resistance changes in capillary lumina, since it is, on
the one hand, continuously controlled by physiological stimuli and, on the
other hand, is related to flow to the fourth power. However, changes in
the microvascular radius occur almost exclusively in the arterial portion
of the microvascular bed, since only the peripheral arteries and arterioles
are both structurally and functionally adapted for active changes in their

width. The capillaries and the smaller veins (especially in the brain)
play a comparatively less significant role in the active control of blood
flow by changing their lumina under physiological conditions. The wall
structure of the microvessels is perfectly adapted to their principal function, i.e., to the transport of various substances across their walls between blood and surrounding tissue. Accordingly there are no specific contractile elements in the capillary walls, like smooth muscle cells, and
their walls do not actively constrict or dilate in order to control the
blood flow in their lumina. The capillary walls, however, are not fully
passive, i.e., devoid of mobility when the active capillaries are transformed into nonactive forms, and vice versa (see Chapter 1 and below, pp.
271-273).

The role of blood viscosity, versus fluidity, in the resistance to
flow in microvessels is a very important factor in determining blood flow
changes in microvessels, especially during various pathological conditions.
In view of its great complexity and the difficulty in understanding the
role of this factor in blood flow in the microvascular bed, it will be considered below in more detail.

Viscosity, Versus Fluidity, of Blood in Microvessels. The viscosity
of blood is its property that offers continued resistance to flow in vessels. Fluidity is the opposite, or the reciprocal, of viscosity. Both
the viscosity and fluidity of blood are dependent on the shear of its particles against each other during flow.

The viscosity, and thus the fluidity, of liquids is significantly dependent on its chemical and physical composition. In homogeneous fluids,
like water, water solutions, or glycerin (called Newtonian fluids) the
particles are exceedingly small in comparison to the lumen of any vessel,
through which the Newtonian fluid is flowing. Therefore, if there is no
turbulence in the flow (this is related to a very high flow rate or a complex form of the vessel) the viscosity remains constant during various flow
velocities. Such homogeneous fluids completely obey Poiseuille's law.
Blood is not a homogeneous fluid due to the presence of blood cells, especially red cells (since their concentration is much greater than that of
the white cells). This complicates the laws of blood flow in microvessels
and creates flow anomalies. Therefore, blood is considered as a fluid having non-Newtonian properties, which are increasingly pronounced as the size
of the vessel lumen through which the blood flows decreases. The most obvious non-Newtonian anomalies of blood appear in the narrowest blood vessels, i.e., in the capillaries, whose luminal diameter is equal to or even
narrower than the size of red blood cells.

However, the fluidity of blood in microvessels is much higher than
that of other suspensions and emulsions with comparable relationships between the particle size and vessel diameters (Fig. 6.5) because of the exceedingly high fluidity of red cells. The erythrocytes are easily adapted
to flow forces and behave like fluid droplets in microvessels. Hence, the
fluidity of normal blood is comparable to the fluidity of red cells. It
has been shown that the fluidity of blood is preserved when concentration
of red cells increases to more than 95%, i.e., almost all red cells are
moving in microvessels (Dintenfass, 1964; Schmid-Schönbein et al., 1969).
The fluidity of blood, in contrast to other suspensions and emulsions with
comparable relationships between particle size and vessel diameter, can be
altered within a wide range between the fluidity of plasma alone and zero
when the fluidity becomes completely abolished in spite of the absence of
blood coagulation.

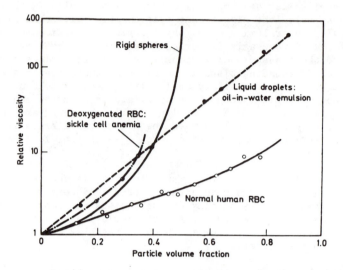

Fig. 6.5. Plots of the relative viscosity (logarithmic scale)
of various suspensions against their particle volume fraction. The viscosity of normal human red
blood cells is considerably lower than liquid droplets (oil-in-water emulsion). The viscosity difference is even greater than that of a suspension
of red cells possessing low deformability, as in
sickle cell anemia or rigid spheres. (Modified
from Fung, 1981.)

Since the fluidity of blood is a very important variable that determines the microcirculation especially under pathological conditions (Dintenfass, 1976), numerous attempts have been made to estimate blood viscosity. However, in spite of the fact that quite different, and sometimes
very complicated, viscometers have been constructed, they could not measure the actual viscosity of blood in microvessels, only some rheological
parameters of the blood, which can either promote or interfere with the
fluidity of blood *in vivo*. Summarizing the perennial task of creating a
satisfactory viscometer, Schmid-Schönbein concluded that the viscosity of
blood is a quantity which cannot be simply defined nor measured by any
single viscometer and that the extrapolation of the measurements made by
viscometers to the behavior of blood *in vivo* is not feasible.

The data obtained from viscometry *in vitro* present values characterizing the blood viscosity (the so-called relative viscosity), but the experimental conditions in any of the existing viscometers are significantly
different from the flow conditions in the actual microvessels. Examples
of such differences include, first, the relationship of the luminal diameter of microvessels to the size of red cells, since blood flows through
microvessels with successively changing diameters in both the arterial and
venous portions; second, the pattern of blood flow (see pp. 243-249) in
living microvessels of different luminal size (which cannot be reproduced
with certainty in any viscometer); and, third, the unique surface properties of the capillary walls, where there is a specific mechanical interaction between the flowing blood and the vessel walls (these surface properties cannot be recreated in any viscometer, either).

In addition, the viscometers cannot reflect the actual situation of blood flow in microvessels *in vivo* because there are vasomotor responses compensating for the changes in blood fluidity and interfering with distur- bances of normal microcirculation in the body. The true viscosity, and fluidity, of blood in microvessels appear *in vivo* only under conditions in which the physiological compensatory mechanisms are exhausted and the ves- sels behave like rigid tubes (as is the case in a viscometer). Under *in vivo* conditions, it is especially dangerous for the organism if the pres- sure gradient in microvessels is significantly reduced due to any cause (arterial obstruction by vasospasm, thrombus, etc., and venous blood stag- nation).

The viscometers also cannot precisely quantify the blood flow proper- ties in microvessels because of the specific rheological anomalies of blood flow *in vivo*. These anomalies manifest themselves particularly in the much lower hematocrit in the vessels in comparison with the macrovessels (see pp. 276-279).

Therefore, it becomes almost impossible to apply the term "viscosity" in the usual sense of continuum mechanics to discussions of hemodynamics in microcirculation. To overcome this conceptual confusion, Schmid-Schön- bein has proposed to apply "relative apparent blood fluidity" in considera- tion of blood rheological properties in microvessels. Using the term fluidity in place of the inverse of viscosity, Poiseuille's law can be re- written in the following manner in which the flow rate through vessels (and vessel networks) is proportional to the driving forces multiplied by fluidity and geometric factors:

$$Q = \Delta P \zeta \, \frac{\pi r^4}{8L} \, ,$$

where Q stands for the flow rate, ΔP stands for the pressure gradient (the driving force) in the vessel, ζ stands for the fluidity, r stands for ves- sel radius, and L stands for the vessel length (Schmid-Schönbein et al., 1980a).

There are two specific rheological phenomena related to the blood flow in the microcirculation (as distinguished from macrocirculation). The first is the so-called Fahraeus-Lindqvist phenomenon which was first ob- served in narrow tubes with a luminal diameter under 300 µm (Fahraeus and Lindqvist, 1931) and then corroborated by many other researchers (Isenberg, 1953; Haynes, 1960; and others). According to this phenomenon, in con- trast to Newtonian fluids, the fluidity of blood increases (and its viscos- ity hence decreases) with decreases in the luminal diameter of the tubes (Fig. 6.6). This represents an opposite relationship to Poiseuille's law (see above), according to which the flow of liquids is directly proportion- al to the fourth power of the vessel radius. This peculiarity of blood fluidity in microvessels is related to the presence of red cells in blood, since a similar relationship has been obtained with other suspensions flow- ing in artificial capillaries with comparable diameters and particle sizes (Isenberg, 1953). However, in the most narrow glass capillaries, in which the red cell diameter exceeds the vessel diameter, an "inversion phenome- non" was observed, namely, a significant increase in the apparent viscosity of blood, when the vessel diameter decreased (Dintenfass, 1967, 1981).

The other rheological phenomenon characteristic of the microvessels is the inverse relationship between the shear rate (i.e., the velocity of flow) and the apparent viscosity of blood (Whitmore, 1968; Brooks et al., 1970). While the viscosity of blood actually remains constant with a re- duction in flow velocity in the larger blood vessels, this relationship

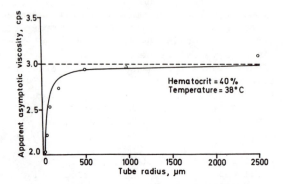

Fig. 6.6.   Fahraeus–Lindqvist effect of vessel radius on blood
            flow viscosity.   In narrow tubes (under about
            300 μm in diameter), the apparent viscosity of blood
            decreases surprisingly (i.e., its fluidity in-
            creases) with a reduction in tube diameter.   This
            is one of the anomalous blood viscosity phenomena
            that contributes considerably to blood flow in the
            narrowest microvessels under normal conditions.
            (Reproduced from Haynes, 1960.)

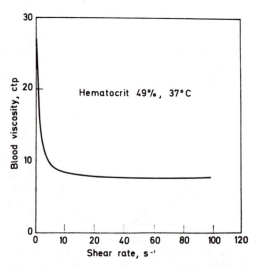

Fig. 6.7.   The effect of flow rate on blood viscosity in micro-
            vessels.   With an increase in shear rate in micro-
            vessels the viscosity of blood decreases.   This is
            another anomalous blood viscosity phenomenon that
            contributes considerably to blood fluidity in
            microvessels.   (Reproduced from Lightfoot, 1974.)

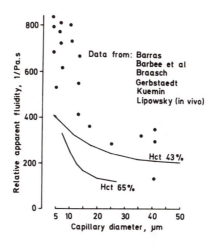

Fig. 6.8.   Effect of capillary diameter and hematocrit
             on blood fluidity. Blood fluidity in-
             creases (i.e., its viscosity becomes re-
             duced) in narrow capillaries, especially
             when their diameter is below 20 µm (the
             data, including *in vivo* data, were taken
             from works of six authors). Because of
             the ideal flow adaptation of mammalian red
             blood cells, the hemotocrit level has neg-
             ligible effects in tubes with small diam-
             eter. (Reproduced with permission from
             Schmid-Schönbein et al., 1980a.)

changes in the microvessels: the blood viscosity increases significantly
when the velocity decreases (Fig. 6.7). This phenomenon is in all probability related to increased red cell aggregation under these conditions
(see below, pp. 253-256) and to specific changes in blood flow patterns in
microvessels when the flow velocity decreases (see pp. 247-249).

    Factors Affecting Blood Fluidity in Microvessels. There are a number
of factors that promote or decrease blood fluidity: the microvessel diameter, the concentration of red cells (hematocrit) in small vessels, the
deformability of the red cells, the specific flow pattern in microvessels
(see pp. 243-249), the tendency of the red cells to aggregate (see pp.
249-256), the blood plasma viscosity related to its concentration of proteins, especially fibrinogen, etc.

    The relative apparent fluidity of blood increases as the microves-
sel's diameter decreases. This is demonstrated in Fig. 6.8, and seems to
be related to the Fahraeus-Lindqvist rheological phenomenon mentioned above.

    The effect of local changes in hematocrit on blood fluidity, and vis-
cosity, has been demonstrated mainly in viscometers. The effect of hematocrit is seen starting with a hematocrit value of 12% (Caro et al.,
1978). The higher the hematocrit, the lower the fluidity, and the higher
the viscosity of the blood in larger blood vessels. But in smaller blood
vessels with rapid blood flow the relative apparent fluidity is almost unaffected by changes in the hematocrit within certain limits (Fig. 6.8).

The effect of hematocrit on blood fluidity is probably important for blood flow in the microvessels where the local hematocrit is usually lower than in the larger vessels of central circulation (see pp. 276-279). However, changes in the systemic hematocrit have been found to have little effect on the blood rheological properties *in vivo*. This has been convincingly demonstrated in earlier studies (Whittacker and Winton, 1933) and confirmed by many subsequent investigations (Schmid-Schönbein, 1977).

Red cell deformability is a very important factor affecting the blood fluidity in microvessels, especially in the capillaries whose luminal diameter is of the same size or even smaller than the diameter of the nondeformed red cells. Because of the unique mechanical properties of the red cell outer membrane, their deformability is exceedingly high. The red cells can be specifically deformed not only in the capillaries but also in microvessels of much larger diameters. Even in arteries which are much wider than the capillaries, the red cells become deformed as prolate ellipsoids when the shear rate is high. Schmid-Schönbein et al. (1980a) have listed the main factors which determine the high deformability of red cells in microvessels. The first of them is the high compliance of the red cell membrane, which results in a tank-treading motion of the membrane around the fluid red cell cytoplasm. The inside of the red cell undergoes a swirling motion along with the surface membrane. This has been experimentally demonstrated by attaching latex particles to the outer side of the membrane and observing the Heinz bodies inside the cells. The high fluidity of the red cell cytoplasm (a concentrated solution of enzymes and hemoglobin with very low viscosity and no significant elastic structures), as well as the favorable surface-area-to-volume relationship of the red cells, are also very important for their deformability in the blood flow in microvessels.

It has been shown in viscometers that the fluidity of a red cell suspension is considerably reduced when the cells are rigidified by glutaraldehyde (Dintenfass, 1964; Schmid-Schönbein et al., 1969; Chien, 1970). But under natural conditions the deformability of red cells is characteristically very changeable. It is known that red cell deformability steadily decreases with aging of the cells (Nash and Meiselman, 1981), and hence interferes with passage of the cells through very narrow capillaries (ranging to 3 μm in diameter) in the reticuloendothelial system. It has been suggested that this aids in the recognition of old cells and in their removal from the circulation. The rigidification of red cells can probably occur in response to various pathogenic factors, for instance lactacidosis, hyperosmolarity, loss of adenosine triphosphate, etc. Because of this, the viscous properties of blood in microvessels change when significant disturbances occur in the microcirculation, manifesting themselves in a primary slowdown of blood flow in microvessels. Red cells become rigidified during various pathological states (heart diseases, diabetus mellitus, cancer, stress and anxiety, etc.) and change significantly the fluidity of blood in microvessels (Dintenfass, 1976, 1981). One compensation for such disorders in blood fluidity is accomplished by regular lowering of the hematocrit in these patients (Dintenfass, 1980).

Red cell aggregation is also a major determinant of blood fluidity. This problem will be considered below (pp. 249-256).

6.2. FLOW CONDITIONS IN MINUTE BLOOD VESSELS

The actual fluidity of blood in microvessels differs from that of homogeneous liquids because of the presence of particles — the red cells —

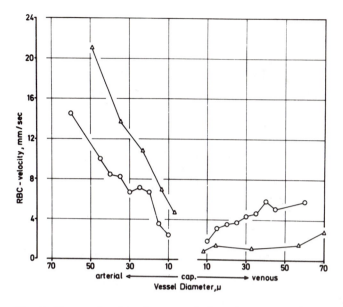

Fig. 6.9.   Blood flow velocity in arterial and venous microvascular
            branches. The red cell velocity steadily decreases with a re-
            duction in arterial microvascular diameter toward capillaries,
            but the velocity increase is less pronounced with an increase
            in the diameter of venous microvessels. The data were obtained
            from cat mesentery (open circles) and rat pial microvessels
            (triangles). (Reproduced with permission of Gaehtgens, 1977.)

rendering it a suspension. However, as we have already mentioned on p. 237
and in Fig. 6.5, the fluidity of the blood in microvessels is significantly higher than that of other suspensions and emulsions with a comparable
ratio of particle size and luminal diameter. These peculiarities of blood
fluidity in microvessels are dependent not only on the high deformability
of red cells (see above) but also on the specific pattern of blood flow in
microvessels, which will be considered below.

    The patterns of blood flow in microvessels is an important determinant
of the viscous properties of the blood. The blood flow pattern seen in
microvessels with a luminal diameter under approximately 100 μm is related
to the presence of red cells in the microvascular lumina of various diameter and to the velocity of blood flow in them. Generally, the flow decreases as the microvascular diameter decreases (Fig. 6.9), but it may
vary considerably under different physiological and, especially, pathological conditions. The blood flow velocity in microvessels determines
the resistance in them but it is also significantly dependent on the
flow pattern in the vessels.

    The blood flow pattern denotes, in this case, the specific distribu-
tion of flowing (not aggregated) red cells, their orientation, deformation,
and position along and across the blood stream inside the microvascular
lumina. The peculiarity of blood flow pattern in the microvessels, as
distinguished from that in larger blood vessels, is naturally most pronounced in the microvessels with the narrowest lumina, i.e., the true
capillaries. Since a reduction in microvascular diameter occurs gradual-

Type I   over 100 μm

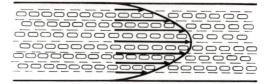

Type II   15-100 μm

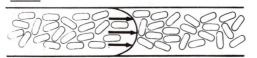

Type III   3-15 μm

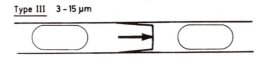

Fig. 6.10.   Three types of blood flow structure in microvessels
             of various diameters. (I) In microvessels larger
             than 100 μm in diameter (comparable to macrovessels);
             (II) in the transient type of microvessels; and
             (III) in true capillaries, where the typical plug
             flow (or the bolus flow) is observed. The main dif-
             ferences of blood flow structure are observed, first,
             in the velocity profile and, second, in the typical
             orientation of red cells; in the transient type (II)
             the orientation of red cells is dependent on their
             velocity. See text for details.

ly from the larger arteries to the capillaries, the structural properties
of blood flow likewise change gradually from the larger arteries and veins
(pertaining to the central circulation) to the capillaries. The anomalous,
i.e., non-Newtonian, viscous properties of blood become most evident when
the red cell size becomes comparable to the microvascular diameter.

    When considering the microvascular flow structure we can classify the
microvessels into the following three types: (I) microvessels with a
luminal diameter of 80-100 μm and more, in which the blood flow conditions are comparable to those in larger arteries and veins; (II) the
microvessels with a luminal diameter under 100 μm but larger than 10-15 μm,
i.e., when the lumen is considerably larger than red cell size; and (III)
the smallest blood vessels whose lumen is equal to or even smaller than the
dimensions of individual red cells, i.e., the true capillaries and the adjacent arterioles and venules. Since the blood flow pattern peculiarities
change gradually from one type of microvessel to another according to the
gradual changes of their diameters, it is impossible to precisely indicate
where this transition takes place.

    In the largest microvessels (Type I) the blood flow is comparable to
homogeneous, or Newtonian fluids. This can be explained by a comparatively

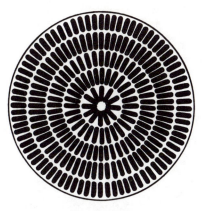

Fig. 6.11.   The unique distribution of red blood
             cells in the lumina of larger arteries.
             In an artery with a diameter of approxi-
             mately 75 μm, the red cells are oriented
             perpendicular to the vessel cross sec-
             tion (i.e., they move in parallel to the
             vessel axis) and are separated in par-
             ticular layers (there are five in the
             present case) which move with different
             velocities, thus forming the specific
             velocity profile in the vessel lumen.
             (Reproduced from Chizhevsky, 1980.)

great difference between the red cell size and the luminal diameter of vessels. The red cells move, as a rule, parallel to the vessel wall. As
shown in Fig. 6.10 I, the velocity profile of the blood layers has a parabolic form, analogous to the laminar flow of homogeneous (i.e., Newtonian)
fluids in narrow tubes, where the velocity of the layers is maximum at the
axis and decreases toward the vessel walls. Accordingly, the specific
shear rate appears between the neighboring layers of fluid. Likewise, the
laminar flow of homogeneous fluids — the flow of blood in larger microvessels (as in almost all macrovessels, excluding the aorta) — has a parabolic velocity profile when the shear rate of individual blood particles is
zero at the axis and increases toward the vessel walls where it attains
its maximum. This distribution of shear rates in vascular lumina results
in a specific orientation of red cells with respect to flow: they move
parallel to the vessel wall in layers. This laminar flow creates a comparatively low resistance to flow in larger blood vessels.

In the microvessels the red cells are oriented parallel to the direction of flow and hence to the vessel axis. The orientation of red cells
in the vessels of the indicated diameter ranges is determined, in particular, by the comparatively fast blood flow in the lumina. The laminar character of blood flow in these microvessels contributes to a specific distribution of blood layers which contain red cells, as schematically drawn
by Chizhevsky in Fig. 6.11.

A different type of blood flow behavior is seen in the microvessels
that possess the narrowest lumen, i.e., in the true capillaries whose luminal diameter is close to that of red cells (type III). The velocity

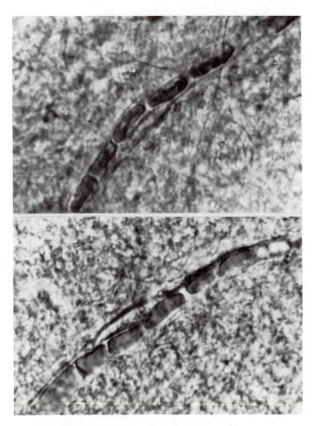

Fig. 6.12. The photomicrographs show two flow patterns of con-
            siderably deformed red blood cells in the capil-
            laries of the parietal cortex of rabbits. The
            photomicrographs have been taken from thick un-
            stained histological slices of the parietal cor-
            tex following *in vivo* fixation by 20% formalde-
            hyde in ethanol. (Investigations by Mchedlish-
            vili and Varazashvili.)

profile of different layers of blood which is characteristic for the microvessels of group I (see above) certainly cannot occur under these conditions, since every blood cell flowing along the microvessels actually occupies almost the whole microvascular lumen. It thus moves as a plug and
carries the respective plasma columns in front of and behind it. That is
why this type of flow, schematically shown in Fig. 6.10 III, has been
called the plug flow or the bolus flow.

    The relationship of the size of red cells to the luminal diameter varies
considerably from organ to organ and may be different even in the same
tissue in different species. But the principal characteristic in the
majority of tissues is a greater diameter of undeformed red cells compared
to the luminal diameter of the capillaries. Thus, in the cerebral cortex,
the luminal diameter of capillaries is approximately 5–10 μm in man
(Blinkov and Gleser, 1968), 5.1 ± 0.84 μm in cats (Pawlik et al., 1981),
and 4.8 ± 0.04 μm (M ± SE) in rabbits (Mchedlishvili and Varazashvili, unpublished data). The mean diameter of red cells is approximately 7.6, 5.6,

and 7.4 μm, respectively (Levtov et al., 1982). Therefore, to pass through the capillary lumina, the red cells must be deformed. The red cell flow conditions in the capillaries of rabbits' cerebral cortex (investigated in unstained histological slices after *in vivo* fixation of the tissue) have been found to be as follows: the capillary diameter ranges from 2.8 to 6.3 μm, with mean values equal to 4.8 ± 0.1 μm. When the flow is preserved, the red cells are regularly deformed, i.e., stretched, in the lumina. Red cells are stretched to such a degree that their length is about 2.2 times greater than their width. Thus, the red cells occupy approximately 80% of the internal diameter of the capillaries, and a parietal plasma layer always remains near the capillary walls (Fig. 6.12), which creates a lubrication layer. It has been stated that without such lubrication at the capillary walls, no blood flow could occur in such narrow blood vessels (Caro et al., 1978).

The remaining group of microvessels, type II, has an intermediate luminal size between types I and III. The red cell flow in them has accordingly characteristics of both type I and III microvessels. An obvious deviation in the parabolic shape of the flow velocity profile was observed in microvessels larger than the capillaries but smaller than 100 μm in diameter; this velocity profile was found to be much blunter than that seen in larger arteries (Thoma, 1910; Berman and Fuhro, 1969; Gaehtgens et al., 1971). In pial microvessels ranging from 15 to 36 μm in diameter, the ratio of red cell velocities in the vicinity of the walls to that at the axis was only 0.8 (Rosenblum, 1972). Hence, in the type II microvessels, the blood flow is, on the one hand, similar to that in larger vessels (type I, see Fig. 6.10), since there is an apparent tendency to form a parabolic flow velocity profile. On the other hand, the profile may be blunted, thus resembling the flow in the smallest microvessels (type III, see Fig. 6.10). This transitional type of flow condition is shown schematically as II in Fig. 6.10.

This transitional type of blood flow is an especially complicated and changeable pattern of red cell flow in microvessels ranging from approximately 15 to 100 μm. The majority of investigations of this problem has been carried out in physical models with flow of various particles, including red cells, in artificial (usually glass) capillaries (Caro et al., 1978). But recently, analysis of red cell flow has become possible in direct studies of living microvessels in the frog mesentery. The frame-to-frame analysis of projected films following cinemicrography provided direct and quantitative data illustrating the factors involved in the formation of flow structure in microvessels of type II (Mamisashvili and Baratashvili, 1980; Mamisashvili et al., 1982).

The red cell orientation in the microvascular flow to a great extent determines the fluidity of blood. The parallel orientation of red cells to the vessel axis creates a considerably lower resistance to flow than their perpendicular orientation. This has been shown in living microvessels during the flow of individual red cells: the cells, which were oriented parallel to the vessel axis (and flow direction) were transported significantly faster than the neighboring red cells, which were oriented perpendicular to the axis (Fig. 6.13). In contrast to the larger arteries, where the orientation is predominantly parallel to the blood flow direction (this is dependent, in particular, on the comparatively high velocity rate under physiological conditions), the orientation of red cells in type II microvessels might be quite variable — from parallel to perpendicular to the direction of flow (Fig. 6.10). The factor determining the red cell orientation in the lumina of such microvessels has been found to be primarily the mean velocity of flow. The relationship between these two vari-

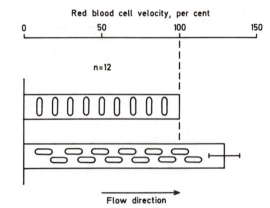

Fig. 6.13.   Resistance to flow of red cells oriented
             either perpendicularly or parallel to
             the microvessel axis. In the same micro-
             vessels of frogs' mesentery individual
             red cells oriented in parallel to the
             vessel axis (i.e., in the direction of
             flow) are moving with a significantly
             higher velocity than the cells having a
             perpendicular orientation. This is
             direct evidence that the resistance to
             flow is significantly lower for the red
             cells oriented in parallel to the flow
             direction. (Reproduced with permission
             from Mamisashvili, unpublished data.)

ables is as follows: the greater the velocity (or the greater the shear
rate), the more parallel to the direction of flow the red cells are
oriented (Mamisashvili and Baratashvili, 1980). This relationship is demonstrated in Fig. 6.14. Thus, a comparatively high velocity of flow promotes the orientation of red cells along the microvessels and hence an increase in blood fluidity. The slowdown of blood flow in such microvessels
results in chaotic orientation of red cells related to the microvessel
axis, and thus to an increased resistance to flow.

     The velocity profile of red cells is another variable related to the
viscosity, versus fluidity, of blood in microvessels. The parabolic velocity profile of homogeneous fluids, characteristic of the laminar flow,
provides the most favorable conditions from the point of view of minimum
resistance. These flow conditions are seen in the majority of large arteries and veins, as well as in the larger microvessels (see pp. 244-245). However, in the transitional microvessels (type II), the profile might be
quite variable — from a parabolic shape to one completely flattened in the
vascular lumina. Recent *in vivo* studies showed that in microvessels with
a luminar diameter of 25-70 μm, the trajectory of red cells is linear in
cases of comparatively high flow rate, but becomes chaotic when the flow
velocity decreases (Fig. 6.15). The velocity profile of red cells is, in
turn, dependent on the blood flow rate. Figure 6.16 shows that when the
mean axial flow velocity is greater than 0.3-0.4 mm/sec, the profile becomes parabolic. This was found to be partly independent of the red cell
concentration (hematocrit) in flowing blood; the red cell orientation is
also predominantly parallel to the blood flow under these conditions. How-

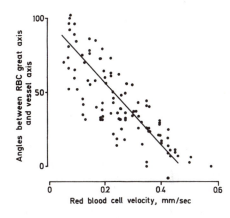

Fig. 6.14. Dependence of red blood cell orientation
            on their velocity in microvessels. The
            smaller the angle is between the frogs'
            red blood cell great axis and the vessel
            axis (i.e., the red cells are predomi-
            nantly oriented along the vessel axis),
            the faster is their flow velocity. These
            data were obtained from frame-to-frame
            analysis of cinemicrographs of frogs'
            mesenterial microvessels of 20-40 μm in
            diameter. (Reproduced with permission
            from Mamisashvili and Baratashvili, 1980.)

ever, when the linear velocity of blood flow is lower than 0.3-0.4 mm/sec,
the orientation of individual red cells becomes chaotic (Mamisashvili et
al., 1982, 1984).

    Consequently, an increase in flow rate in the microvessels causes the
red cell flow to resemble the laminar flow of Newtonian fluids, which is
usually characteristic of the larger blood vessels where the resistance is
comparatively lower. However, the red cell flow becomes irregular (pseudo-
turbulent) with an ensuing increase in resistance as soon as the velocity
of blood decreases.

    Red Cell Aggregation as a Factor Disturbing Blood Flow Structure with
Ensuing Reduction in Blood Fluidity in Microvessels. We have seen above
that, under normal conditions, blood flow has a specific pattern in microvessels. One of the conditions necessary to maintain this structure is
the presence of dissociated red cells in the flowing blood. Such cells
can behave with relative independence inside the vascular lumina. But
even under normal conditions the slowing-down of flow rate (because of a
reduction in driving force) induces red cell aggregation. But the red
cells dissociate again as soon as the flow accelerates. However, the red
cell aggregation may be significantly enhanced under pathological conditions when blood changes from an emulsion of red cells with high fluidity
into a reticulated suspension with very low fluidity. Thus the disturbances
in normal blood flow structure in the microvessels result in significant
changes in the viscous properties of blood and a drop in its fluidity. The
fluidity can be reduced to a critical level when the normal driving forces
(i.e., the pressure gradient) can no longer maintain blood flow in the
microvessels.

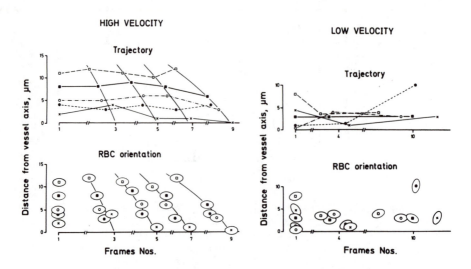

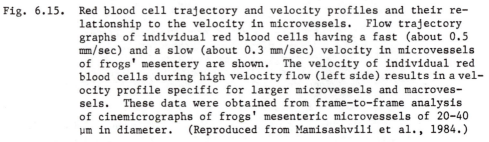

Fig. 6.15.   Red blood cell trajectory and velocity profiles and their re-
             lationship to the velocity in microvessels. Flow trajectory
             graphs of individual red blood cells having a fast (about 0.5
             mm/sec) and a slow (about 0.3 mm/sec) velocity in microvessels
             of frogs' mesentery are shown. The velocity of individual red
             blood cells during high velocity flow (left side) results in a vel-
             ocity profile specific for larger microvessels and macroves-
             sels. These data were obtained from frame-to-frame analysis
             of cinemicrographs of frogs' mesenteric microvessels of 20-40
             μm in diameter. (Reproduced from Mamisashvili et al., 1984.)

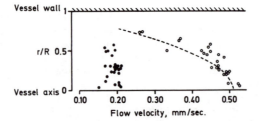

Fig. 6.16.   Velocity profile in frogs' mesenteric
             microvessels with respect to red blood
             cell flow. When the red blood cell
             velocity in microvessels is low, the
             velocity profile is blunt, but with an
             increase in velocity the profile be-
             comes typical of that seen in larger
             microvessels and macrovessels. These
             data were obtained from frame-to-frame
             analysis of cinemicrographs of frogs'
             mesenteric microvessels of 20-40 μm in
             diameter. (Reproduced from Mamisash-
             vili et al., 1984.)

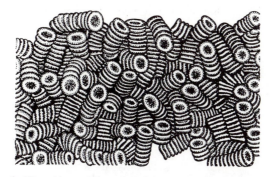

Fig. 6.17.   Mammalian red blood cell aggregation *in
vitro*, where the individual red cells
have joined together and formed rouleaux,
which adhere to each other. (Reproduced
from Chizhevsky, 1980.)

Aggregation of red cells occurs when individual cells become loosely associated and gather into masses. This phenomenon has been observed *in vitro*
under the microscope for many years: the red cell membranes join together
and form rouleaux, and then other red cells and other rouleaux adhere to them
(Fig. 6.17). Aggregate formation is a normal property of cells and can be
enhanced by various agents affecting the physical properties of the membrane
(Fahraeus, 1929).

Through the 19th century and in the course of the first half of this
century there existed at least three relatively separate characteristics
of red cell behavior which were not understood: (A) the blood stasis observed in living capillaries, (B) the red cell sedimentation rate *in vitro*
as a diagnostic means, and (C) the red cell aggregation observed both *in
vitro* and *in vivo*. Subsequently, these three problems merged and became
transformed into the single problem of red cell aggregation, which can, on
the one hand, occur intravascularly and interfere with the blood rheological properties and, on the other hand, affect the extravascular red cells
and determine their sedimentation rate *in vitro*. These problems, schematically presented in Fig. 6.18, will be considered in more detail below.

A. Blood stasis, i.e., the sharp local slowdown to complete stoppage
of blood flow in capillaries, was regularly observed starting in the 19th
century in numerous biomicroscopical studies of transparent tissues (e.g.,
the swimming and retrolingual membrane of frogs, the mesentery of amphibians and mammals, etc.). The great significance of this microcirculatory
phenomenon for disturbance of blood supply to tissues has always been well
understood. But the immediate cause of blood flow arrest during capillary
stasis was not properly analyzed in experiments until the 1950s. Several
hypotheses were then proposed to explain why blood flow could stop during
this pathological phenomenon of microcirculation.

Some researchers proposed that the causes of blood flow stoppage in
capillaries during stasis were the microvascular luminal changes, namely,
spasm of the afferent arterioles and expansion of the capillaries (Brücke,
1850; Ricker and Regendanz, 1921). However, this assumption contradicted
the experimental data and therefore was reasonably criticized (Danilov,
1940; Illig, 1955; Mchedlishvili, 1958). Blood stasis in capillaries was

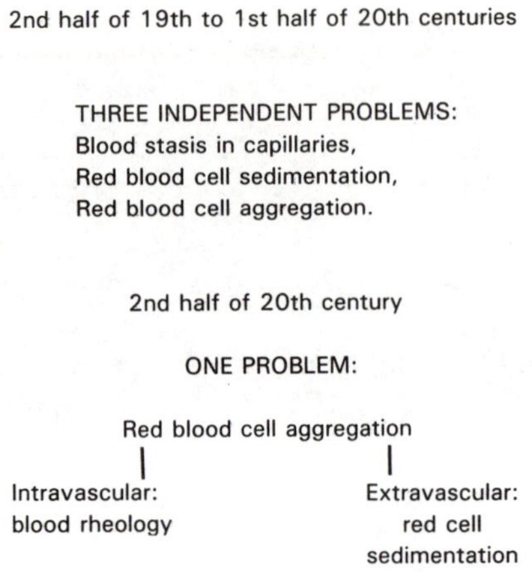

2nd half of 19th to 1st half of 20th centuries

THREE INDEPENDENT PROBLEMS:
Blood stasis in capillaries,
Red blood cell sedimentation,
Red blood cell aggregation.

2nd half of 20th century

ONE PROBLEM:

Red blood cell aggregation

Intravascular: Extravascular:
blood rheology   red cell
                                  sedimentation

Fig. 6.18. The 19th and 20th century concepts of
red blood cell aggregation problems.
See text for details.

also suggested to result from primary hemoconcentration in the microvessels (Weber, 1852; Schuler, 1854; Recklinghausen, 1883; Illig, 1955), although substantial evidence contradicted this assumption (Mchedlishvili,
1958). As long ago as the 1850s some authors suggested that the stasis
in capillaries is due to an increased stickiness of red cells (Jones,
1851; Lister, 1857-1858), but later this assumption was abandoned. The
red cell aggregation during stasis was further described at the beginning
of this century as a secondary occurrence following the stoppage of blood
flow in capillaries (Natus, 1910; Ricker and Regendanz, 1921; Illig, 1955)
and as a cause of homogenization of capillary contents during stasis (Tannenberg and Fischer-Wasels, 1927), but not as the cause of blood flow arrest. It has also been speculated that the blood stasis depends on
changes in the friction of blood against the capillary walls (Cohnheim,
1873), although it is known that a lubricating plasma layer is always
present between the red cells and microvascular walls, and the blood fluidity is determined not by blood friction forces at the walls but by the
blood viscosity in microvessels. There was also an assumption that the
immediate cause of blood flow stoppage in capillaries during stasis is the
loss of elasticity of the red cells (Gubler, 1951) but the evidence was
then indirect (i.e., altered staining properties of red cells). Thus, the
scientific literature prior to the 1950s contained speculations about immediate causes of blood flow arrest in capillaries during stasis providing
no convincing experimental evidence.

     B. The sedimentation of red cells in blood removed from the body is
probably one of the most ancient diagnostic methods (this technique was
applied even when the existence of the red cells in blood was still unknown). It was practiced as far back as in the eras of the ancient Greeks
and Romans, or even earlier, and through the entire medieval epoch. The
application of this method in medical practice was, up to the middle of
the 19th century, related to "phlebotomy," i.e., removal of a certain
amount of blood from veins, which was customary and even popular throughout known medical history (Schmid-Schönbein, 1981).

     In the first half of this century red cell sedimentation was carefully
investigated by Fahraeus (1929). At that time it became known that the
sedimentation rate is dependent on the degree of red cell aggregation,

which begins after 5-25 minutes. The sedimentation rate is initially slow (before the appearance of the aggregates), then accelerated (when the aggregates are formed), and finally slows down. The mechanism of this phenomenon was thought by Fahraeus to be dependent on factors enumerated in the Stokes' formula. In particular, the sedimentation rate of solids in a liquid medium is directly proportional to the diameter of the solid being sedimented. Therefore the rate of red cell sedimentation increases with an increased speed of aggregate formation. In addition, Fahraeus studied the factors that affect red cell aggregation and attempted to understand the mechanism of these effects. He found (and this has been corroborated by many researchers) that red cell aggregation is related mainly to the properties of the interface between the red cell surface layer and the plasma. This was proved by the following experiment: if the washed red cells of a healthy person are placed in the plasma of a sick person, the sedimentation rate increases. The composition of plasma proteins is very important in this respect, especially the concentration of fibrinogen and to a lesser extent globulins, in the plasma. Increases in protein contribute considerably to red cells aggregation and to acceleration of their sedimentation. We will not study the details of the mechanism of red cell aggregation and their sedimentation, which has been thoroughly investigated by Thorsen and Hint (1950), Chizhevsky (1980), and many others. The mechanism of red cell aggregation has been recently reviewed by Levtov et al. (1982).

Fahraeus (1929) has assumed that under pathological conditions red cell aggregates might impede blood flow in narrow blood vessels. In his experiments, blood with increased red cell aggregation flowed through narrow glass tubes, which often became stopped by the aggregates. Later, Voronin (1947) made computations based on Stokes' formula and proved that with sharply increased sedimentation of red blood cells, aggregates should reach the size that would impede blood flow in capillaries. The reality of this phenomenon, however, can be proved only in direct investigations during normal, *in vivo* conditions of blood flow in microvessels.

C. Red cell aggregation inside microvessels was observed in the 1920s in *in vivo* studies of the capillaries of nailfolds of human digits during a primary slowdown in blood flow rate. The red cells gathered into aggregates which moves slowly, separated by comparatively large plasmatic intervals, toward the venules (Nesterov, 1929). The intravascular aggregation of red cells was also observed in other studies both in man and animals during a decrease in the capillary flow rate. The aggregation was manifested as a granular flow of red cells in microvessels (Fahraeus, 1929; Chizhevsky, 1953; Thuranszky, 1957).

The extensive studies of microvessels in the human conjunctiva which were carried out in the 1950s showed that the intravascular aggregation of red cells often occurs in pathological conditions (Knisely et al., 1947; Matteis et al., 1955; Madow and Bloch, 1956). This phenomenon was found to be coincident with an increased sedimentation rate of red cells in blood samples taken from the same patients. Thus, it became evident that red cell aggregation occurred in the whole blood of these patients but not locally in the microvessels under investigation. The intravascular aggregation of red cells was always found to be associated with simultaneous slowing down of blood flow in the conjunctival microvessels. This was interpreted as follows: the red cell aggregates in the patients' blood obstruct the lumina of the terminal arterioles and hence impede the blood inflow to the capillary networks, disturbing the microcirculation. However, evidence for this assumption has not been conclusive. In particular, detailed studies of the retina showed that if the systemic arteri-

1. Microvascular diameter unchanged:

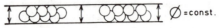

$\emptyset$ =const.

2. Pressure difference unchanged:

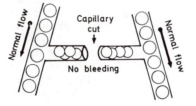

Fig. 6.19. Blood flow arrest in capillaries dependent on obstruction of the microvascu-
lar lumina by red cell aggregates is
shown during two conditions: (1)
the microvascular diameter remains unchanged and the pressure gradient is
preserved; (2) dissection of the capillary with stasis does not result in exsanguination from their lumina despite
the preservation of normal blood flow,
and consequently of intracapillary
pressure, in the neighboring microvessels. (Data from Mchedlishvili, 1953.)

al pressure was not lowered, the red cell aggregates seldom obstructed a
large number of arterioles, since they are usually destroyed in the microvessels of this caliber, so that only separate red cells entered the capillaries (Thuránszky, 1957).

Thus, although intravascular red cell aggregation has been observed
in a number of studies in the 1950s, its role in microcirculatory disturbances had not then been clarified enough. To solve this problem it seemed
more promising to carry out investigations under the conditions of red
cell aggregation in specific microvascular regions, e.g., during local
capillary stasis and inflammation. The analysis of the immediate cause of
local blood stasis development provided much evidence concerning the role
of intravascular red cell aggregation in the reduction of blood fluidity
and local blood flow arrest in microvessels (Mchedlishvili, 1952, 1953,
1957). The main experimental data obtained during direct biomicroscopical
investigation in the frogs' retrolingual membranes are schematically summarized in Figs. 6.19 and 6.20.

Following the local application of agents producing blood stasis in
capillaries (for example, a concentrated solution or a small crystal of
sodium chloride), blood flow stops locally while the luminal diameter remains unchanged all along the microvessel, and the pressure gradient in it
is still preserved (Fig. 6.19). This proves that blood flow slowdown and
full arrest in the capillaries is determined by a significant local decrease in blood fluidity inside the microvascular lumina.

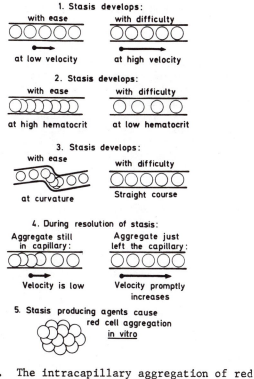

Fig. 6.20. The intracapillary aggregation of red blood cells is the immediate cause of blood flow slowing down and of complete arrest in capillaries during primary capillary stasis. (Data from Mchedlish-vili, 1953.) See text for details.

Further data have shown that the immediate cause of the reduction in blood fluidity is the enhanced intravascular red cell aggregation, which is evidently the requisite cause of the capillary obstruction during the development of primary stasis. The evidence listed schematically in Fig. 6.20 is as follows: (1) stasis develops readily when the actual flow rate in the capillary is reduced; stasis occurs with considerably more difficulty when the flow is accelerated; (2) blood stasis occurs with ease when the local hematocrit is high, but is far less likely to develop when the local hematocrit is reduced; (3) stasis develops first at the sites of additional local resistance in the capillaries, e.g., at curvatures, where the red cells are readily retained and come in contact with each other; (4) during the resolution of stasis, the flow velocity in the capillary is slow as long as the red cell aggregates are still inside the vascular lumina, but as soon as the aggregate leaves the microvessel into a larger vessel (the venule) the flow rate immediately accelerates; (5) the agents producing stasis, including a high concentration of sodium chloride, enhance red cell aggregation *in vitro* (Mchedlishvili, 1953, 1958).

In the period after the 1950s, no additional direct evidence was added to the listed data. On the other hand, no proof against the conclusion that increased intravascular red cell aggregation caused local blood flow resistance during capillary stasis was described in special literature.

As mentioned above, red cell aggregation *in vivo* is dependent on the interaction of the red cell surface with chemical ingredients of the extracellular red cell environment (Fahraeus, 1929; Levtov et al., 1982). The blood plasma proteins possessing the highest molecular weight (as well as high molecular weight dextrans) are of great importance in this respect. Fibrinogen and some of the globulins dissolved in blood plasma contribute to red cell aggregation in blood and thus affect its fluidity. Therefore, filtration of water from the capillary lumina across the capillary walls into the surrounding tissue might contribute considerably to intravascular red cell aggregation and blood flow arrest during capillary stasis. Therefore, it does not seem surprising that flow stasis more readily develops in the venous portions of the capillaries (where the wall permeability is considerably higher) (Danilov, 1940; Gubler, 1951; Mchedlishvili, 1953; Illig, 1955).

Consequently, during the 1950s, convincing evidence was obtained that the intravascular aggregation of red cells is the factor which decreases the blood fluidity and contributes to blood flow slowdown and the development of full capillary stasis. The significance of this phenomenon in blood fluidity in the microvessels is now commonly accepted and has been interpreted in more detail (Schmid-Schönbein et al., 1980a).

6.3. SPECIFIC PHENOMENA RELATED TO BLOOD FLOW RATES IN THE CAPILLARY CIRCULATION

Specific circulatory phenomena in blood capillaries are related to their unique structure and function. These phenomena include: (a) the dependence of the rate of capillary circulation on active diameter changes in the feeding arteries and arterioles; (b) the variable distribution of the blood stream among all the capillaries in their networks; (c) the physiological mechanism that transforms active into inactive capillaries, and vice versa, thus determining changes in the number of active capillaries. All these phenomena will be considered below.

The Functional Arrangement of the Microvascular Bed. The microvascular bed of the brain, similar to everywhere else in the body, consists of at least three types of microvessels: (a) the bifurcating terminal arteries with a diameter decreasing from approximately 100 μm* to the precapillary arterioles 6-10 μm wide; (b) the branching capillaries, devoid of specific contractile elements — smooth muscle cells — in the walls forming the main microvascular networks; (c) the draining veins whose diameter is initially similar to that of the capillaries, but gradually increases as the venular vessels join each other. The microvascular bed of the cortex supplied by the surface pial arterial network thus possesses microvessels which are distributed partly on the brain surface and partly inside the cerebral substance. The surface network consists of smaller pial ramifications of 100 to 20 μm in diameter, including the active vascular segments controlling the microcirculation in minute areas of the cerebral cortex

---

*The vascular diameter of 100 μm is approximate. It has been used as a discrimination point in discussion of the structural and functional differences of pial arteries which are larger and smaller than 100 μm (see pp. 104-107) and the differences in blood flow conditions in arterial vessels which are larger and smaller than 100 μm (see pp. 143-149).

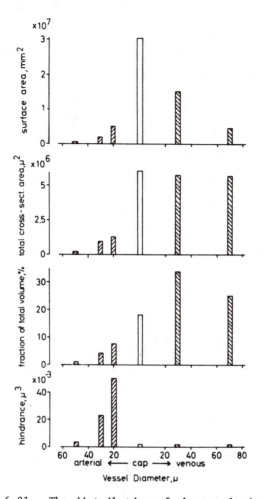

Fig. 6.21. The distribution of the total microvascular area, total cross-sectional
area, fraction of total microvascular
volume, and vascular hindrance along
the microvascular bed from small arteries to small veins obtained from the
analysis of morphometric data. (Reproduced with permission from Gaehtgens,
1977.)

(see Chapter 4). As for the microcirculation of the subcortical brain
structures, all appropriate arterial branches are completely distributed
within the brain substance.

While the organization of the pial microvascular system on the brain
surface has been well investigated, there are so far no generalized quantitative descriptions of the microvascular bed inside the brain substance
(the cross-sectional areas, the length and number of microvessels, etc.),
as has been established for some flat organs like the mesentery, omentum,
etc. Therefore, we can only extrapolate to cerebral tissue the data ob-

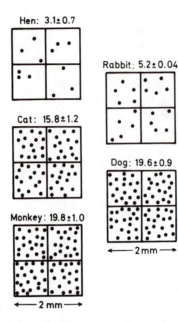

Fig. 6.22. The increasing number of radial arteries originate from the pial arterial network and feed the cerebral cortex (parietal region) per unit of brain surface in the evolutionary process. This provides evidence for the significance of the pial arterial branches in the regulation of blood supply to the cerebral cortex, as demonstrated in Chapter 4. (Reproduced from Mchedlishvili and Kuridze, 1984.)

tained in some organs other than the brain, supposing that there is some resemblance between them. The present-day knowledge of the microvascular system is mainly based on morphometric measurements made in histologic preparations of canine intestinal tissue by Mall (1888). By comparing different levels of microvascular branching it has been established that total cross-sectional area increases gradually toward the capillary network, reaches a maximum, and then decreases again on the venous side of the microvascular bed. The intravascular blood volume, which is comparatively low within the arteriolar ramifications, increases toward the capillaries and even to a greater extent in the smaller veins; hence the latter contain almost 50% of total blood volume of the microvascular bed. Calculations of the impedance to blood flow, made on the basis of morphometric data and Poiseuille's equation, revealed that the vascular resistance is maximal in the precapillary arterioles, but is low in capillaries and in veins (Fig. 6.21). A commonly accepted conclusion from these data has suggested that the arterial part of the microvascular bed causes a relatively high resistance to blood flow, while its venous portion is characterized by the largest storage capacity for blood in the peripheral vascular bed.

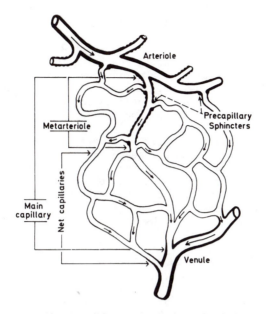

Fig. 6.23.   Diagram of an ideal capillary bed according to Chambers and Zweifach. The
distribution of smooth muscle in vascular walls is indicated by thicker
lines. Individual muscle cells are
distributed along metarterioles and offshoots of capillary side branches (the
"precapillary sphincters"). Arrows
show the direction of blood flow in
microvessels. (Modified from Chambers
and Zweifach, 1944.)

The ability of the arterial portion of the microvascular bed to control the microcirculation is related to the presence of smooth muscle
cells in the vessel walls supplied with adrenergic, cholinergic, and other
types of nerves. Arterial muscle responds to vasomotor impulses and the
action of various vasoactive substances, both from blood and from the surrounding tissue, by changing the vascular lumina within large limits.
Thus, the peripheral arterial branches function as the vascular effectors
controlling capillary circulation. The significance of the pial arterial
ramifications in the control of microcirculation of the cerebral cortex is
demonstrated by the increase in the number of precortical arteries feeding
progressively reduced areas of cortical tissue as the evolutionary development of animal species increases (Fig. 6.22).

The distribution of smooth muscle cells in terminal arterial branches
is shown in the schematic drawing of a microvascular bed in Fig. 6.23.
Originally this figure represented mesenteric microvessels (Chambers and Zweifach, 1944) but it probably characterizes the microvascular beds of any
organ, including the brain. The smooth muscle cell layer is uninterrupted
in the larger arterial and arteriolar branches, but the cells are rarely
encountered in the transient portions of arterioles to capillaries. Those
portions having separate smooth muscle cells are called metarterioles.

Single muscle cells have been found surrounding the offshoots of individual capillaries from the metarterioles. Such vessels are called precapillary sphincters (Chambers and Zweifach, 1947). These single muscle cells have been observed to react independently to direct electrical or mechanical stimulation with a micromanipulator, resulting in changes in the microvascular lumina; and, therefore, they were thought to be the device controlling blood flow in individual capillaries. But the precapillary sphincters have not been confirmed in further studies to be a specifically functioning structure in the microvascular bed (see below).

The capillary networks of different parts of the brain are quite diverse. The density, distribution, shape, and size of cerebral capillaries, as in other organs, depend on the structure and the metabolic rate of surrounding tissue. It has been shown that the density of the capillary network increases as the intensity of the metabolism in the brain tissue increases (Lierse, 1963). Embryological investigations have also shown that the formation of capillary networks is determined by metabolism, structure, and the intensity of blood flow (Thoma, 1893). Therefore, the gray matter of the brain which is rich in cell elements is far more abundantly supplied with capillaries than the white matter, built mostly of nerve fibers. The capillary networks are, in turn, quite variable throughout the brain (Pfeifer, 1940; Klosovsky, 1951; Lierse, 1963), as are the metabolic rate and local blood flow (see pp. 99-101). In addition, the capillary networks can undergo sharp changes under different experimental conditions as well as in pathology.

In histological preparations of tissues where the capillary networks were filled with contrast media beforehand, the microvascular density and the shape of the networks are visible, but it is impossible to differentiate the functional aspects of individual capillaries. However, attentive examination of the capillary blood flow in living tissues enabled some researchers to identify functionally different microvessels in the capillary networks. However, because of the considerable difficulties in direct *in vivo* microscopic examination of the blood flow in cerebral capillary networks, the flow peculiarities in individual microvessels of the brain have not been detected so far. This has usually been attained only in organs where the microvessels are distributed in one plane. Thus, Dubois (1841) was probably the first who described capillaries of two types: those of the first order, or dendritic capillaries, which form direct connections between the arterioles and venules; and the capillaries of the second order, or reticular capillaries, which form the capillary networks (the latter were thought not to have their own walls, according to the concept of that time, as if a part of blood capillaries were formed only by the organs' own structural elements). Jacobj (1920) has accordingly differentiated flow capillaries (Stromcapillaren) and net capillaries (Netzcapillaren) in the swimming membrane of frogs. In numerous studies by Zweifach and his associates (Zweifach, 1939, 1940a; Chambers and Zweifach, 1944, 1947) these two types of capillaries were described in great detail. The most direct arteriovenous pathways have been called "arterio-venous capillaries," "arterio-venous bridges," "muscular capillaries," "thoroughfare channels," and "preferential channels." The authors attempted to find an anatomical basis for their differentiation from other microvessels in the capillary networks. However, in further investigations, proceeding from their functional features two types of capillaries have been distinguished in capillary networks (Mchedlishvili, 1957, 1985). Schmid-Schönbein (1976, 1977) also regards the various capillary types as functionally different microvessels and calls them "main arteriovenous pathways." We shall refer to the types of capillaries below as the main capillaries and the second-order type, the net capillaries. In the capillary networks where a

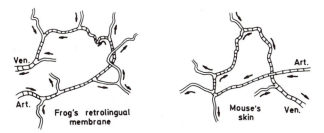

Fig. 6.24. Patterns of main capillaries with side branches in
            amphibia (left) and mammal (right) made with a
            drawing device under a microscope (magnification:
            left, 56×; right, 280×). Arrows show the direc-
            tion of blood flow. (Reproduced from Mchedlish-
            vili, 1958.)

number of microvessels are positioned in parallel between the arterioles
and venules, the main capillaries are merely those which have the least
hydraulic resistance. In all probability, these capillaries should exist
in the cerebral microvascular bed as well. But since the capillary networks have not been examined *in vivo* so far in the brain from this viewpoint, we should consider the distribution of flow in the capillary networks of flat organs as a model of the microcirculation in cerebral tissue.

The principal feature of the main capillaries is that they form the
shortest and the most direct route between arterioles and venules and have
a faster flow rate. Other capillaries branch off from the initial portion
of main capillaries, forming side branches that branch further and finally
merge with the distal part of the same or a neighboring main capillary
(Fig. 6.24). Usually the side branches shoot off from the main capillaries
at more or less right angles. Due to further branching and interanastomos-
ing of the side branches, they form the capillary networks as such,
i.e., the basic mass of the blood capillaries. Estimation of the
microvascular diameter and the blood flow velocity in both the main capillaries and the adjacent side branches (Mchedlishvili, 1951, 1958) has
shown that both values are usually greatest at the origin and the end of
the main capillaries, and the least in their middle portion, between the
last offshooting and the first joining capillaries (Fig. 6.25). Both vascular diameter and flow velocity are always greater in the main capillaries than in the adjoining side branches. For instance, in the frog's retrolingual membrane the diameter of main capillaries is larger than that of
their adjoining side branches by an average of 24%, the linear velocity of
flow by a mean of 36%, and the volume velocity (calculated from those
values) by 65%.

The initial portion of main capillaries — usually about 1/7 to 1/5 of
their length both in frogs' retrolingual membrane and in mice skin — represent the transient portion of the arterioles into the capillaries (i.e.,
the metarterioles, according to Zweifach). The walls here contain isolated
muscle cells which cause rhythmic fluctuations of the vessel diameter (a
type of vasomotion). The remainder of the main capillaries, up to their
transition into venules, i.e., over most of their length, has a wall structure generally identical to that of the true capillaries, i.e., devoid of
true muscle cells. Some of the side branches offshooting from the initial
part of main capillaries contain isolated muscle cells, while the rest
originate from nonmuscular capillaries (Mchedlishvili, 1958).

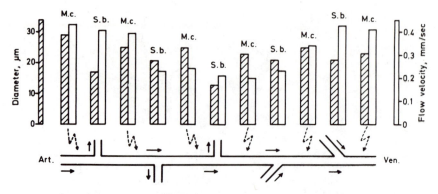

Fig. 6.25. Diameters and flow velocities in the main capillary and its
            side branches in frogs' retrolingual membrane. The diameter
            and blood flow velocity along the main capillary (M.c.) de-
            crease peripheral to the offshooting of each side branch (S.b.),
            but the diameter and velocity increase when other side branches
            have joined its venous portion. The least diameter and slow-
            est blood flow is between the last offshooting and the first
            joining side branches. On the bottom is a schematic drawing
            of a main capillary with its side branches. (Data from Mched-
            lishvili, 1958.)

     Existence of the main capillaries, with their specific length, diam-
eter, and blood flow velocity, does not, however, provide evidence for the
presence of specific "structural units" in the capillary networks, as had
been assumed by Zweifach. It seems to be more reasonable to suppose that
the main capillaries appear in the course of formation of capillary networks either in embryonic or in postnatal periods. The blood flow then becomes greater in those microvessels which form the shortest and most direct
route from the arterioles to the venules and therefore possess the least
hydraulic resistance to blood flow (Mchedlishvili, 1958; Schmid-Schönbein,
1976). Consequently, these capillaries play the functional role of main
capillaries. The other capillaries, which offshoot from them as side
branches, are longer and have more bifurcations and therefore have greater
resistance and slower flow rate. Thus, the proper capillary network forms.

     However, if the physiological conditions were altered (e.g., if the
feeding arterioles, draining venules, or main capillaries became obstructed), one of the neighboring microvessels could take over the functions of
the main capillaries. This type of transformation has been repeatedly observed in experiments by this author (Mchedlishvili, 1958). Schmid-
Schönbein stated more recently that such a vessel could be, but need not
always be, anatomically defined; moreover, it need not always be exactly
the same vessel. Vessels may take turns in performing this function,
adapting to different physiological effects. Obviously, long, narrow
capillaries are unlikely candidates for this function, whereas any type of
short arteriovenous pathways, especially those with a larger diameter, is
predisposed to operate as a main arteriovenous channel, i.e., a main capillary (Schmid-Schönbein, 1976, p. 46).

     The question arises: How can the structural characteristics of the
main capillaries mentioned by Zweifach, particularly the distribution of

muscle cells in the arteriolar portion, be explained? This seems to be related to the rate of blood flow in these vessels. A similar dependence of
structural transformation of blood vessels on the blood flow rate was
noted long ago by Thoma (1893). In addition, this phenomenon has been confirmed by Clark and Clark (1940) in direct observations of the transparent
chambers of rabbit ears. Following an increase in blood flow in newly
formed microvessels, the adventitial cells change into muscle cells.
Thus, the appearance of the structural characteristics in the walls of the
main capillaries is undoubtedly dependent on the functional characteristics
of the blood flow inside them.

Although experimental data on the presence of the main and the net
capillaries in the microvascular beds have not been obtained so far in the
brain, the results of studies in flat organs may nevertheless serve as a
model for the more complicated, three-dimensional capillary networks of the
cerebral tissue. Undoubtedly during the embryonic formation of capillary
networks, or when the tissue structure or the microcirculation become
altered in the postnatal period, some capillaries form in privileged hemodynamic conditions, i.e., when there is a minimum hydraulic resistance to
blood flow. These capillaries usually have: (a) the shortest distance
for blood flow from the arterioles to venules, (b) comparatively larger
luminal diameters, and (c) minimum curvatures along their course. Hence,
the blood flow in these capillaries becomes notably higher than in the
neighboring microvessels with higher resistance. The latter must be the
offshoots of the arterial part of the main capillaries, which branch further on (creating, in turn, supplementary hindrance to the blood flow at
each bifurcation), and ultimately merge with the venous portion. If the
blood flow conditions in the capillary network change, other capillaries,
having advantageous hemodynamic conditions, will transform into main capillaries. The principle of general hemodynamics in the capillary network,
however, should always remain the same; this is very important for the
mechanisms of distribution of blood flow in capillary networks.

Changeable Distribution of Blood Streams in Capillary Networks. In
view of the fact that the microvessels are organized into variously shaped
networks of capillaries, i.e., a number of parallel microvessels situated
between arterioles and venules, the rate of microcirculation in a given
tissue ultimately depends on the distribution of blood in the networks.
Thus it seems evident that blood flowing from the feeding arteries to the
capillary networks first reaches the "main capillaries," or "main arterio-
venous pathways" (Schmid-Schönbein, 1976) that form the shortest path to
the venules. But these capillaries represent only a small part of the
microvessels in the networks. The major part of the networks consists of
the capillaries which branch off from the initial portion of main capillaries, branch further, and finally join the main capillaries in their
venous portion. Therefore, from the point of view of both the flow rate
at a given moment and the changes in microcirculation, primary consideration must be given to the problem of the determinants of blood flow in the
side branches of the main capillaries.

Zweifach (1939) has noted that blood flow is more constant in the
main capillaries than in the side branches which form the capillary networks. According to this view (Chambers and Zweifach, 1944), it is the
precapillary sphincters (see p. 260) that control the blood flow from the
main capillaries into their side branches. Constriction of the sphincters
results in restriction of the blood flow into the branches up to their
complete exclusion from circulation. However, the perennial investigations of microcirculation during increases and decreases in flow in both
the retrolingual membrane of frogs and the skin of white mice showed that

the precapillary sphincters do not play an important part in distribution
of blood in capillary networks. In particular, the changes in distribution of blood in the microvascular bed are not related to any isolated
constriction of precapillary sphincters. Therefore, the "precapillary
sphincters" cannot be considered as a universal mechanism which determines
the flow rate in single capillary offshoots of main capillaries (as well
as in further branches of the net capillaries) because the majority of the
side branches originate from nonmuscular portions of main capillaries, and
accordingly have no muscle cells, or "sphincters," at their origin. It
was inferred from these considerations that the hemodynamic phenomena in
the capillary networks play a crucial role in the distribution of blood in
the capillary networks, which are primarily dependent on flow conditions
in the feeding arteries and the main capillaries (Mchedlishvili, 1958).

Periodic fluctuations in the diameter of the feeding arteries, called
vasomotion (Chambers and Zweifach, 1947), has recently been demonstrated
in the pial arteries of various diameter (Auer, 1981). Vasomotion alone
can result only in periodic fluctuations of capillary blood flow which do
not exceed about 10% of the given level. Thus, changes in blood distribution in capillary networks, due to significant physiological or pathological processes, are more affected by the mean diameter of the feeding
arterial vessels.

Because the side branches of main capillaries form the basic capillary networks, the question arises concerning what factors actually determine the rate of blood flow in those side branches. In order to flow into
the branches, the blood has to overcome the frictional forces resisting
blood flow along the entire span of these branches and their ramifications,
particularly: (a) at the side of their offshooting from the main capillaries, (b) all along the span of the branches including their subsequent
bifurcations and interconnections, and (c) at the joining site to the
venular portion of main capillaries. It stands to reason that all these
resistances are overcome by the pressure difference between the origin
and the end of these capillaries. Since they are actually side branches
of main capillaries, shooting off from their arterial and joining their
venous portions, the total resistance along the net capillaries is overcome by the arteriovenous pressure differences in respective main capillaries, that is, the pressure difference between the A and V in Fig. 6.26.
The greater the pressure difference $(P_A - P_V)$, the higher the blood flow
rate in the side branches of main capillaries and in the whole capillary
network. If the pressure difference $(P_A - P_V)$ is not enough to overcome
the resistance all along the side branches, blood flow should stop in
these branches.

The next problem considered by the author (Mchedlishvili, 1951, 1958)
was the following: What determines the arteriovenous pressure difference
$(P_A - P_V)$ in the main capillaries of a microvascular network? In general,
it should depend on the resistance along the main capillaries, i.e., between the points A and V in Fig. 6.26. If we consider an isolated main
capillary, the high resistance along its course results in a great expenditure of energy and hence a considerable pressure drop. Thus, the
pressure in the venous end (P_V) will be much lower than in its arterial
portion (P_A), and the pressure gradient $(P_A - P_V)$ will be large. Conversely, if the resistance along the main capillary is small, the pressure difference in the main capillary will decrease. It is known that the resistance in any blood vessel, including the main capillaries, depends on a
number of factors. These are the distance between the given points, the
microvessel diameter, the velocity of flow, and the viscosity of the flowing blood. Since the distance between two points in a capillary network

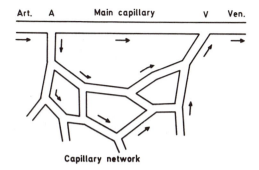

Fig. 6.26.   Main capillary with side branches form-
             ing capillary networks. The blood flow
             velocity in the capillary network is
             determined by the pressure gradient be-
             tween the arterial and venous portions
             of the main capillary, i.e., $(P_A - P_V)$.
             See text for details. (Reproduced from
             Mchedlishvili, 1970.)

remains constant and the diameter of true capillaries does not change primarily during acute changes in microcirculation (see pp. 269-270), it seems
doubtful that these factors would play an essential role in the changes of
blood distribution in capillary networks. Therefore, two other factors,
i.e., the velocity of blood flow and the viscosity of flowing blood, probably have a decisive role in the distribution of blood in capillary networks.

     Evidence for this conclusion has been obtained in experiments where
the perfusion of the whole capillary network was attained only when the
flow velocity was sufficiently high to overcome the resistance in the whole
capillary network (Gontscharoff, 1935; Gedevanishvili and Javrishvili, 1948).
In addition, the dependence of the distribution of blood, or other perfusing fluids, in capillary networks on their viscosity, has been shown in
the experiments by Zweifach (1940b). Perfusion of frogs' tongues with
Ringer's solution allowed the solution to pass only through the main capillaries, without entering their side branches, while colloid solutions
and suspensions flowed both in the main capillaries and their side
branches. The latter phenomenon is certainly dependent on a comparatively high viscosity of the perfusing fluids, creating sufficient resistance in main capillaries, so that the arteriovenous pressure difference along them (i.e., $P_A - P_V$ in Fig. 6.26) becomes sufficient to overcome resistance in the side branches of the entire capillary network.

     The assumption that the blood flow rate in the capillary networks,
formed by the side branches of the main capillaries, depends on the arterio-
venous pressure difference along the main capillaries has been examined in
studies of blood distribution in capillary networks after experimentally
produced increases (arterial hyperemia) and decreases (ischemia) in microcirculation (Mchedlishvili, 1951). Enhancement of blood circulation in
capillary networks has been produced by dilatation of the feeding arteries
(e.g., by local administration of acetylcholine or histamine) in frogs'
retrolingual membranes or the skin of white mice. The diameter of the
capillaries does not appreciably change under these conditions, but the

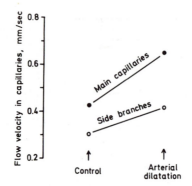

Fig. 6.27. Blood flow velocity changes (average
            values) in main capillaries and their
            adjacent side branches following ar-
            terial dilatation. Following dilata-
            tion of the feeding arteries (in frogs'
            retrolingual membrane), the increase in
            the arteriovenous pressure difference
            along the main arteriovenous pathways
            causes a greater increase in blood flow
            velocity in main capillaries than in
            their side branches, which form capil-
            lary networks. This is evidence that
            an enhanced distribution of blood in
            the capillary networks is determined by
            flow conditions in the main capillaries.
            See text for details. (Reproduced from
            Mchedlishvili, 1958.)

velocity of blood flow in the capillaries increases. However, the velocity increase in the main capillaries is considerably more pronounced than
that seen in their side branches (Fig. 6.27). The increase in blood velocity in the main capillaries is a direct consequence of the increased
arteriovenous pressure difference along these microvessels; this essential-
ly means that the pressure difference between the inlet and outlet points
of the side branches (i.e., the $P_A - P_V$ in Fig. 6.26) undergoes respective
increases, giving rise to an enhancement of blood flow in these capillary
branches, and ultimately in the whole capillary networks.

Diverse changes have been detected in capillary networks following a
sharp decrease in microcirculation. Upon gradual narrowing of the feeding
arteries, which causes ischemia, the blood flow rate decreases both in the
main capillaries and in their side branches. Figure 6.28 shows the average reduction in the blood flow velocity associated with varying degrees
of ischemia. The velocity reduction is more pronounced in the main capillaries than in their side branches. The reduction of flow in the main
capillaries indicates decreases in the arteriovenous pressure difference
along their course, since the diameter of capillaries remains constant.
This means that the pressure gradient between points A and V, i.e., $P_A -$
P_V in Fig. 6.26, decreases. Since this is the case, the difference in
the inlet and outlet pressures of the side branches, forming the capillary
network, correspondingly decreases. This in turn results in a decrease in
the blood flow in the side branches, but this is less pronounced than that
seen in the respective main capillaries. When ischemia reaches a certain

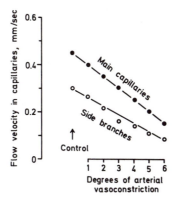

Fig. 6.28.   Blood flow velocity changes (average
             values) in main capillaries and their
             adjacent side branches following ar-
             terial constriction. Following gradual
             obstruction of the feeding arteries
             (in frogs' retrolingual membrane), the
             decrease in the arteriovenous pressure
             difference along the main arteriovenous
             pathways causes a greater decrease of
             blood flow velocity in main capillaries
             than in their side branches, which form
             capillary networks. This is evidence
             that a reduced distribution of blood in
             the capillary networks is determined by
             flow conditions in the main capillaries.
             See text for details. (Reproduced from
             Mchedlishvili, 1958.)

stage, the side branches of the main capillaries gradually transform into
plasmatic capillaries, devoid of red cell flow. This phenomenon is considered below (see pp. 269-271). All of these hemodynamic events occur in
spite of the fact that the luminal size of capillaries does not change
considerably.

     The blood distribution shifts between the main capillaries and their
branches during obstruction of the draining veins. Slowing down of blood
flow is more pronounced in the main capillaries than in their side branches,
so that the blood velocity in the latter can become even greater than in
the main capillaries (Fig. 6.29). This phenomenon can be explained by the
increased resistance to blood outflow into venules, while blood is still
flowing into their side branches and then possibly into collateral venous
routes. Therefore, experimental results on the typical changes in microcirculation confirm the initial hypothesis that the distribution of blood
flow in capillary networks depends on the arteriovenous pressure difference in the main capillaries, which in turn depends on resistance changes
in the feeding arteries (during cases of arterial hyperemia and ischemia)
and the blood outflow into the veins (venous blood stagnation).

     Active and Nonactive Capillaries. It has long been demonstrated that
a significant portion of capillaries is always cut off from the microcirculation. This means that the number of active capillaries is changeable;
this significantly affects the efficiency of both enhancements and reduc-

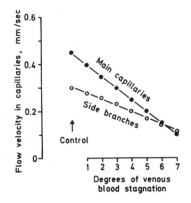

Fig. 6.29. Blood flow velocity changes (average
values) in main capillaries and their
adjacent side branches during venous
blood stagnation. The figure shows the
same relationship as in Fig. 6.28, but
the flow in the side branches of main
capillaries is less decreased than during ischemia due to blood outflow
through the side branches into collateral pathways. (Data from Mchedlishvili, 1958.)

tions in the rate of microcirculation. In particular, the more capillaries that are active in a microvascular bed, the less distance the metabolic substances must diffuse in order to reach tissue elements, and back.

Direct evidence for changes in the number of active capillaries in
tissues was obtained as far back as the beginning of the 19th century.
Kaltenbrunner (1826) observed a sharp augmentation of active capillaries
during inflammation, and this was further confirmed by other researchers.
A rich network of previously invisible capillaries is always seen during
inflammation (Voronin, 1959). A significant increase in the number of
active capillaries has been shown in skeletal muscle following contraction
(Krogh, 1922; Martin et al., 1932; Sjöstrand, 1935). Alterations in the
number of active capillaries have been demonstrated in rabbits' cerebral
cortices (Mchedlishvili, 1956b) during various experiments (Table 1).

The ability of blood vessels to be cut off from the circulation is
particularly characteristic of the capillaries, although this is somewhat
characteristic of the smaller arteries and veins as well. This ability of
the capillaries is, in all probability, related first to the actual luminal diameter of the true capillaries, which is equal to or even smaller
than the red cell (see pp. 245-247). Therefore, the capillary lumen can no
longer contract without disturbing the blood flow; the diameter of true
capillaries also cannot be significantly increased, especially in the
brain, since there is no free space surrounding the capillary wall to expand (the interstitial spaces in the brain are rather small). Second, the
structure of the capillary walls is perfectly adjusted to transport various substances between the blood and surrounding tissue, but is not adapted for producing dynamic changes in the vascular diameter. There are no
specific contractile elements, such as smooth muscle cells, to change
actively the vascular tone in the capillaries.

Table 1. Changes in the Number and Diameter of Active Capillaries in Rabbits' Cerebral Cortices (parietal region) under
Various Experimental Conditions.*

Experimental conditions	Mean number of active capil- laries (per 0.1 mm^2 of slices)	Mean diameter of capillaries (microns)
Obstruction of both carotid arteries	23	6.2
Breathing a gas mixture rich in carbon dioxide	29	7.1
Asphyxia (occlusion of tracheotomy tube)	39	8.6
Purulent leptomeningitis	39	7.6
India ink injection into brain vessels	53	—
Silver impregnation of capillary walls	53	—

*The data were obtained from transverse histological slices
following tissue fixation *in situ* (the depth of focus was
standard).

The changes in number of active capillaries is a very effective means
for the optimal performance of their function. With the changes in number
of active capillaries, the total area of their walls, through which all
essential substances are transported from blood to tissue and vice versa,
changes correspondingly. Further, the changes in the number of active
capillaries is the most effective means to change the cross-sectional area
of the microvascular bed for enhancing or reducing the blood flow rate in
microvessels without altering the velocity of blood flow significantly.
The latter would inevitably lead to significant changes in resistance in
the capillaries, which have a very small luminal diameter and hence a
great resistance to blood flow (Lipowsky et al., 1978).

Careful investigation of the process of transformation of the active
capillaries into nonactive forms, and vice versa, has led to the conclusion
that blood capillaries can exist in the following three functional states:
(a) active capillaries filled with flowing blood, including both plasma
and cells, (b) plasmatic capillaries whose diameter remains normal, but
only blood plasma without cells flows through them, and (c) closed capillaries with completely, or almost completely, contracted lumen (Mchedlishvili, 1958). Every capillary can take on one of these forms during changes
in microcirculation. One can observe in the process of these changes
transitional forms of blood capillaries, such as plasmatic capillaries,
through which individual red cells flow, or capillaries with a partially
contracted lumen. The presence of these transitional forms confirms that
these capillaries may readily be transformed from one form into another.
The lumen of blood capillaries is typically either open or closed, but
never dilated or contracted, which is typical for arteries and veins of
various caliber (see below).

The significance of the plasmatic capillaries in the process of transformation of active capillaries into the nonactive forms, and vice versa,
was directly shown in the early 1950s during an investigation of microcirculatory events in the course of the development of ischemia and ar-

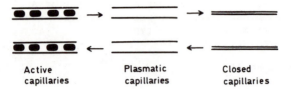

Active   Plasmatic   Closed
capillaries   capillaries   capillaries

Fig. 6.30. Stages of transformation of active capil-
            laries into closed forms, and vice versa.
            During cutoff of the active capillaries
            from microcirculation, they transform in-
            to plasmatic capillaries and only then do
            they close. When the process of capil-
            lary transformation goes in the opposite
            direction, the closed capillaries first
            become plasmatic capillaries, i.e., their
            lumen opens and fills with plasma without
            red cells, and only then do they trans-
            form into active capillaries. (Repro-
            duced from Mchedlishvili, 1969b.)

terial hypermia (Mchedlishvili, 1951). The plasmatic capillaries are an
intermediate stage between the active and closed capillaries. When cut
off from the circulation, an active capillary always changes first into a
plasmatic form and closes. The opposite occurs when the closed capillaries
start to open. They are first filled with pure plasma, i.e., they transform into plasmatic capillaries, and only afterwards do they fill with
whole blood (Fig. 6.30).

The brain capillaries have not yet been investigated in detail. There
is indirect evidence that the nonactive capillaries usually remain open,
i.e., plasmatic. In microscopic preparations of hundreds of capillaries,
impregnated with silver by Klosovsky's technique, only a small amount of
"closed" (i.e., considerably narrowed) capillaries have been found. If
the majority of the nonactive capillaries in the brain are indeed plasmatic, this might be of great physiological importance for the brain; the
need for transformation of nonactive capillaries into active capillaries
can arise suddenly, and the opening of previously closed capillaries could
slow down this process (Mchedlishvili, 1956b). Direct observation in the
retina (where the circulation is probably similar to the cerebral circulation) has shown that only some capillaries (about 30%) contain flowing
blood and all the rest are plasmatic (Thuránszky, 1956).

The transformation of active capillaries into plasmatic capillaries,
and vice versa, during increases and decreases in circulation occurs in
spite of the fact that the vascular lumina actually remains unchanged along
all microvessels. In this case the occurrence of plasmatic capillaries is
by no means related to local narrowing of any part of the microvascular
bed, where the red cells could be trapped but the plasma could still flow
(as had been supposed by earlier researchers: Jacobj, 1920; Nesterov,
1929; Zweifach and Kossman, 1937; Clark and Clark, 1943). The pure hemo-
rheological nature of this phenomenon has recently been confirmed (Mchedlishvili and Varazashvili, 1981a, 1982b).

The mechanism of transformation of active capillaries into plasmatic
forms, and vice versa, involves red cell:plasma ratio changes in microcir-

culation, which is considered in more detail below. The main cause of transformation of a great number of active capillaries into plasmatic forms during decreasing microcirculation is the reduction of the red cell:plasma ratio in blood flowing into the capillary network from the feeding arteries. The transformation of individual capillaries into the plasmatic form is, in turn, dependent on the blood flow velocities in the branches formed at capillary bifurcations and on the angles of capillary offshoots from the feeding capillaries (see pp. 286-289).

Thus, the plasmatic capillaries play an important role in changing the number of active capillaries. They represent an intermediate stage between active and closed capillaries, and in some instances can be considered as a form of nonactive capillaries. During the cutoff of the capillaries from circulation, their initial transformation into plasmatic forms is important since it creates the necessary conditions for complete closing of capillaries; trapped red cells have never been observed under these conditions.

The "closure" and opening of blood capillaries are somewhat different from the constriction and dilatation of arteries, although in both cases changes in vascular lumina occur. The principal difference between the capillary and arterial diameter changes is related to differences in vessel wall tension due to structural differences. The specific contractile elements of the arterial walls, smooth muscle cells, possess an active tone which is continually controlled by neurogenic and humoral stimuli. The capillary walls contain no specific contractile elements, but this does not mean that the endothelial cells and the surrounding connective tissue, or glial, structures are completely passive with respect to their mobility in response to some physiological stimuli.

Vascular diameter, regardless of the type of vessel, is primarily dependent on the relationship between wall tension and intravascular pressure. The narrowing and complete closure of the capillary lumina should occur when the vessel wall tension prevails over the intravascular pressure, and vice versa. The lower the intracapillary pressure, the more readily the capillaries are closed. The factors which determine changes in intracapillary pressure have already been considered (see pp. 234-236). It is only during a reduced rate of microcirculation, caused by the constriction of feeding arteries, that the microvascular pressure decreases and creates favorable conditions for closing of the capillary lumina. An opposite situation is seen during enhanced microcirculation caused by arterial dilatation: the intracapillary pressure increases and promotes the opening of previously closed capillaries.

The tension of capillary walls, the "contractility of the capillaries," has been investigated over the last 100 years. When the intravascular pressure is low (live tadpole tails in early stages of development or isolated nictitating and swimming membranes of frogs), direct electrical, mechanical, and chemical stimulation of capillary walls results in protrusion of the endothelial cell nuclei into the vessel lumen (Golubew, 1869; Tarchanoff, 1874; Tarkanoff, 1875; Stricker, 1877; Kahn and Pollak, 1931; Field, 1935). In recent studies (Lübbers et al., 1979) the contraction of capillary endothelial cells in frog mesenteries following direct electrical stimulation was observed, but not in all cells. However, in mammals, under conditions in which the blood flow in capillaries is preserved, local stimulation of the capillary walls results only in an insignificant protrusion of the endothelial cells into the lumina without notable change in blood flow (Zweifach, 1934; Zweifach and Kossman, 1937). Careful studies in rabbits' ear transparent chambers led to the conclusion that the contractility of the capillary walls is so weak under natural conditions that it cannot independently regulate the blood flow in microvessels (Sandison, 1932; Clark and Clark, 1932, 1939, 1940, 1943). Only in cases when the blood flow in capillaries has been reduced due to constriction of feeding arterioles do the endothelial nuclei protrude into the capillary lumina, hence contributing to their narrowing. These experimental findings have demonstrated that the structural components of capillary walls possess the capacity to contract. This property can be seen only when the intracapillary pressure is low; under natural conditions this is usually due to constriction of the feeding arteries.

The problem as to which of the structural elements of capillary walls are responsible for this contractility cannot as yet be considered solved. The endothelial protrusion into the capillary lumina has led some investigators to propose that the luminal contraction is due to active constriction of the endothelial cells themselves. However, the contraction of the structural elements surrounding the endothelial cells could also cause the endothelial thickening. This was convincingly proved in computations by Hutt and Wick (1954). Furthermore, Kolossov (1893) has observed endothelial contraction during inflammation, with concomitant sharp dilatation of capillaries, thus proving that the constriction of the endothelial cell itself does not necessarily result in luminal contraction. In this case, however, the contraction of endothelial cells certainly plays an important part in increasing the capillary permeability.

The comparative role of the endothelial cells and the surrounding connective tissue structures (covering the cells from the outside) in the expansion of the capillary lumina was carefully investigated by Voronin (1897), who came to the conclusion that only the outside structures determine the mechanical properties of the capillary walls and are hence responsible for significant dilatation in the focus of inflammation. This has been confirmed in further investigations (Nagel, 1934; Burton, 1954). Summarizing the present evidence for the distensibility of capillary walls, Fung (1978) has concluded that the distensibility of capillary blood vessels with respect to blood pressure depends almost completely on the surrounding media and only about 1% is dependent on the capillary wall itself.

The adventitial cells of the capillaries, usually called pericytes, are connective tissue elements with all their specific properties. Clark and Clark (1940) have directly observed in rabbits' ear transparent chambers the way in which the adventitial cells transform into smooth muscle cells when the capillaries transform into arterioles. In addition, the adventitial cells have been shown to take part in the formation of endothelial cells during growth of capillaries in the brain (Klosovsky, 1951). On the other hand, some histologists classify the adventitial cells of capillaries as specific contractile elements of these microvessels (Rouget, 1873, 1874, 1879; Mayer, 1902; Vimtrup, 1922). This concept was widely admitted in the 1920's thanks to August Krogh's popular works (Krogh, 1920, 1921, 1922); the cells became known as the Rouget cells at this time. However, convincing evidence against the specific contractile properties of the adventitial cell of capillaries (comparable to smooth muscle cells of larger blood vessels) was obtained in the 1930s: they reacted in various ways to direct stimulation with a micromanipulator, but never caused contraction of the capillaries (Zweifach, 1934; Rogers, 1935; Zweifach and Kossman, 1937). Changes in the form of the capillary pericytes following the administration of vasoconstrictor drugs have been found in newer studies with electron microscopy (Tilton et al., 1979), but whether this contributes significantly to changes of the vessel lumina, particularly during closing of the capillaries, remains unsolved. It has also been proposed that the contractility of neuroglial cells might affect the luminal changes in the brain capillaries (Monro, 1979), but this has not been proved convincingly. Thus, in spite of the fact that the investigation of the problem of the contractility of capillary walls, contributing to closure of the lumina during their cutoff from the microcirculation, has a long history, our knowledge is still incomplete.

Two main factors are involved in the mechanism of blood capillary closure and opening: the intravascular pressure and the wall tension. These two factors are interrelated in the law of Laplace: $T \approx Pr/d$, where T stands for vessel wall tension, P stands for intravascular pressure, r stands for luminal radius, and d stands for vessel wall thickness (see pp. 191-192 in Chapter 5). According to this relationship the actual vessel radius, as well as the wall thickness, is important in changes in capillary lumina. The intravascular pressure is always multiplied by the luminal radius and divided by the wall thickness. It follows that when a capillary starts to narrow and its radius decreases, the value of Pr/d becomes smaller than that of T, thus resulting in a disturbance of the balance in the Laplace relationship. Hence the wall tension promotes further narrowing of the microvessel until the lumen closes completely. Conversely, when the previously closed capillary has already started to open by the intravascular pressure, the luminal radius increases and this promotes further widening of the lumen (because of the increase in the radius and the decrease in wall thickness) until the lumen opens to a maximum. This maximal luminal size corresponds to the structure of the vessel wall and the surrounding connective tissue or glial elements. Therefore, the capillaries are primarily in one of the two extreme states: open or closed (Voronin, 1947).

The closing of the blood capillary lumina has its peculiarities. The narrowing of their lumina never starts immediately following a decrease in intravascular pressure. This was observed in studies of isolated tissues (Roy and Brown, 1879) and then during ischemia caused by obstruction or tangible constriction of the feeding arteries (Mchedlishvili, 1951, 1958; Mchedlishvili and Varazashvili, 1981a). It is not yet clear why the closing of capillaries has such a long latent period. This may be related to the structural and functional characteristics of capillary walls, which respond to stimuli differently than the muscle elements of the larger vessels. Three conclusions can be drawn from these findings. First, the capillary walls are devoid of elastic properties in the usual sense. Second, the "critical closing pressure" of the vessels, which is important for small arteries in some cases (Burton, 1951), does not play an essential role in the capillaries. Third, a certain time period is probably necessary to accumulate vasoactive substances near the capillary walls to cause their contraction. Following the lowering of pressure in the capillaries, which have become plasmatic, adrenaline promotes their closing (unpublished data by Andjaparidze in the author's laboratory). This is evidence that some physiological stimuli and the specific "contractility" of the capillary walls are involved in their closure following a drop in intravascular pressure. The responsibility of physiological stimuli for the contraction of capillary walls is of great importance. These stimuli may be the effects of physiologically active substances which diffuse to the capillary walls, i.e., neurotransmitters from nerve fibers and terminals near the arterioles or active substances originating in the surrounding tissue as "local hormones," as well as some metabolic substances (catecholamines, acetylcholine, histamine, prostaglandins, vasoactive peptides, etc.). Furthermore, the capillaries seem never to be closed when even a single red cell is still inside their lumina. It is uncertain whether the lowering of oxygen tension or some other factor, occurring in the absence of red cells inside the capillary lumina, might be involved in the process of capillary closing.

Even if the "mobility," or "contractility," of capillary walls is dependent only, or mostly, on the endothelium, connective tissue, or the glial cells surrounding the vessel walls, complete closure of the vessel lumen is possible only as a result of endothelial cell thickening (since the perimeter's length can never reach zero). Following shortening of the adventitial perimeter, the endothelium inevitably thickens and protrudes into the vessel lumen, thus promoting complete closure of the capillaries.

Thus, in spite of the fact that the capillary wall contractility is very weak, it is sufficient to close the capillary lumen. At first, the capillaries transform into plasmatic forms, keeping their initial lumen unchanged, and then the lowered intracapillary pressure creates the necessary conditions for contraction of their walls, resulting in closure of their lumen. The opening of the blood capillaries also goes through a plasmatic stage and then the capillaries become filled with flowing blood, including red cells and plasma, indistinguishable from the neighboring active capillaries.

6.4. RED CELL:PLASMA RATIO (RED CELL CONCENTRATION, LOCAL HEMATOCRIT) IN BLOOD FLOWING THROUGH MICROVESSELS

The relationship of red cells to plasma in blood flowing in peripheral, including cerebral, vascular beds is highly significant for the following reasons: First, the red blood cells, as oxygen carriers in the blood, determine the oxygen supply to respective tissue regions. Second, the red cell concentration determines the viscosity and fluidity of the blood in microvessels (see pp. 241-242). Third, the red cell:plasma ratio is one of the determinants of transformation of active capillaries into the inactive forms (plasmatic and closed capillaries), and vice versa, in microvascular beds (see pp. 269-271).

The first observations of local changes in the red cell:plasma ratio were probably the descriptions of the plasmatic capillaries appearing in the microvascular beds. The early reports date from the first half of the 19th century (Müller, 1837) and, in addition, the plasmatic capillaries have been described by other researchers, particularly in the classical works of the 1920s through the 1940s (Krogh, 1922; Clark and Clark, 1943; Zweifach et al., 1944). The decrease in the red cell:plasma ratio in microvessels, and the appearance of plasmatic capillaries in particular, have been interpreted by earlier researchers to be a consequence of the luminal contraction of the smallest arterioles, or precapillary sphincters, where red cells could be trapped while plasma could still flow (Jacobj, 1920; Nesterov, 1929; Zweifach and Kossman, 1937; Clark and Clark, 1943). However, virtually none of the researchers has observed an accumulation of trapped blood cells in the arteriolar lumina, including the precapillary sphincters, under such conditions. At present this conception has only a historic significance. It is generally agreed today that the red blood cells can be distributed in vascular branches independent of the blood plasma.

The arterial blood, which is pumped by the left ventricle of the heart to the aorta, initially contains a specific red cell:plasma ratio. However, the blood, distributed among the largest branches of the aorta and then via the arterial branching sequence into the thousands of microvascular regions, may attain a varying red cell:plasma ratio in different microvessels. This phenomenon may be interpreted as being relatively independent of the plasma and red cell distribution in blood throughout the

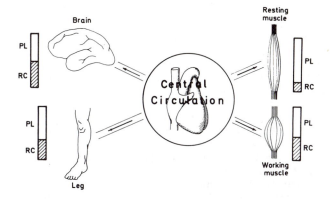

Fig. 6.31. The red cell:plasma ratio, or local hematocrit, in
            various regions of the peripheral circulation. The
            hematocrit, which is specific in arterial blood ex-
            pelled from the heart left ventricle into the aorta,
            becomes different in the peripheral circulation.
            The values of the local hematocrit are high in tis-
            sues with a high metabolic rate, e.g., in the brain
            compared to the hind leg (left side), as well as in
            working versus resting muscles (right side).

vascular system, or the separation (or screening) of red cells from plasma
during circulation (Fig. 6.31).

    The parameters which demonstrate the changeable red cell:plasma ratio
in the vascular bed are the red cell number per unit of blood volume in
the vessels and the local hematocrit value, i.e., the corpuscular volume
percentage, estimated by direct methods (centrifugation) or any indirect
method described below.

    <u>Methods for estimating the red cell:plasma ratio in the circulation</u>
must be specially considered because comparatively little is known about
them. Since each of the proposed methods has both advantages and limitations, these methods may be used only under specific experimental circumstances.

    The most direct method is the count of red cells relative to a known
plasma volume inside the vascular lumen (Mchedlishvili and Varazashvili,
1981a). However, this may be done only when all the red cells can be
seen in microvessels either in microfilms, or in microscopic preparations
where the blood flow has been suddenly stopped by *in situ* tissue fixation
(Mchedlishvili, 1958; Mchedlishvili and Varazashvili, 1981a). Another
direct and quantitative method is the red cell count or determination of
hematocrit value in blood samples taken from some vascular system or individual blood vessels under specific experimental conditions (Kostiurin,
1880; Mchedlishvili and Varazashvili, 1980). While doing this, however,
it is necessary to be certain that the obtained samples contain blood
identical to that actually flowing in the vessels at the moment of samp-
ling. For instance, the flow velocity in various capillaries, each
having a distinct hematocrit, always differs significantly; therefore, when
the blood is sampled from a cutting of tissue with a number of microvessels, only an average red cell:plasma ratio in the blood circulating in the
microvascular bed can be obtained.

Variations in the red cell:plasma ratio in microcirculation may be investigated directly in living tissue by microscopy, like that done when the
plasmatic capillaries were detected (Müller, 1837; Clark and Clark, 1943;
Zweifach et al., 1944; Mchedlishvili, 1951, 1958; Palmer, 1959; Svanes and
Zweifach, 1968). However, this has not provided researchers in the majority of cases with quantitative data on the red cell:plasma ratio in the
microvasculature under study.

The red cell:plasma ratio in the larger arteries and veins has been
estimated by determination of the red cell axial flow relative volume,
i.e., with respect to the volume of the vascular lumen. This may be done
either in photomicrographs (or cinemicrographic films) or in the microscopic preparations made after *in situ* tissue fixation (Mchedlishvili,
1956a, 1958). However, there are limitations to this method: the cross-
sectional area of the vascular lumen is considered to have a circular
shape; the width of the red cell axial flow can change with alterations in
blood flow velocity; and a certain amount of plasma is always present within the red cell axial flow.

There are several optical methods which have made it possible to determine the red cell:plasma ratio, or hematocrit, in the blood vessels.
One method permits determination of the hematocrit in relative units by
automatic counting of red cells passing through individual capillaries
placed under a phototube (Johnson et al., 1971). The red cell:plasma ratio
has also been estimated by recording the blood opacity or relative density
of capillaries measured with phototubes placed above the microvessels
(Johnson, 1971; Lipowsky et al., 1980). These methods can measure changing red cell concentrations in individual microvessels, but they yield only
qualitative or semiquantitative data on the parameter under investigation.
A modification of the optical method that provides the investigators with
quantitative data due to special calculations has been used recently, but
this requires temporary stoppage of blood flow in the vessels (Klitzman
and Duling, 1979).

Another indirect method which has been used largely for estimation of
the red cell:plasma ratio, or local hematocrit, in blood vessels is the
labeling of blood constituents with isotopes. The red cells are usually
labeled with ^{51}Cr, ^{59}Fe, or ^{32}P, and the plasma albumins are labeled with
^{131}I or with the dye T-1824 (see Lawson, 1962, for references). The main
limitation of these techniques is that the obtained results are related
not to specific microvessels but to the whole vascular bed of an organ or
a considerably large mass of tissue. In addition, it is very difficult
to obtain sufficiently accurate quantitative data on the red cell:plasma
ratio in the microcirculation using this method (Lawson, 1962).

Red Cell:Plasma Ratio or Local Hematocrit in Large and Small Blood
Vessels. Even in the 19th century, some researchers commented on the relative paucity of red cells in microvessels (Cohnstein and Zuntz, 1888).
Furthermore, Fahraeus (1929) has demonstrated the dependence of the red
cell:plasma ratio on the tube diameter in his classical experiments with
narrow glass tubes. According to the obtained results, in comparatively
narrow tubes with a lumen less than 0.3 mm, the red cell:plasma ratio decreases and the relative flow velocity of cells (as compared with plasma)
increases with a reduction in tube diameter.

The comparatively low red cell:plasma ratio in minute blood vessels
has been further demonstrated in *in vivo* experiments in which the blood
constituents were labeled with isotopes or dyes. The red cell: plasma
ratio has thus been found to be much less in the peripheral vascular beds

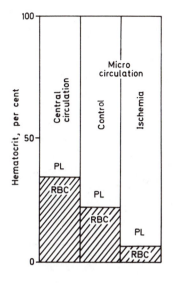

Fig. 6.32. The mean values of local hematocrit, estimated by direct counting of red cells in
microvessels with subsequent computation,
in the retrolingual membrane of frogs.
The microvascular hematocrit is considerably smaller than that in the central
circulation. The hematocrit in capillaries undergoes further decreases during
reduced microcirculation, while it is unchanged in the central circulation. (Data
from Mchedlishvili and Varazashvili, 1981a.)

of the kidneys, heart, and skeletal muscles, as well as other tissues,
than in arterial blood (Gibson et al., 1946; Dunn et al., 1958). Similar
results also have been obtained with several other techniques (Pappenheimer
and Kinter, 1956). Thus, the small peripheral blood vessels are thought
to be cell-poor in comparison with the larger vessels. However, it has
been difficult to obtain sufficiently accurate quantitative results with
these methods because of their inherent limitations (Lawson, 1962).

In the microvascular research of the 1970s, researchers, using advanced experimental techniques, have demonstrated that the amount of red
cells in the microvessels of transparent tissues (mesenterium, omentum) is
approximately one-third of that in the systemic circulation (Johnson et al.,
1971; Schmid-Schönbein and Zweifach, 1975). Further studies by Klitzman
and Duling (1979) have shown an even greater difference in hematocrit between the resting cremaster muscle capillaries and the systemic circulation, by an average of 10% and 50%, respectively. However, the difference
decreased when the muscular blood flow increased. The local hematocrit
reached ≈18.5% during working hyperemia and even ≈39.8% when the hyperemia
was enhanced by adenosine, yet the systemic hematocrit remained unchanged.
In another study (Mchedlishvili and Varazashvili, 1981a) a hematocrit of
≈23% under control conditions in the capillaries of frogs' retrolingual
membranes decreased considerably — to ≈6.7% — with a reduction in peripheral blood flow (caused by partial obstruction of the lingual arteries),
while the systemic hematocrit, ≈39%, was not changed appreciably (Fig.

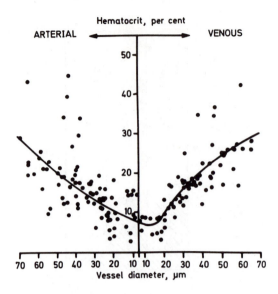

Fig. 6.33. Arteriovenous distribution of microvessel
hematocrit. For microvessels larger than
20 μm in diameter, the hematocrit was determined by the optical density method.
In smaller microvessels, the hematocrit
was determined by microocclusion. (Reproduced with permission from Lipowsky
et al., 1980.)

6.32). The gradual decrease in hematocrit in microvessels of decreasing
diameter has been clearly demonstrated in the cat mesentery (Fig. 6.33)
by estimating the optical density with a subsequent computation of the obtained data (Lipowsky et al., 1980). Further, estimations of the hematocrit in the parent and daughter branches of vascular bifurcations in the
cat's mesentery (the vascular diameter ranged from 20 to 99 μm) showed
that the daughter-to-parent ratios of local hematocrit average 0.917,
i.e., it regularly decreases following each arterial bifurcation (Lipowsky
et al., 1981).

The red cell:plasma ratio in the cerebral capillaries has been determined recently by calculating the red cell number in microscopic sections
of the parietal cortex of rabbits after *in situ* fixation (Mchedlishvili
and Varazashvili, unpublished data). Thus, the number of red cells in the
cortical capillaries has been found to be about 5,296,000 per 1 mm^3 and
the hematocrit 31%, while in the pial veins draining blood from the same
areas of the cortex the values were 6,179,000 per 1 mm^3 and 36%, respectively. The differences in the red cell:plasma ratio in the capillary and
venous blood persisted during cerebral ischemia.

Consequently, there is sufficient experimental evidence to prove that
the hematocrit is considerably smaller in the minute blood vessels, especially in capillaries, than in the larger blood vessels. The hematocrit
can also change substantially when the peripheral blood flow changes (for
further details, see below).

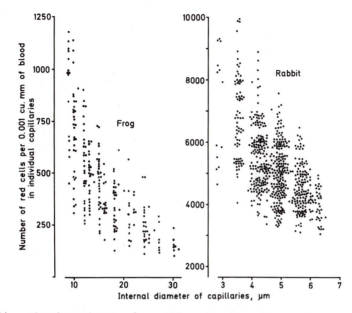

Fig. 6.34.   The dependence of capillary hematocrit on microvessel diameter.
The hematocrit in the frog retrolingual membrane (left) and the
rabbit cerebral cortex (right) increases with decreasing vessel
diameter, in contrast to larger blood vessels. This phenomenon
is presumably dependent on the flux of red cells in narrow blood
vessels in single file, since the marginal plasma layer is narrower
in the thin capillaries. (The data with amphibia are reproduced
from Mchedlishvili and Varazashvili, 1981a, and the mammals' data,
by the same authors, have not been published.)

One of the causes of this phenomenon is, in all probability, the hemodynamic effect demonstrated by Fahraeus (see p. 239). This effect was confirmed later by several researchers and further investigated in model experiments with small glass tubes perfused with human red cells (Albrecht
et al., 1979). The authors confirmed that this effect is seen only in
tubes with a considerable cell-free marginal plasma layer; in addition,
they found that in very narrow glass tubes with a diameter under 20 μm,
the relationship of the diameter to the hematocrit reverses, i.e., a further
decrease in the diameter causes an increase in the hematocrit. This phenomenon has recently been substantiated in both amphibian and mammalian
capillaries (Mchedlishvili and Varazashvili, 1981a) with a comparable size
relationship between red cells and vessel diameters (Fig. 6.34). Such a
relationship seems to be dependent chiefly on the movement of red cells in
single file at the capillary axis and, therefore, the plasma volume decreases proportionally to the thickness of the marginal cell-free plasma
layer when the microvessel diameter decreases.

This comparatively reduced hematocrit in microvessels, ranging approximately from 300 to 15 μm in diameter, is related chiefly to their luminal
sizes and less significant from the standpoint of regulation of oxygen
supply to tissues than other specific changes in the red cell:plasma ratio
in microcirculation related to the blood flow rate. The latter is considered below.

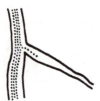

Fig. 6.35. "Plasma skimming" into an arteriolar
            branch. The arteriolar branch, which
            is narrowed at the periphery, transforms
            into a plasmatic vessel due to "plasma
            skimming" from the parent vessel. (Re-
            produced from Krogh, 1922.)

Changes in the Red Cell:Plasma Ratio Related to Flow Rate in the Peripheral Circulation. This phenomenon is of great importance from the
standpoint of both physiology and pathology, since it determines the rate
of oxygen supply to tissue and the fluidity of the blood in microvessels
(see pp. 241-242). These changes in the red cell-to-plasma ratio in circulation usually appear with changes in the microcirculation rate, which
are related to the level of tissue metabolism and activity. The phenomenon has attracted attention only recently, although evidence for it has
been gradually accumulating. In 1880, Kostiurin reported that the red
cell levels in samples of blood taken from various regions of animal and
human skin may be different. Proceeding from his animal experiments, the
author proposed that this is related to the blood flow rate. In the well-
known observation by Krogh (1922) an arteriolar branch transformed into a
plasmatic vessel after a considerable decrease in blood flow velocity. The
phenomenon of "plasma skimming" from the parent artery to the arteriolar
branch has been postulated to explain Krogh's results (Fig. 6.35). However, the actual significance of changes of red cell:plasma ratio in microcirculation could not be sufficiently understood during that period because of the paucity of available experimental data. Conclusive evidence
about the relationship between the red cell:plasma ratio and rate of regional blood flow has only been obtained in the 1950s.

The author investigated the circulatory events in the capillary bed
during considerable reductions and enhancements of peripheral circulation
(i.e., ischemia and arterial hyperemia). The issues were published in a
series of articles (Mchedlishvili, 1951, 1953, 1956a, 1957) and summarized
in a monograph (Mchedlishvili, 1958). The results were not publicized in
Western research literature and, therefore, are cited below in some detail.

In experiments with retrolingual membranes of frogs and ears of white
mice, a large number of associated capillaries were found to become converted into plasmatic forms following increases in the resistance in the
feeding arteries, although the microvascular lumina were not contracted
to a great degree and mechanical impedance for red cell transportation along
the vessels was not created. When the arterial lumen was partially obstructed
by a micromanipulator along a small portion, both the upstream and down-
stream segments of the artery became pale because of a significant reduction in red cell concentration in the blood. The red cell number could
decrease to such an extent that some arterial branches transform into plasmatic vessels. An example is shown in Fig. 6.36, where an arterial branch
became completely deprived of red cells.

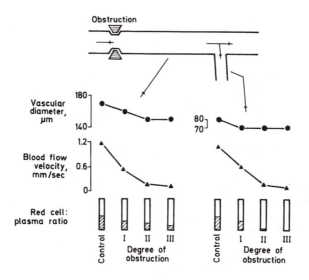

Fig. 6.36.   Decrease in the red cell:plasma ratio in arterial
             vessels during ischemia. During ischemia produced
             by gradual obstruction of the feeding artery (the
             lumen remains wide enough for red cell transporta-
             tion), the red cell:plasma ratio in the arterial
             bifurcation decreases considerably so that trans-
             formation of a side branch into a plasmatic vessel
             occurs. This is related to decrease in blood flow
             velocity, although the vessel diameter does not
             change appreciably. (Data from Mchedlishvili,
             1958.)

     In contrast, with dilatation of the feeding arteries, i.e., with ar-
terial hyperemia, a considerable number of new active capillaries, which
were previously invisible, become apparent in the microvascular region
where the blood flow is rich in red cells. However, the rather high velocity of blood flow has impeded a detailed study of the red cell:plasma
ratio in the microcirculation. This difficulty has been overcome by the
application of *in situ* tissue fixation with subsequent determination of
the red cell:plasma ratio within the blood vessels in microscopic preparations.

     The relative volume of red cell axial flow in the feeding arteries
and draining veins has been determined in the mesentery of white rats and
guinea pigs during ischemia and arterial hyperemia. The obtained data
are presented in Figs. 6.37 and 6.38. Thus, with a slowing down of the
peripheral circulation during ischemia, the concentration of red cells, or
hematocrit, in blood flowing into and out of the microvascular bed has
proved to be considerably less than during the enhanced flow rate seen in
arterial hyperemia. In these cases, the actual changes in the local hematocrit in the vessels have been detected, since the red cell axial flow
width is inversely correlated to the blood flow velocity (i.e., the axial
flow should be relatively increased during ischemia, and vice versa).
Therefore, the red cell:plasma ratio in feeding arteries and draining
veins should differ even more sharply than is shown in Figs. 6.37 and 6.38.
The quoted experimental results have been summarized in the following way:

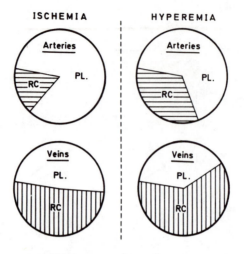

Fig. 6.37.   Changes of red cell:plasma ratio in feeding arteries and draining veins under
conditions of reduced and enhanced peripheral circulation. The mean values of
red cell axial flow (RC) and parietal
plasma layer (PL) relative volumes (relative to the total luminal volume of the
vessels) in mesenteric arteries and veins
of guinea pigs during arterial hyperemia
(due to local application of histamine or
acetylcholine) and ischemia (due to local
application of adrenaline or neurogenic
vasoconstriction) are presented. (Data
from Mchedlishvili, 1956a.)

"Consequently, with constriction of the feeding arteries (ischemia), the
blood containing relatively few red cells and much plasma is flowing across
the vascular bed, that is, from arteries into the capillaries and then into
the veins. On the contrary, with dilatation of the feeding arteries (arterial hyperemia) the blood contains, respectively, more red cells and a
small amount of plasma" (Mchedlishvili, 1958, p. 98). The obtained results are summarized in Fig. 6.39.

The following problem consequently arises: What determines the red
cell:plasma ratios in individual active capillaries? Observations (Mchedlishvili, 1958) have provided direct evidence that the factors, schematically presented in Fig. 6.40, are: (a) the angle of capillary offshoots
(inverse correlation), (b) the ratio of red cells to plasma in the feeding microvessels (direct correlation), and (c) the ratio of blood flow
velocities in branches at bifurcations (direct correlation). These blood
flow phenomena are considered in more detail below.

Several studies dealing with the unequal distribution of red cells
in microvascular bifurcations in transparent tissues have been conducted
in the late 1960s and early 1970s with different techniques (Svanes and
Zweifach, 1968; Johnson, 1971; Johnson et al., 1971). The authors obtained conclusive results confirming the principle of red cell distribution in the microvascular bifurcations. They showed convincingly that

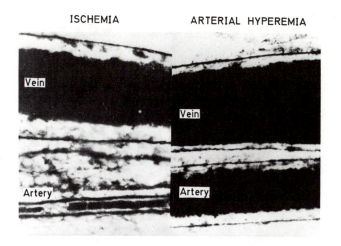

Fig. 6.38. Red cell axial flow width in mesenteric arteries and
            veins related to microcirculation rate are shown in
            these unretouched photomicrographs (the mean values
            are given in Fig. 6.37). The left figure shows a
            low red cell:plasma ratio during ischemia and the
            right figure shows a high red cell:plasma ratio dur-
            ing arterial hyperemia. To the top are veins and to
            the bottom, arteries. (Reproduced from Mchedlish-
            vili, 1969b.)

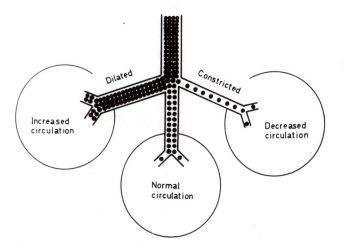

Fig. 6.39. Changes in red cell:plasma ratio in regional circu-
            lation. The concentration of red cells in blood
            flowing to regional vascular beds is related to the
            functional state of the feeding arteries. The red
            cell concentration in blood increases with an en-
            hancement of flow rate due to vasodilatation and de-
            creases with a reduction in flow due to vasocon-
            striction. (Reproduced from Mchedlishvili, 1979b.)

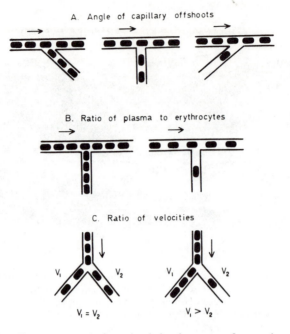

A. Angle of capillary offshoots

B. Ratio of plasma to erythrocytes

C. Ratio of velocities

V_1 V_2 V_1 V_2

$V_1 = V_2$ $V_1 > V_2$

Fig. 6.40.   Factors correlated with the transformation of indi-
             vidual capillaries into plasmatic forms are: (A)
             the angle of capillary offshoots (inverse correla-
             tion), (B) the red cell:plasma ratio in the feeding
             vessel (direct correlation), and (C) the blood flow
             velocity in the capillary branch relative to the
             other (direct correlation). See text for details.
             (Reproduced from Mchedlishvili, 1979b.)

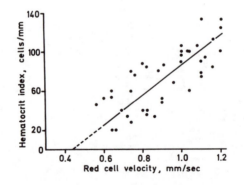

Fig. 6.41.   The linear relationship between the he-
             matocrit index and red cell velocity in
             blood capillaries showing periodic vari-
             ations in both factors. The hematocrit
             pattern is shifted forward in time to
             coincide with the velocity factor. (Re-
             produced with permission from Johnson,
             1971.)

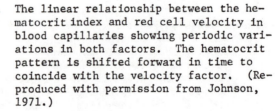

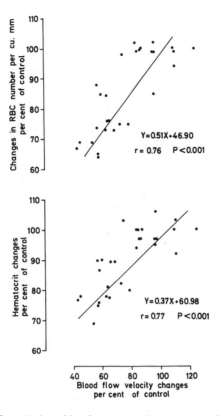

Fig. 6.42.   Red cell:plasma ratio versus the flow
              velocity in the common carotid artery.
              Changes in blood flow velocity in the
              common carotid artery (produced by
              partial obstruction of the initial por-
              tion of the vessel) in rabbits is direct-
              ly correlated with the red cell:plasma
              ratio, estimated as red blood cell num-
              ber per mm^3, and the hematocrit in the
              blood flowing through the artery. The
              blood flow velocity has been recorded
              with a Doppler ultrasound blood veloc-
              ity meter, and the red cell number and
              hematocrit have been determined direct-
              ly in blood samples from the vessels.
              See text for details. (Data of Mched-
              lishvili and Varazashvili.)

the capillary hematocrit, i.e., the red cell:plasma ratio, is dependent on
the blood flow velocity in the various branches. Johnson (1971) has demonstrated the linear relationship between the capillary hematocrit and the
blood flow velocity in the microvessel (Fig. 6.41). A linear relationship
of intravascular hematocrit and blood flow velocity has also been seen in
the large blood vessels (Fig. 6.42). Thus, it has been convincingly demonstrated that the red cell and plasma separation in the circulation occurs
not only in the microvascular bed (Mchedlishvili, 1958; Svanes and Zwei-

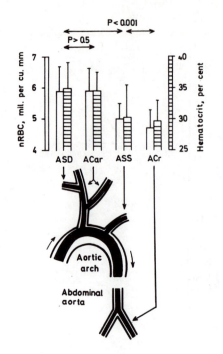

Fig. 6.43. Red cell:plasma ratio in blood distributed to different branches from the
aorta. From the aortic arch the head
and the right forelimb are supplied
with blood having a higher red cell:plasma
ratio than the left forelimb and
hind legs. ASD — arteria subclavia
dextra, ACar — the carotid arteries,
ASS — arteria subclavia sinistra, and
ACr — arteria cruralis. Explanation
in the text on p. 287.

fach, 1968; Johnson, 1971), but also in the larger arterial bifurcations
(Mchedlishvili, 1956; Klitzman and Duling, 1979; Mchedlishvili and Varazashvili, 1981b), including the largest branches of the aorta (Mchedlishvili and Varazashvili, 1981b, 1982a).

Consequently, there is convincing evidence at present that the red
cell:plasma ratio, or the local hematocrit, changes considerably in individual parts of the peripheral circulation, and this phenomenon is due to
red cell and plasma separation in the arterial branching sequence.

The mechanism of irregular red cell and plasma distribution in vascular bifurcations has not been completely understood so far. In all probability, it basically consists of biomechanical phenomena, which, in turn,
are closely related to the anatomical characteristics of the vascular bifurcations and to physiological blood flow changes.

To analyze the factors that actually determine the red cell and
plasma separation in the circulatory bed, it is necessary first to find
out at which level of arterial branching sequence this phenomenon can take

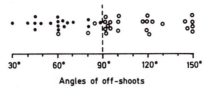

Fig. 6.44.   The distribution of angles between parent
             main capillaries and their side branches
             determines which vessels remain active,
             i.e., with red cell flow (black circles),
             or transform into plasmatic capillaries
             (white circles) during a reduction in
             microcirculation rate due to partial ob-
             struction of the feeding artery in the
             retrolingual membranes of frogs. (Re-
             produced from Mchedlishvili and Varazash-
             vili, 1982b.)

place. The separation occurs not only in the peripheral circulation, and
in microvascular bifurcations in particular, but is in evidence even in
the largest arteries, such as the main branches of the aorta. The red
cell concentration in blood distributed via the common carotid arteries to
the brain is about 20-25% higher than in the blood flowing via the abdominal aorta and crural arteries to the hind limbs (Mchedlishvili and
Varazashvili, 1981a, 1982a). In addition, the red cell concentration in
blood flowing through the right subclavian artery to the right forelimb
was found to be significantly higher than in the blood flowing through the
contralateral subclavian artery to the left forelimb (Fig. 6.43). This
unequal distribution of red cells among the different branches of the
aortic arch could contribute, first, to a preferential supply of the brain
with oxygen (Mchedlishvili and Varazashvili, 1980, 1982) and, second, to
the functional asymmetry of the body.

    Two factors seem to be primarily involved in the red cell and plasma
separation in vascular bifurcations: the anatomical arrangement of vascular branches and the related biomechanical events in the red cell and
plasma flow at the vascular bifurcations. However, the effect of anatomical vascular arrangements is different in the case of the aortic branches
and the additional arterial and microvascular branching sequences.

    Blood is expelled at every systole from the heart ventricle into the
aorta with a great velocity (ranging up to 120 cm per sec in rabbits) and
has its greatest inertia near the convexity of the aortic arch. It can be
speculated that because of the difference between the specific gravity of
red cells and plasma (the former is about 7% higher than the latter; see
Diem, 1962), the red cell axial flow is shifted to the outside wall of the
aorta (Fig. 6.43). The right subclavian and the carotid arteries (via the
brachiocephalic artery, which is variable in different species) offshoot
from the top of the aortic arch. Thus, blood with a higher hematocrit is
distributed into the right subclavian and carotid arteries.

    The angles of the arterial offshoots and the relative diameter of the
feeding and daughter arteries, which are significant in the smaller arterial bifurcations (see below), have been found to be insignificant with respect to blood distribution in the case of the aortic branches. In rab-

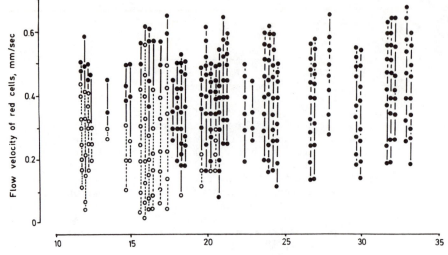

Fig. 6.45. Slowing down of blood flow velocity without changes in vessel
            diameter and transformation of some capillaries into plasmatic
            forms during ischemia. During the development of ischemia in
            the frogs' retrolingual membranes (caused by partial obstruc-
            tion of the lumen of the feeding artery) primarily those capillar-
            ies whose diameter is initially smaller (16 ± 3 μm) transform
            into plasmatic forms (white circles), but the larger ones
            (24 ± 7 μm) maintain red cell flow (black circles) at the same
            velocity. (Reproduced from Mchedlishvili and Varazashvili,
            1982b.)

bits, the red cell concentration in blood flowing in carotid arteries is
considerably higher than in crural arteries, although the angle of offshoot of the brachiocephalic artery is about 2.5 times greater and the relative diameter is about 2 times smaller in the cephalic than in the crural
artery (Mchedlishvili and Varazashvili, in preparation).

    The importance of the angles of offshoot and relative diameters of
feeding and daughter vessels for red cell distribution in microvascular
bifurcations has been demonstrated in the earlier studies (Mchedlishvili,
1958, 1969b). This was later quantified under conditions of reduced blood
inflow to the capillary networks from the feeding artery whose lumen was
narrowed in steps (Mchedlishvili and Varazashvili, 1982b). It has appeared that only those capillary side branches whose angles are right or
obtuse relative to main capillaries transform into plasmatic capillaries, but
those having an acute angle usually remain active during decreases in blood
flow in the capillary networks (Fig. 6.44). When the red cell velocity
progressively decreases in capillaries, the luminal diameter of the capillaries remains unchanged, but only the narrower capillaries transform into
plasmatic microvessels, while the larger capillaries remain active with
undisturbed red cell flow (Fig. 6.45).

    The principal biophysical mechanism responsible for the specific
red cell separation from plasma in vascular bifurcations is, in all

probability, the inertia of red cells (which have a higher specific weight than plasma) in the blood stream. Inertia drives the red cells to the outside wall of the aortic arch resulting in a higher hematocrit in blood flowing into the right subclavian and both carotid arteries (Fig. 6.43). Again, the inertia of red cells causes their more ready entrance into the capillary side branches that shoot off the main capillaries at an obtuse or right angle (Fig. 6.44).

The comparative blood flow velocity in the vascular branches formed at the bifurcations at the periphery of the aortic arch is the most important factor determining the red cell and plasma separation in the flowing blood of the arterial branching sequence. The greater the comparative blood flow velocity in a branch, the higher the concentration of red cells, and hematocrit, in blood flowing into it. Such a relationship has been demonstrated in the 1950s through the 1970s (see pp. 287-288) and has been recently confirmed in newer investigations with the living blood vessels as well as in the physical and mathematical models (Schmid-Schönbein et al., 1980b; Pries et al., 1981; Cokelet, 1982). Thus, the separation of red cells and plasma which gradually occurs along the arterial branching sequence is primarily dependent on the blood flow velocity differences at the bifurcations as well as on the angle of offshoot from parent vessels.

The biomechanical phenomena in vascular bifurcations were considered by numerous researchers in the 1970s (for references, see Gaehtgens, 1977). An important point in the unequal distribution of red cells and plasma in vascular bifurcations is thought to be the nonuniform dispersion of red cells over the cross section of the vascular lumen. The presence of an axial red cell flow and a parietal cell-free plasma layer produces favorable conditions for "plasma skimming" into the smaller side branches from the parent arteries. The slower the blood flow velocity in a side branch, the more plasma (from the marginal layer) and the fewer red cells (from the axial flow) are drawn into the branch. In experiments conducted both *in vitro* and *in vivo*, Gaehtgens (1977) explains the affect of flow rate differences in two branches on red cell flow fractionation by the division of the streamlines (isovelocity lines) causing a net surface traction and forcing the cells into the branch with the higher flow rate (Fig. 6.46).

Another factor may also be significant for the red cell and plasma separation in vascular bifurcations: the axial red cell flow contracts more than the parietal plasma layer when the arterial branch becomes constricted, while with arterial dilatation it is the axial flow that widens. This results in the respective changes in the axial flow relative volume in the arteries shown in Fig. 6.38 (Mchedlishvili, 1956b, 1958). In model experiments with glass tubes, the discharge hematocrit (the red cell:plasma ratio in blood flowing out of a glass capillary) is always lower than the tube hematocrit (Albrecht et al., 1979). Thus, there is an "adherence" of the plasma marginal layer to the vessel wall, when the layer of plasma is closely bound to the vascular wall surface. This plasma marginal layer undergoes less change during alterations in arterial diameter than in axial red cell flow. Therefore, when an artery is constricted, the corresponding vascular region gets relatively cell-poor blood, while with dilatation the opposite occurs (Mchedlishvili, 1958).

Significance of the phenomenon of the changeable red cell:plasma ratio in microcirculation seems considerable from different standpoints:

(a) The oxygen supply to tissues is only a function of the number of red cells reaching the microvessels per unit time. Therefore, a positive correlation between the red cell:plasma ratio and the blood flow rate

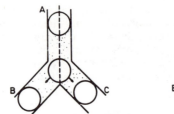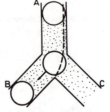

Fig. 6.46. Causes of unequal distribution of red
cells among branches in a simplified
model. Fluid is streaming from a parent trunk A into the branches B and C.
The arrows represent force vectors acting on the spheres. In case of equal
flow rate in both branches the probability for the spheres to enter any of
the branches is equal (left panel).
But if the flow rate in branch B is
higher than in branch C, this causes a
traction force directing the flowing
spheres into the branch B (right panel).
(Reproduced from Svanes and Zweifach,
1968.)

should be of great significance from this point of view. This was understood as soon as the actual existence of such a correlation became evident.
In the earliest article (Mchedlishvili, 1956a), it was concluded: "It is
well known that an increase in functional activity of an organ is regularly followed by dilatation of its arteries. We have shown that this immediately causes red cell enrichment of blood flowing through the capillaries, and this increases the oxygen delivery to the tissue elements. On
the contrary, when the organs' activity decreases, their arteries become
constricted, and the capillaries are then supplied with blood containing
comparatively less red cells and more plasma. The red cells redistribute
to other tissues with a higher oxygen requirement or become retained in
the depots" (p. 89). Therefore it should not be surprising that even
under resting conditions blood with a higher concentration of red cells is
distributed to tissues with a higher metabolic rate, e.g., to the brain as
opposed to the hind leg of the same animal (Mchedlishvili and Varazashvili,
1980, 1982a).

    (b) When the regional blood flow changes with a tissue's metabolic
needs, a decrease in metabolic demand usually results in red cell-poor
blood flow in the microvessels. This is always related to transformation
of some capillaries into the plasmatic form. Since the latter have been
shown to be the intermediate state of the microvessels between active and
closed capillaries (Mchedlishvili, 1958, 1969b, 1970), the change in
the red cell:plasma ratio contributes to the cutoff of many capillaries
from circulation. In contrast, when the arteries undergo dilatation resulting in an enhanced blood supply to tissues having an increased metabolic demand, many previously inactive capillaries become active, and all
of them become perfused with the red cell-rich blood.

    (c) When the arteries supplying an appropriate microvascular bed be-
come considerably narrowed, from vasospasm or any other cause, this inevit-

ably entails a corresponding decrease in blood flow therein. This in turn results in a reduction in the red cell:plasma ratio in blood flowing to the microvascular area. A three- to fourfold drop in the capillary hematocrit with a simultaneous fifty percent decrease in blood velocity has been found in microvessels in our studies of ischemia (Mchedlishvili and Varazashvili, 1981a). This should certainly result in more pronounced hypoxic damage to the respective tissues than would occur if the blood contained a normal hematocrit. Thus, the phenomenon of a changeable red cell:plasma ratio in the microcirculation, which has positive significance under physiological conditions, results in negative sequences during pathological states in the peripheral circulation. On the other hand, the reduction of the red cell:plasma ratio in blood flowing in the larger and especially in the minute blood vessels during ischemia should promote higher fluidity of blood, which is very important for microcirculation under ischemic conditions (Schmid-Schönbein and Riegel, 1981).

6.5. FLOW CONDITIONS IN MINUTE BLOOD VESSELS FOLLOWING VASOMOTOR DISORDERS

A very complicated problem, which is still for from being solved, is the relative role of the rheological properties of the blood in microvessels (considered above in this chapter) and of the vasomotor changes (considered in previous chapters of this book). The most interesting events from both physiological and medical points of view are probably those which occur in the ischemic vascular bed, i.e., behind an arterial stenosis. In this case it is actually unimportant whether stenosis has appeared as a result of functional disorders, such as vasospasm (see the previous chapter), or is related to morphologically detectable changes either inside the vascular lumina (e.g., thrombi, emboli) or in the vascular wall (e.g., sclerosis of any kind). The principal hemodynamic change occurring in the peripheral microvascular bed following an arterial obstruction (whether the obstruction is complete or only partial) is the drop in intravascular pressure and in the pressure gradient, i.e., reduction of the driving force of blood flow in microvessels.

This disturbance is usually compensated for by dilatation of the arterial bed located in the periphery of the arterial stenosis. This vascular response is certainly a manifestation of the regulation of adequate blood supply to tissue which is accomplished by the physiological mechanisms considered in Chapter 4 of this book. However, the compensatory vasodilatation, directed toward improving the blood supply to the ischemic area of tissue, has certain limits and therefore cannot always fully compensate for the rise in vascular resistance at the arterial stenosis. Therefore, any changes in the rheological properties of the blood in the respective microcirculatory bed are of primary significance in the ischemic area.

One of the important factors influencing the blood fluidity in microvessels which undergoes change under these conditions is the peripheral hematocrit. The latter is dependent, on the one hand, on the central hematocrit, but, on the other hand, is to a certain degree independent of it (see above). These specific changes in the peripheral hematocrit are determined, first, by the red cell separation in the arterial branching sequence carrying blood to the given microvascular bed and are certainly also dependent on the increased water transport across the microvascular walls from the capillary lumina into the surrounding tissue spaces.

When the resistance increases considerably in a peripheral artery (irrespective of the cause of luminal stenosis) not only is there a reduced blood volume flowing into the peripherally located microvascular ramifications, but the red cell concentration in blood flowing in these microvessels is also reduced. Therefore, the local hematocrit in the ischemic microvascular area is considerably lowered (Mchedlishvili and Varazashvili, 1981a). This can be considered as a compensatory event maintaining the blood flow in the ischemic region, since it promotes a higher fluidity of blood in the microvascular ramifications, where the driving force of blood flow, i.e., the pressure gradient, has been considerably reduced. Thus, it is a self-protecting, or a compensatory, physiological mechanism that promotes blood flow in microvessels which are affected by ischemic circulatory disturbances (Schmid-Schönbein and Riegel, 1981).

On the other hand, microcirculatory disturbances, which affect blood fluidity in an opposite direction, occur simultaneously in the ischemic area, i.e., fluidity in the microvessels is reduced. These disturbances are: (a) the primary reduction in blood velocity, which changes the structure of the flow in microvessels of 15-100 μm so that its fluidity decreases (see pp. 247-249); (b) the enhanced water transfer from the microvessels into the tissue spaces, which induces an increase in red cell concentration and hence an increase in the local hematocrit, and decreases blood fluidity in respective capillaries; (c) the increased red cell aggregation inside the vascular lumen which is due to the slowdown of blood velocity in microvessels, and to an increased concentration of plasma proteins (because of enhanced water transfer to the tissue); (d) the rigidification of red cells due to local lactacidosis and depletion of adenosine triphosphate that always occurs because of a deficient oxygen supply to tissue. All these factors decrease blood fluidity in the ischemic region and are especially dangerous when the blood flow has already been stopped. Even then the recovered pressure gradient, because of partial or complete reestablishment of arterial blood supply (due to collateral blood supply), becomes unable to drive the flow of blood, which stagnates in the microvessels subjected to ischemia.

Furthermore, when the blood supply via the collateral pathways to the ischemic area is sufficient and can compensate, at least partly, for a deficient blood supply to tissue, the flowing blood should contain a relatively high red cell concentration, or hematocrit, due to an enhanced blood flow in all the arterial branching sequences which carry blood through collateral pathways to the ischemic area. Thus, blood with a high hematocrit flows to the microvascular bed subjected to ischemia, where the abovementioned conditions which disturb blood fluidity are in evidence. Therefore, the use of a collateral blood supply, which is certainly a positively significant event for blood supply to the ischemic region, can become a negative event. It can cause further lowering of the blood fluidity in the ischemic microvascular bed as well as further slowing of blood flow therein, thus enhancing deficiency of the blood supply to the tissue. Certainly, the "red infarcts" and the red boundary zone surrounding the "white infarcts," frequently seen by pathologists in postmortem sections of the brain, occur due to these changes in blood fluidity following obstruction of the feeding arteries.

To remove these disturbances in microcirculation in the ischemic regions due to disturbed blood fluidity in microvessels, it is necessary first to delete the immediate cause of the arterial stenosis and promote the collateral blood supply by increasing, if possible, the arteriovenous pressure gradient to induce local vasodilatation. It is also necessary to improve the rheological properties of the systemic blood by hemodilution, decreasing fibrinogen concentration, and by prevention of platelet aggregate embolization; this induces increases in the fluidity of blood in the ischemic microvascular area.

In managing the circulatory phenomena in the peripheral microvascular bed which is subject to ischemia, it is always necessary to control, if possible, the actual effects of the therapeutic maneuvers. The therapeutic effect may have a dual significance — it can be positive from one point of view, but also provoke harmful pathological events in the microcirculation.

6.6. SUMMARY

This chapter deals with the circulatory phenomena which occur in microcirculation and hence relate the cerebral blood flow to metabolic events in brain tissue. These phenomena are mainly dependent on the cerebral arterial behavior described in previous chapters. The specificity of the microcirculatory phenomena is dependent, in particular, on the flow of blood, a non-Newtonian fluid, in microvessels, i.e., in small arterial ramifications (down from ≈100 μm in diameter), in capillary networks, and in venous ramifications (up to ≈100 μm in diameter). The flow rate in microvessels is determined by the pressure gradient (related to peripheral arterial behavior and venous outflow) and by the blood fluidity, versus viscosity, in microvessels (based on the blood flow structure in microvessels described in this chapter). Specific circulatory phenomena in the capillaries are further associated with the arrangement of microvascular beds and the blood flow conditions in specific arteriolo-venular main capillaries, which represent important functional units in the capillary beds; these determine the distribution of the blood stream in capillary networks and hence the actual rate of microcirculation. A peculiar phenomenon, which was the object of considerable attention in recent years, is the changeable red cell:plasma ratio (the hematocrit), particularly in microvascular beds, where the red cell concentration is usually smaller than in the larger blood vessels. A unique phenomenon, which is significant from both physiological and pathological viewpoints, is a specific, and partly independent, distribution of red cells and plasma in vascular bifurcations. This phenomenon is determined by the anatomical arrangement of the bifurcations and by the velocity of blood flow in branches formed at the bifurcations, and has been found throughout the whole arterial branching sequence, starting from the largest arteries in the body (the branches of the aorta) down to the capillary ramifications. This phenomenon is of great significance for adequate oxygen supply to tissues and for transformation of active capillaries into nonactive forms, and vice versa, as well as for the actual fluidity changes of blood in the microvascular beds.

Concluding Remarks

Although significant progress has been made in the research of cerebral circulation, much is still unknown. It is the lack of our knowledge in the field that creates limitations for the efficient control of the circulatory events in the normal brain and for the efficient elimination of disturbances in cerebral blood flow, which, unfortunately, develop with increasing frequency in the modern mode of life.

Thus, cerebral blood flow in health and disease has been extensively investigated by both researchers and clinical workers. Many of the factors thought to determine the progress in accumulation of genuine knowledge in this field are certainly questionable, but insight into such factors is surely important since it might facilitate augmentation of the level of our knowledge of the physiology and pathology of cerebral circulation. Various points of view are available in this case and they might be very different.

Probably no one would doubt that advances in research techniques are very important in providing progress in scientific research in biomedical fields. However, careful insight into the history of the gradual progress in our knowledge in the field of cerebral circulation provides evidence that the effect of new ideas related to new approaches to research was considerably more important. However, this was inseparable from the fundamental research work whose purpose was to find conclusive evidence as to whether or not the ideas and hypotheses are correct.

In the case of normal and pathological physiology of cerebral circulation, the progress in our knowledge, described in this book, was significantly related to findings on the specific functional behavior of particular subdivisions of the cerebral arterial bed. These are the "vascular mechanisms" of the brain — the specific vascular effectors pertaining to particular types of regulation of cerebral circulation.* We can see in this book that the finding of these specific vascular mechanisms of the brain which control cerebral blood flow under various conditions has con-

---

*The phenomenon of regulation of cerebral circulation by specific vascular effectors was recorded in the "Register of Discoveries of USSR" in 1981. The author of the discovery was acknowledged to be George Mchedlishvili, and the priority date was fixed as April 1959 (when the manuscript of the first article was submitted to a scientific periodical).

tributed significantly to the elucidation of: (a) all types of cerebral
blood flow regulation; (b) the characteristics of the myogenic responses
of the specific vascular effectors, compared to the actual responses of
cerebral blood flow during changes of the systemic arterial pressure; (c)
the involvement of metabolic factors in cerebral blood flow regulation,
their distribution in the brain, and their specific effects on walls of
vascular effectors during normal blood flow regulation; (d) the neurogenic
mechanism controlling the major, pial, and parenchymal cerebral arteries,
including receptors, afferent and efferent nervous pathways, as well as
specific neurotransmitters; and (e) the criteria of efficiency of the controlling system of different types of regulation of cerebral blood flow.

Was it purely technical problems that hindered the discovery of the
vascular effectors of cerebral blood flow regulation during the 1950s and
1960s? From the point of view of experimental techniques, these could
have been found much earlier. Thus, it was certainly the shortage of new
ideas and related new approaches in research that restricted the progress
of accumulation of new knowledge in the field.

The same conclusion can be drawn concerning the progress of our knowledge of the mechanisms of microcirculation described in Chapter 6 of this
book. The main topics in this field — the role of the feeding arteries in
the distribution of the blood stream in capillary networks, the mechanisms
of transformation of active capillaries into inactive forms, the regulari-
ties of the distribution of red cells and plasma in arterial and capillary
bifurcations, the role of intracapillary aggregation of red cells for blood
fluidity, etc. — could have been discovered considerably earlier than they
actually were. The factor that slowed down real progress in the field was
not the lack of technical opportunities for investigation, but the absence
of new ideas and of new approaches in research, which have in turn restricted the progress of accumulation of new knowledge. Technical progress was
a secondary factor that only facilitated the actual findings.

An important theoretical point allowing for progress in our knowledge
was the determination of the actual difference between the physiological
and pathological events in the cerebral circulatory system. Indeed,
changes in cerebral circulation may be both physiological, i.e., related
to the functioning of the organism during health, and pathological, representing deviations from normal function. The physiological and pathological events in the cerebral circulation (as in any other system in the
living body) are sometimes difficult to differentiate. First, both represent biological processes utilizing the same morphological substrates and
driven by the same physiological, biochemical, and biophysical mechanisms
which are unique to the circulatory system. Second, every physiological
and pathophysiological event results in some disturbance that activates
the regulatory mechanisms. Thus, any pathological disturbance involves
the physiological mechanisms of regulation, which compensate for the disturbance. These control systems operate during pathological disturbances
even more extensively than during physiological changes. Therefore,
it is informative to use pathological models in experimental research on
the physiological control systems of cerebral circulation.

However, physiological experimentation requires a lot of time from
researchers. All the phenomena of life, and of cerebral circulation in
particular, are carried out by rather complicated systems, which are to be
studied by morphological, physiological, biochemical, and biophysical methods. Such multidisciplinary studies are certainly inaccessible for individual scientists and even for research teams. Scientists all over the
world are participating in this complex work. But a very complex problem

arises: how to plan, how to coordinate, how to cooperate, how to discuss, and how to appraise the work with maximum efficiency.

Thorough consideration of this problem over the course of many years led the author to believe that the systems approach could facilitate the solution of this seemingly insoluble problem. The systems approach should be applied not only to analyze the regulation of cerebral circulation, but also to formulate the problem to be investigated so that it fits the requirements of a multidisciplinary approach and organizes the structure of the biomedical experiments needed for efficient investigation (Mchedlishvili, 1982). An application of the systems approach to the solution of the problem was first made at the Fourth Tbilisi Symposium on Cerebral Circulation, which was devoted to the regulation of cerebral blood flow (April 19–21, 1978); the proceedings were published elsewhere (Mchedlishvili, Purves, et al., 1979; Mchedlishvili, 1980b). The systems approach was further applied to the solution of the problem of the pathophysiological mechanisms of brain edema development at the Fifth Tbilisi Symposium on Cerebral Circulation, held on April 20–23, 1983. But these were only the first steps. Additional steps need to be taken to further the accumulation of our knowledge of cerebral blood flow.

References

Adelstein, R. S., 1980, Regulation and kinetics of the actin-myosin-ATP interaction, Annu. Rev. Biochem., 49:921-956.

Albrecht, K. H., Gaehtgens, P., Pries, A., and Heuser, M., 1979, The Fahraeus effect in narrow capillaries (i.d. 3.3 to 11.0 μm), Microvasc. Res., 18:33-47.

Aleksandrovskaya, M. M., 1955,"Vascular Changes in Brain during Various Pathological States," Medgiz, Moscow.

Allen, G. S., Henderson, L. M., Chou, S. N., and French, L. A., 1974, Cerebral arterial spasm. 1. *In vitro* contractile activity of vasoactive agents on canine basilar and middle cerebral arteries, J. Neurosurg., 40:433-441.

Amashukeli, G. V., 1969, Analysis of circulatory changes in the brain in hemorrhage and hemotransfusion, Patol. Fiziol. Eksp. Ter., No. 3:29-32.

Antoshkina, E. D., and Naumenko, A. I., 1960, Changes in blood supply of the cortical ends of the visual and auditory analyzers during stimulation, Fiziol. Zh. SSSR, 46:1305-1311.

Arutiunov, A. I., Baron, M. I. A., Dobrovolsky, G. F., Kornienko, V. N., and Majorova, N. A., 1975, Prolonged arterial spasm at the base of brain during experimental fibrinolysis in subarachnoid space, Vopr. Neirokhirurg., No. 5:5-11.

Arutiunov, A. I., Baron, M. A., and Majorova, N. A., 1970, Experimental and clinical study of the development of spasm of the cerebral arteries related to subarachnoid hemorrhage, J. Neurosurg., 32:617-625.

Arutiunov, A. Baron, M., and Majorova, N., 1974, The role of mechanical factors in the pathogenesis of short-term and prolonged spasm of cerebral arteries, J. Neurosurg., 40:459-471.

Arutiunov, A. I., Konovalov, A. N., Shakhnovich, A. R., Dadiani, L. N., Salalykin, V. I., Fedorov, S. N., and Filatov, Yu. M., 1972, Autoregulation of cerebral blood flow and its disturbances after surgical operations, Vopr. Neirokhirurg., No. 1:3-6.

Ask-Upmark, E., 1935, "The Carotid Sinus and the Cerebral Circulation," Munskgaard, Copenhagen.

Astrup, J., Heuser, D, Lassen, N. A., Nilsson, L., Norberg, K., and Sjesjö, B. K., 1978, Evidence against H^+ and K^+ as main factors for the control of cerebral blood flow: a microelectrode study, in: "Cerebral Vascular Smooth Muscle and Its Control," M. J. Purves, ed., Elsevier, Amsterdam, pp. 313-332.

Astrup, J., Symon, L., Branston, N. M., and Lassen, N. A., 1977, Cortical evoked potential and extracellular K^+ and H^+ at critical levels of brain ischemia, Stroke, 8:51-57.

Auer, L. M., 1981, Rhythmic patterns of pial vessels to neurogenic and metabolic stimuli and blood pressure changes, in: "Cerebral Microcirculation and Metabolism," J. Cervós-Navarro and E. Fritschka, eds., Raven Press, New York, pp. 271-277.

Auer, L. M., and Johansson, B. B., 1980, Dilatation of pial arterial vessels in hypercapnia and in acute hypertension, Acta Physiol. Scand., 106:249-251.

Auer, L. M., and Johansson, B. B., 1981, Reaction of pial arteries and veins to sympathetic stimulation in the cat, Stroke, 12:528-531.

Auer, L. M., Kuschinsky, W., Johansson, B. B., and Edvinsson, L., 1982, Sympatho-adrenergic influence on pial veins and arteries in the cat, in: "Cerebral Blood Flow: Effects of Nerves and Neurotransmitters," D. D. Heistad and M. L. Marcus, eds., Elsevier/North-Holland, pp. 291-300.

Ayala, G. F., and Himwich, A. W., 1965, Middle cerebral and lingual artery pressure in the dog, Arch. Neurol., 12:435-442.

Azin, A. L., 1981, Role of pH in the action mode of CO_2 on smooth muscles of the cerebral arteries, Byull. Eksp. Biol. Med., 91:385-512.

Bader, H, 1963, The anatomy and physiology of the vascular wall, in: "Handbook of Physiology," Section 2: Circulation, W. F. Hamilton, ed., Vol. 2, American Physiological Society, Washington, DC, pp. 865-889.

Baldy-Moulinier, M., and Frèrebeau, Ph., 1969, Blood flow in cases of coma following severe head injury, in: "Cerebral Blood Flow. Clinical and Experimental Results," M. Brock, C. Fieschi, D. H. Ingvar, N. A. Lassen, and K. Schürmann, eds., Springer-Verlag, Berlin-Heidelberg-New York, pp. 216-218.

Baramidze, D. G., 1979, Pathological responses of the cerebral arterial system from the point of view of its functional behaviour, in: "Regulation of Cerebral Circulation," G. I. Mchedlishvili, M. J. Purves, and A. G. B. Kovách, eds., Akadémiai Kiadó, Budapest, pp. 171-176, 189-193.

Baramidze, D. G., Gadamski, R., Gordeladze, Z. T., and Mamaladze, A. A., 1982a, Effect of sympathectomy on pial arterial responses under conditions of cerebral blood flow deficiency, Fiziol. Zh. SSSR, 68:1381-1391.

Baramidze, D. G., Gadamski, R., and Szumańska, G., 1981, Histochemical studies of the microvascular effectors of the cerebral cortex blood supply regulation, Byull. Eksp. Biol. Med., 91:228-231.

Baramidze, D. G., and Gordeladze, Z. T., 1980, Further studies of active segments of pial microvessels controlling microcirculation of the cerebral cortex, Neuropatol. Pol., 18:554-567.

Baramidze, D. G., Khananashvili, M. M., Mchedlishvili, G. I., and Gordeladze, Z. T., 1980, Responses of pial microvascular effectors regulating adequate blood supply to the cerebral cortex under conditions of its neuronal isolation, Byull. Eksp. Biol. Med., 79:265-267.

Baramidze, D. G., Levkovich, Yu. I., and Mchedlishvili, G. I., 1983, Dynamics of local vascular responses under conditions of increased activity of cerebral cortex, Fiziol. Zh. SSSR, 69:1158-1164.

Baramidze, D. G., and Mchedlishvili, G. I., 1970, Arrangement and responses of smooth muscle cells in arterial walls of the cerebral cortex, Byull. Eksp. Biol. Med., 70:No. 11, 110-112.

Baramidze, D. G., and Mchedlishvili, G. I., 1977, Functional behaviour of microvascular mechanisms in the pial, precortical, and cortical arteries under experimental conditions, in: "Brain Blood Supply," G. I. Mchedlishvili, A. G. B. Kovách, and I. Nyáry, eds., Akadémiai Kiadó, Budapest, pp. 55-64.

Baramidze, D. G., Reidler, R. M., Gadamski, R., and Mchedlishvili, G. I.,
    1982b, Pattern and innervation of pial microvascular effectors which
    control blood supply to cerebral cortex, Blood Vessels, 19: 284-291.
Baramidze, D. G., and Zelman, I. B., 1974, Histochemical study of nucleo-
    side phosphatase activity in rabbit brain following circulatory
    hypoxia. Neuropatol. Pol., 12:617-624.
Bates, D., Weinshilboum, R. M., Campell, R. J., and Sundt, T. M., 1977,
    The effect of lesion in the locus coeruleus on the physiological re-
    sponses of the cerebral blood vessels in cats. Brain Res., 136:431-
    443.
Berman, H. J., and Fuhro, R. L., 1969, Effect of rate of shear on the
    shape of the velocity profile and orientation of red cells in arteri-
    oles. Bibl. Anat. (Basel), 10:32-37.
Berntman, L., Dahlgren, N., and Sjesjö, B. K., 1979, Cerebral blood flow
    and oxygen consumption in the rat brain during extreme hypercapnia.
    Anesthesiology, 50:299-305.
Betz, E., 1972, Cerebral blood flow: its measurement and regulation.
    Physiol. Rev., 52:595-630.
Betz, E., Kok, N., Mchedlishvili, G., Meyer, J. S., and Pocchiari, F.,
    1974, Influence on the EEG of certain physiological states and other
    parameters, in: "Handbook of Electroencephalography and Clinical Neuro-
    physiology," A. Remond, ed., Vol. 7, Part B, 7B-7-7B-71, Elsevier,
    Amsterdam.
Bevan, J. A., 1981, A comparison of the contractile response of the rabbit
    basilar and pulmonary arteries to sympathomimetic agonists: Further
    evidence for variation in vascular adrenoreceptor characteristics.
    J. Pharmacol. Exp. Ther., 216:83-89.
Bevan, J. A., and Bevan, R. D., 1977, Sympathetic control of the rabbit
    basilar artery, in: "Neurogenic Control of Brain Circulation,"
    C. Owman and L. Edvinsson, eds., pp. 285-293. Pergamon Press, Oxford
    and New York.
Bevan, J. A., Bevan, R. D., Buga, G., Florence, V. M., Jope, C. A., and
    Moritoki, H., 1981a, The cranial neural vasodilator outflow, in:
    "Vasodilatation," P. M. Vanhoutte and I. Leusen, eds., pp. 19-26,
    Raven Press, New York.
Bevan, J. A., Bevan, R. D., and Duckles, S. P., 1980, Adrenergic regula-
    tion of vascular smooth muscle, in: "Handbook of Physiology." Sec.
    2: The Cardiovascular System, Vol. 2: Vascular Smooth Muscle, D. F.
    Bohr, A. P. Somlyo, and H. V. Sparks, eds., pp. 515-566, American
    Physiological Society, Bethesda, Maryland.
Bevan, J. A., Buga, G. M., Snowden, A., and Said, S. I., 1981b, Is the
    neural vasodilator mechanism to cerebral and extracerebral arteries
    the same? in: "Proceedings of the Symposium on Cerebral Blood Flow:
    Effect of Nerves and Neurotransmitters, Iowa City, Iowa, June 15-18,
    1981," D. D. Heistad and M. L. Marcus, eds., Elsevier, New York.
Bicher, H. I., 1974, Brain oxygen autoregulation: a protective reflex to
    hypoxia? Microvasc. Res., 8:291-313.
Biedl, A., and Reiner, M., 1900, Studien über Hirncirculation und Hirnödem,
    Pflügers Arch., 79:158-194.
Biscoe, T. J., Purves, M. J., and Sampson, S. R., 1970, The frequency of
    nerve impulses in single carotid body chemoreceptor afferent fibres
    recorded in vivo with intact circulation, J. Physiol. (London), 208:
    121-132.
Blaustein, M. P., 1977, Sodium ions, calcium ions, blood pressure regula-
    tion and hypertension: a reassessment and a hypothesis, Am. J.
    Physiol., 232:C165-C173.
Blinkow, S. M., and Gleser, I. I., 1968, "Das Zentralnervensystem in Zahlen
    und Tabellen," Gustav Fischer Verlag, Jena.

Bohr, D. F., and Elliott, J., 1963, 5-Hydroxytryptamine and the contraction of smooth muscle from resistance vessels, in: "Metabolismus parietis vasorum," B. Prusik, Z. Reinis, and O. Riede, eds., pp. 337-345, Státni zdravotnické nakladatelstvi, Praha.

Bohr, D. F., Somlyo, A. P., and Sparks, H. V., eds., 1980, "Handbook of Physiology," Sec. 2: The Cardiovascular System, Vol. 2: Vascular Smooth Muscle, American Physiological Society, Bethesda, Maryland.

Boisvert, D. P. J., Gregory, P. C., and Harper, A. M., 1978, Effect of decreased arterial P_{CO_2} on pial arteriolar response to adenosine. Advances in Neurology, Vol. 20, "Pathology of Cerebral Microcirculation," J. Cervós-Navarro, E. Betz, G. Ebhardt, R. Ferszt, and R. Wüllenberger, eds., pp. 50-63, Raven Press, New York.

Borgström, L., Johansson, H., and Sjesjö, B. K., 1975, The relationship between arterial PO_2 and cerebral blood flow in hypoxia, Acta Physiol. Scand., 93:423-432.

Born, G. V. R., 1970, 5-Hydrotryptamine receptors, in: "Smooth Muscle," E. Bülbring, A. F. Brading, A. W. Jones, and T. Tomita, eds., pp. 418-450, Edward Arnolds (Publishers), London.

Borodulya, A. V., 1965, Morphology of the nervous apparatus of the normal human internal carotid artery, Zh. Neiropatol. Psikhiat., 65:379-385.

Borodulya, A. V., and Pletchkova, E. K., 1973, Distribution of cholinergic and adrenergic nerves in the internal carotid artery, Acta Anat., 86:410-425.

Bouckaert, J. J., and Heymans, C., 1933, Carotid sinus reflexes, influence of central blood pressure and blood supply on respiratory and vasomotor centres, J. Physiol. (London), 79:49-66.

Bouckaert, J. J., and Heymans, C., 1935, On the reflex regulation of the cerebral blood flow and the cerebral vasomotor tone, J. Physiol. (London), 84:367-380.

Brain, S. R., 1957, Order and disorder in the cerebral circulation, Lancet, No. 7001:857-862.

Brandt, L, Andersson, K.-E., Bengtsson, B., Edvinsson, L., Ljundgren, B., and MacKenzie, E. T., 1979, Effects of nifedipine on pial arteriolar calibre: an *in vivo* study, Surg. Neurol., 12:349-352.

Brandt, L., Andersson, K.-E., Bengtsson, B., Edvinsson, L., Ljundgren, B., and Mackenzie, E. T., 1980, Effects of a calcium antagonist on cerebrovascular smooth muscle *in vitro* and *in vivo*, in: "Cerebral Vascular Spasm," R. H. Wilkins, ed., pp. 604-607, Williams and Wilkins, Baltimore.

Branston, N. M., Strong, A. J., and Symon, L., 1977, Extracellular potassium activity, evoked potential and tissue blood flow. Relationships during progressive ischemia in baboon cerebral cortex, J. Neurol. Sci., 32:305-321.

Brock, M., Fieschi, C., Ingvar, D. H., Lassen, N. A., and Schurmann, K., 1969, "Cerebral Blood Flow. Clinical and Experimental Results," Springer-Verlag, Berlin-Heidelberg-New York.

Brooks, B. E., Goodwin, J. W., and Seaman, G. V. F., 1970, Interaction among erythrocytes under shear, J. Appl. Physiol., 28:174-182.

Brown, A. M., 1980, Receptors under pressure. An update on baroreceptors, Circ. Res., 46:1-10.

Brücke, 1850, Bemerkungen über die Mechanik des Entzündungsprozesses, Arch. Physiol. Heilk., 9:493-499.

Bülbring, E., Brading, A. F., Jones, A. W., and Tomita, T., eds., 1970, "Smooth Muscle," Edward Arnolds, London.

Bulter, H. M., and Davies, R. E., 1980, High-energy phosphates in smooth muscle, in: "Handbook of Physiology," Sec. 2: The Cardiovascular System; Vol. 2, Vascular Smooth Muscle, D. F. Bohr, A. P. Somlyo, and H. V. Sparks, eds., pp. 237-252, American Physiological Society, Bethesda, Maryland.

Burnstock, G., 1975, Purinergic transmission, in: "Handbook of Psycho-
    pharmacology," L. L. Iversen, S. D. Iversen, and S. H. Snyder, eds.,
    pp. 131-194, Plenum, New York.
Burnstock, G., 1980, Cholinergic and purinergic regulation of blood ves-
    sels, in: "Handbook of Physiology," Sec. 2: The Cardiovascular Sys-
    tem; Vol. 2: Vascular Smooth Muscle, D. F. Bohr, A. P. Somlyo, and
    H. V. Sparks, eds., pp. 567-612, American Physiological Society,
    Bethesda, Maryland.
Burton, A. C., 1951, On the physical equilibrium of small blood vessels,
    Am. J. Physiol., 164:219-229.
Burton, A. C., 1954, Relation of structure to function of the tissues of
    the wall of blood vessels, Physiol. Rev., 34:619-642.
Burton, A. C., 1972, "Physiology and Biophysics of the Circulation," Year
    Book Med. Publishers, Inc., Chicago.
Busija, D. W., Heistad, D. D., and Marcus, M. L., 1980, Effects of sympa-
    thetic nerves on cerebral vessels during acute, moderate increases in
    arterial pressure in dogs and cats, Circ. Res., 46:696-702.
Busija, D. W., Marcus, M. L., and Heistad, D. D., 1982, Pial arterial
    diameter and blood flow velocity during sympathetic stimulation in
    cats, J. Cereb. Blood Flow Metab., 2:363-367.
Butler, T. H., and Davies, R. E., 1980, High-energy phosphates in smooth
    muscle, in: "Handbook of Physiology," Sec. 2: Cardiovascular System,
    D. F. Bohr, A. P. Somlyo, and H. V. Sparks, eds., Vol. 2, pp. 237-252,
    American Physiological Society, Bethesda, Maryland.
Capon, A., 1975, Effect of acute sections of the brain stem on hypercapnic
    vasodilatation in cerebral and spinal vessels, in: "Blood Flow and
    Metabolism in the Brain," A. M. Harper, B. Jenett, D. Miller, and
    J. Rowan, eds., pp. 1.16-1.18, Churchill Livingstone, Edinburgh,
    London, and New York.
Carlyle, A., and Grayson, J., 1956, Factors involved in the control of the
    cerebral blood flow, J. Physiol. (London), 133:10-30.
Caro, C. G., Pedley, T. J., Schroter, R. C., and Seed, W. A., 1978, "The
    Mechanics of the Circulation," Oxford University Press, Oxford-New
    York-Toronto.
Carpi, A., 1972, Drugs related to chemical mediators, in: "Pharmacology
    of the Cerebral Circulation," Vol. 1, pp. 87-124, Pergamon Press,
    Oxford-New York-Toronto.
Carpi, A., and Giardini, V., 1972, Drugs acting on muscular receptors, in:
    "Pharmacology of the Cerebral Circulation," Vol. 1, pp. 125-148,
    Pergamon Press, Oxford-New York-Toronto.
Cervós-Navarro, J., 1977, The structural basis of an innervatory system
    of brain vessels, in: "Neurogenic Control of Brain Circulation,"
    Ch. Owman and L. Edvinsson, eds., pp. 75-89, Pergamon Press, Oxford
    and New York.
Cervós-Navarro, J., and Matakas, F., 1974, Electron microscopic evidence
    for innervation of intracerebral arterioles in the cat, Neurology,
    24:282-286.
Cervós-Navarro, J., and Rozas, J. I., 1978, The arteriole as a site of
    metabolic exchange, in: Advances in Neurology, Vol. 20, "Pathology
    of Cerebral Microcirculation," J. Cervós-Navarro, E. Betz, G. Ebhardt,
    R. Ferszt, and R. Wüllenweber, eds., pp. 17-24, Raven Press, New York.
Chambers, R., and Zweifach, B. W., 1944, Topography and function of the
    mesenteric capillary circulation, Am. J. Anat., 75:173-205.
Chambers, R., and Zweifach, B. W., 1947, Intercellular cement and capil-
    lary permeability, Physiol. Rev., 27:436-463.
Chien, S., 1970, Shear dependence of effective cell volume as a determi-
    nant of blood viscosity, Science, 168:977-979.
Chizhevsky, A. L., 1953, Orientation and kinematics of erythrocytes in
    blood flow, Izv. Akad. Nauk SSSR, Ser. Biol., No. 5:72-97.

Chizhevsky, A. L., 1980, "Biophysical Mechanisms of Erythrocytes Sedimentation Reaction," Nauka, Novosibirsk.

Chorobski, J., and Penfield, W, 1932, Cerebral vasodilator nerves and their pathways from the medulla oblongata with observations on pial and intracerebral vascular plexus, Arch. Neurol. Psychiat., 28:1257-1289.

Christ, E. J., and Van Dorp, D. A., 1972, Comparative aspects of prostaglandin biosynthesis in animal tissues, in: International Workshop on Prostaglandins," S. Bergstroem, ed., pp. 35-38, Pergamon Press, New York.

Clark, E. R., and Clark, E. L., 1932, Observations on living blood vessels as seen in a transparent chamber inserted into the rabbit's ear, Am. J. Anat., 49:441-477.

Clark, E. R., and Clark, E. L., 1939, Microscopic observations on the growth of blood capillaries in the living mammal, Am. J. Anat., 64:251-302.

Clark, E. R., and Clark, E. L., 1940, Microscopic observations on the extraendothelial cells of living mammalian blood vessels, Am. J. Anat., 66:1-49.

Clark, E. R., and Clark, E. L., 1943, Caliber changes in minute blood vessels observed in the living mammal, Am. J. Anat., 73:215-250.

Cobb, S., and Finesinger, J. E., 1932, Cerebral circulation: XIX. The vagal pathway of the vasodilator impulses, Arch. Neurol. Psychiat., 28:1243-1256.

Cohen, P. H., and Alexander, S. C., 1967, Effects of hypoxia and normocapnia on cerebral blood flow in conscious man, J. Appl. Physiol., 23:183-189.

Cohnheim, J., 1873, "Neue Untersuchungen über die Entzündung," Berlin.

Cohnstein, J., and Zuntz, N., 1888, Untersuchungen über den Flüssigkeits-Austausch zwischen Blut und Geweben unter verschiedenen physiologischen und pathologischen Bedingungen, Pflügers Arch., 42:303-341.

Cokelet, G. R., 1982, Speculation on a cause of low vessel hematocrits in the microcirculation, Microcirculation, 2:1-18.

Cooper, R., Crow, H. J., Walter, W. G., and Winter, A. L., 1966, Regional control of cerebral reactivity and oxygen supply in brain, Brain Res., 3:174-191.

Corday, E., Rothenberg, S. F., and Putnam, T. J., 1953, Cerebral vascular insufficiency. An explanation of some types of localized cerebral encephalopathy, Arch. Neurol. Psychiat., 69:551-570.

Courtice, F. C., 1941, The effect of oxygen lack on the cerebral circulation, J. Physiol. (London), 100:198-211.

Dacey, R. C., and Duling, B. R., 1982, Mechanics and reactivity of rat intracerebral arterioles, in: "Cerebral Blood Flow. Effect of Nerves and Neurotransmitters," D. D. Heistad and M. L. Marcus, eds., pp. 57-64, Elsevier, New York.

Damask, A. C., 1978, "Medical Physics," Vol. 1: Physiological Physics, External Probes, Academic Press, New York-San Francisco-London.

Danilov, M. G., 1940, On development of capillary stasis. Trans. Milit. Med. Acad., 23:3-16.

Daugherty, R. M., Scott, J. B., Emerson, Th. E., and Haddy, F. J., 1968, Comparison of iv and ia infusion of vasoactive agents on dog forelimb blood flow, Am. J. Physiol., 214:611-619.

de la Torre, E., Mitchell, O. C., and Netsky, M. G., 1962, The seat of respiratory and cardiovascular responses to cerebral air emboli, Neurology, 12:140-147.

Demchenko, I. T., 1979, Discussion on mechanisms regulating cerebral circulation with changes in content of blood gases, in: "Regulation of Cerebral Circulation," G. Mchedlishvili, M. G. Purves, and A. G. B. Kovách, eds., p. 123, Akadémiai Kiadó, Budapest.

Denn, M. J., and Stone, H. L., 1976, Cholinergic innervation of monkey
    cerebral vessels, Brain Res., 113:394-399.
Dickinson, C. J., 1965, "Neurogenic Hypertension," Blackwell Scientific
    Publications, Oxford.
Dieckhoff, D., and Kanzow, E., 1969, Über die Lokalisation des Strömungs-
    wiederstandes im Hirnkreislauf, Pflügers Arch., 310:75-85.
Diem, E., ed., 1962, "Documenta Geigy, Scientific Tables," 6th ed., J. R.
    Geigy, Basel, Switzerland.
Dinsdale, H. B., Robertson, D. M., and Haas, R. A., 1974, Cerebral blood
    flow in acute hypertension, Arch. Neurol., 31:80-87.
Dintenfass, L., 1964, Rheology of the packed red blood cells containing
    hemoglobins A-A, S-A, and S-S, J. Lab. Clin. Med., 64:594-600.
Dintenfass, L., 1967, Inversion of the Fahraeus-Lindqvist phenomenon in blood
    flow through capillaries of diminishing radius, Nature, 215: 1099-1100.
Dintenfass, L., 1976, "Rheology of Blood in Diagnostic and Preventive
    Medicine," Butterworths, London-Boston.
Dintenfass, L., 1980, Autoregulation of blood viscosity in health and
    disease, Vasc. Surg., 14:227-237.
Dintenfass, L., 1981, The clinical impact of the newer research in blood
    rheology: An overview, Angiology, 32:217-229.
Dobrovolsky, G. F., 1975, Electron microscopic studies of the innervation-
    al apparatus of large arteries at base of brain under conditions of
    subarachnoid hemorrhage following rupture of aneurisms, Vopr. Neiro-
    khirurg., No. 1:15-21.
Donders, F. C., 1851, Die Bewegungen des Gehirns und die Veränderungen
    der Gefässfüllung der Pia Mater, Schmid's Fahrbucher, 69:16-20.
Dóra, E., and Kovách, A. G. B., 1982, Effect of acute arterial hypo- and
    hypertension on cerebrocortical NAD/NADH redox state and vascular
    volume, J. Cereb. Blood Flow Metab., 2:209-219.
Dubois, E. F., 1841, "Prélecons de pathologie expérimentale. I Partie.
    Observations et expériences sur l'hyperemie capillaire," Paris.
Duckles, S. P., 1979, Neurogenic dilator and constrictor responses of pial arte-
    ries in vitro. Difference between dogs and sheep, Circ. Res., 44: 482-490.
Duckles, S., and Bevan, J. A., 1976, Pharmacological characterization of
    adrenergic receptors of a rabbit cerebral artery in vitro, J.
    Pharmacol. Exp. Ther., 197:371-378.
Dunn, D. R., Deavers, S., Huggins, R. A., and Smith, E. L., 1958, Effect
    of hemorrage on the red cell and plasma volume of various organs in
    the dog, Am. J. Physiol., 195:69-72.
Duvernoy, H. M., Delon, S., and Vannson, J. L., 1981, Cortical blood ves-
    sels of the human brain, Brain Res. Bull., 7:519-579.
Echlin, F. A., 1942, Vasospasm and local cerebral ischemia. An experimen-
    tal study, Arch. Neurol. Psychiat., 47:77-96.
Edvinsson, L., Högestätt, E. D., and Auer, L. M., 1983, Cerebral veins:
    fluorescence histochemistry, electron microscopy, and in vitro re-
    activity, J. Cereb. Blood Flow Metab., 3:226-230.
Edvinsson, L., Lindvall, M., Nielson, K. C., and Owman, Ch., 1973, Are
    brain vessels innervated also by central (nonsympathetic) adrenergic
    neurons? Brain Res., 63:496-499.
Edvinsson, L., and MacKenzie, E. T., 1977, Amine mechanisms in the cere-
    bral circulation, Pharmacol. Rev., 28:275-348.
Edvinsson, L., Nielsen, K. C., Owman, Ch., and Sporrong, B., 1972, Cholin-
    ergic mechanisms in pial vessels. Histochemistry, electron micros-
    copy and pharmacology, Z. Zellforsch., 134:311-325.
Edvinsson, L., and Owman, Ch., 1975, Pharmacological identification of
    adrenergic (alpha and beta), cholinergic (muscarinic and nicotinic),
    histaminergic (h_1 and h_2), and serotonergic receptors in isolated
    intra- and extracranial vessels, in: "Blood Flow and Metabolism in
    the Brain," M. Harper, B. Jenett, D. Miller, and J. Rowan, eds., pp.
    1.18-1.25, Churchill Livingstone, Edinburgh.

Edvinsson, L., and Owman, Ch., 1976, Amine receptors in brain vessels, in: "Cerebral Vessel Wall," J. Cervos-Navarro, E. Betz, F. Matakas, and R. Wüllenweber, eds., pp. 197–206, Raven Press, New York.

Edvinsson, L., Owman, C., and Sjesjö, B., 1976, Physiological role of cerebrovascular sympathetic nerves in the autoregulation of cerebral blood flow, Brain Res., 117:519–523.

Eidelman, B. H., McCalden, Th. A., and Rosendorff, C., 1975, The role of the carotid body in mediating the cerebrovascular response to altered $PaCO_2$, in: "Blood Flow and Metabolism in the Brain," A. M. Harper, B. Jenett, D. Miller, and J. Rowan, eds., pp. 2.35–2.36, Churchill Livingstone, Edinburgh.

Ekström-Jodal, B., Häggendal, E., Nilsson, N. J., and Norbäck, B., 1969, Changes of the transmural pressure – the probable stimulus to cerebral blood flow autoregulation, in: "Cerebral Blood Flow," M. Brock, C. Fieschi, D. H. Ingvar, N. A. Lassen, and K. Schürmann, eds., pp. 89–93, Springer-Verlag, Berlin.

Endo, S., and Suzuki, J., 1979, Experimental cerebral vasospasm after subarachnoid hemorrhage. Participation of adrenergic nerves in cerebral vessel wall, Stroke, 10:703–711.

Esipova, I. K., Kaufman, O. Ya., and Migulina, T. V., 1967, About morphology of vasomotor reactions of mesenteric vessels, Arkh. Patol. (Moscow), 29, No. 12:14–20.

von Essen, C., 1973, "Effects of Monoamines on Cerebral Blood Flow in Dogs," Elanders Baktrycheri Aktiebolag, Göteborg.

Fahraeus, R., 1929, The suspension stability of the blood, Physiol. Rev., 9:241–274.

Fahraeus, R., and Lindqvist, T., 1931, The viscosity of the blood in narrow capillary tubes, Am. J. Physiol., 96:562–568.

Falck, B., Mchedlishvili, G. I., and Owman, Ch., 1965, Histochemical demonstration of adrenergic nerves in cortex-pia of rabbit, Acta Pharmacol., 23:133–142.

Fang, H. C. H., 1961, Cerebral arterial innervation in man, Arch. Neurol., 4:651–656.

Fenske, A., Hey, O., Theiss, R., Reulen, H. J., and Schürmann, K., 1975, Regional cortical blood flow in the early stage of brain stem edema, in: "Blood Flow and Metabolism in the Brain," A. M. Harper, B. Jenett, D. Miller, and J. Rowan, eds., pp. 1.12–1.15, Churchill Livingstone, Edinburgh.

Ferrari, M., and Carpenado, F., 1968, Antagonism between calcium ions and some myolytic agents on depolarized guinea-pig taenia coli, J. Pharm. Pharmacol., 20:317–318.

Field, E., 1935, The reactions of the blood capillaries of the frog and rat to mechanical and electrical stimulation, Scand. Arch. Physiol., 72:175–191.

Finnerty, F. A., Witkin, L., and Fazekas, J. F., 1954, Cerebral hemodynamics during cerebral ischemia induced by acute hypotension, J. Clin. Invest., 33:1227–1232.

Fitch, W., Ferguson, G. G., Sengupta, D., Garibi, J., and Harper, A. M., 1976, Autoregulation of cerebral blood flow during controlled hypotension in baboons, J. Neurol., Neurosurg., Psychiat., 39:1014–1022.

Fitch, W., MacKenzie, B. T., and Harper, A. M., 1975, Effects of decreasing arterial blood pressure on cerebral blood flow in the baboons, Circ. Res., 37:550–557.

Florence, V. M., and Bevan, J. A., 1979, Biochemical determinations of cholinergic innervation in cerebral arteries, Circ. Res., 45:212–218.

Florey, H., 1925, Microscopical observations on the circulation of the blood in the cerebral cortex, Brain, 48:43–64.

Fog, M., 1937, Cerebral circulation. The reaction of the pial arteries to a fall of blood pressure, Arch. Neurol. Psychiat., 37:351–364.

Fog, M., 1939, Cerebral circulation. II. Reaction of pial arteries to increase in blood pressure, Arch. Neurol. Psychiat., 41:260-268.

Folkow, B. W., 1962, Transmural pressure and vascular tone: some aspects of old controversy, Arch. Int. Pharmacol. Ther., 139:455-469.

Forbes, H. S., 1940, Physiologic regulation of the cerebral circulation, Arch. Neurol. Psychiat., 43:804-814.

Forbes, H. S., and Cobb, S., 1938, Vasomotor control of cerebral vessels, Brain, 61:221-233.

Forbes, H. S., Nason, G. L., and Wortman, R. C., 1937, Cerebral circulation. XLIV. Vasodilatation in the pia following stimulation of the vagus, aortic and carotid sinus nerves. Arch. Neurol. Psychiat., 37:334-350.

Forbes, H. S., and Wolff, H. G., 1928, Cerebral circulation. III. The vasomotor control of cerebral vessels, Arch. Neurol. Psychiat., 19: 1057-1086.

Freeman, J., 1968, Elimination of brain cortical blood flow autoregulation following hypoxia, Scand. J. Lab. Clin. Invest., Suppl. 102, V:E.

Friedman, L., and Friedman, M., 1963, Effects of ions on vascular smooth muscle, in: "Handbook of Physiology," Sec. 2: Circulation, W. F. Hamilton, ed., Vol. 2, pp. 1135-1166, Williams and Wilkins, Washington, DC.

Frolkis, V. V., 1970, "Regulation, Adaptation, and Aging," Nauka, Leningrad.

Fujiwara, S., Suzuki, H., and Kuriyama, H.,1981, Membrane properties and adrenergic innervation of smooth muscle of the dog brain arteries, Blood Vessels, 18:212-213.

Fulton, J. F., ed., 1955, "Textbook of Physiology," 17th edn., W. B. Saunders Co., Philadelphia and London.

Fung, Y.-Ch. C., 1978, Mechanical properties of blood vessels, in: Peripheral Circulation," P. C. Johnson, ed., pp. 45-79, John Wiley and Sons, New York.

Fung, Y. C., 1981,"Biomechanics. Mechanical Properties of Living Tissues," Springer-Verlag, New York.

Gabashvili, V. M., and Mchedlishvili, G. I., 1965, Reflex influences from the carotid sinus receptor zone on the internal carotid arteries, in: "Vascular Diseases of the Brain," Proceedings of the 4th Soviet Congress of Neuropathologists and Psychiatrists, Vol. 2, pp. 355-363, Meditsina, Moscow.

Gaehtgens, P., 1977, Hemodynamics of the microcirculation. Physical characteristics of blood flow in the microvasculature, in: "Handbuch der allegemeinen Pathologie," III/7 Microcirculation, H. Meesen, ed., pp. 231-287, Springer-Verlag, Berlin.

Gaehtgens, P., Wayland, H., and Meiselman, H. J., 1971, Velocity profile measurements in living microvessels by a correlation method, in: "Theoretical and Clinical Hemorheology," H. Hartet and A. L. Copley, eds., pp. 381-385, Springer-Verlag, Berlin.

Gannushkina, I. V., 1958, Aftereffects of closure of the intracerebral arteries and veins of the cerebral cortex, Zh. Neuropat. Psikhiat., 58:1025-1031.

Gannushkina, I. V., 1973, "Collateral Blood Circulation in the Brain," Meditsina, Moscow.

Gannushkina, I. V., 1975, The physiology and pathophysiology of cerebral circulation, in: "Vascular Diseases of Nervous System," E. V. Schmidt, ed., pp. 65-100, Meditsina, Moscow.

Gannushkina, I. V., 1979, Mechanisms of pathological dilation of the cerebral arteries, in: "Regulation of Cerebral Circulation," G. I. Mchedlishvili, M. J. Purves, and A. G. B. Kovách, eds., pp. 183-188, Akadémiai Kiadó, Budapest.

Gannushkina, I. V., Galayda, T. V., Shafranova, V. P., and Rjassina, T. V., 1977a, Further study of the role of geometry of arterial system of the brain in "breakthrough" of cerebral blood flow autoregulation, in: "Cerebral Function, Metabolism and Circulation," D. H. Ingvar and N. A. Lassen, eds., pp. 292-293, Munksgaard, Copenhagen.

Gannushkina, I. V., and Shafranova, V. P., 1975, The differences of arterial autoregulation in gray and white matter in acute hypertension, in: "Blood Flow and Metabolism in the Brain," M. Harper, B. Jenett, D. Miller, and J. Rowan, eds., pp. 5.31-5.35, Churchill Livingstone, Edinburgh.

Gannushkina, I. V., and Shafranova, V. P., 1976, Morphological evidence and pathogenesis concerning the spotty nature of brain tissue damage in experimental hypertensive encephalopathy, in: "Cerebral Vascular Disease," 7th International Conference, Salzburg, 1974, J. S. Meyer, H. Lechner, and M. Reivich, eds., pp. 61-65, G. Thieme Publishers, Stuttgart.

Gannushkina, I. V., and Shafranova, V. P., 1977, Analysis of the causes of predominant localization of maculate lesions of cerebral vessels and tissue during acute rise in arterial pressure, Zh. Neiropat. Psikhiat. Psikhiat. (Moscow), 77:214-221.

Gannushkina, I. V., Shafranova, V. P., and Riasina, T. V., 1977b, "Functional Angioarchitectonics of the Brain," Meditsina, Moscow.

Garbuliński, T., Gosk, A., and Mchedlishvili, G. I., 1963, Photohemotachometric investigations of functions of the neuromuscular apparatus of the internal carotid arteries. Report 1. Experimental method and effects of certain physiologically active substances, Byull. Eksp. Biol. Med., 55, No. 1:6-11.

Gedevanishvili, D. M., and Javrishvili, T. D., 1948, Analysis of sympathetic effect on skeletal muscle. Chap. 2: Amount of blood in vessels of exsanguinated preparation of hind limb, in: "On Biological Significance of Animals' Mucus," pp. 255-277, Gruzmedgiz, Tbilisi.

Gershon, M. D., 1970, The identification of neurotransmitters to smooth muscle, in: "Smooth Muscle," E. Bülbring, A. F. Brading, A. W. Jones, and T. Tomita, eds., pp. 496-524, Edward Arnolds, London.

Gibson, J. G., Seligman, A. M., Peacack, W. C., Aub, J. S., and Evans, R. D., 1946, The distribution of red cells and plasma in large and minute vessels of the normal dog, determined by radioactive isotopes of iron and iodine, J. Clin. Invest., 25:848-857.

Goldby, F. S., and Beilin, L. J., 1972, How an acute increase in arterial pressure damages arterioles, Cardiovasc. Res., 6:569-584.

Golubew, A., 1869, Beiträge zur Kenntniss des Baues und der Entwicklungsgeschichte der Capillargefässe des Frosches, Arch. Mikr. Anat., 5: 49-89.

Gontscharoff, P. P., 1935, Beobachtungen über den Blutkreislauf an "Salzfröschen," Z. Ges. Exp. Med., 97:405-414.

Gotoh, F., Nagai, H., and Tazaki, Y., eds., 1977, "Cerebral Blood Flow and Metabolism," Munksgaard, Copenhagen.

Gregory, P. C., Anderson, M., and Harper, A. M., 1977, Coupling of cerebral blood flow and metabolism following somato-sensory stimulation in rabbit, in: "Cerebral Function, Metabolism and Circulation," D. H. Ingvar and N. A. Lassen, eds., pp. 254-255, Munksgaard, Copenhagen.

Gubler, E. V., 1951, On erythrocyte damage during capillary stasis, Vopr. Eksp. Biol. Med., Issue 1:133-139.

Gurevich, M. I., and Bernstein, S. A., 1972, "Vascular Smooth Muscle and Vessel Tone," Naukova Dumka, Kiev.

Häggendal, E., 1968, Elimination of autoregulation during arterial and cerebral hypoxia, in: International Symposium on CBF and CSF, Scand. J. Lab. Clin. Invest., Suppl. 102, V:D.

Häggendal, E., and Johansson, B., 1965, Effects of arterial carbon dioxide tension and oxygen saturation on cerebral blood flow autoregulation in dogs, Acta Physiol. Scand., 66:Suppl. 258, 27-53.

Hamer, J., Hoyer, S., Alberti, E., and Weinhardt, F., 1976, Cerebral blood
    flow and oxidative brain metabolism during and after moderate and
    profound arterial hypoxemia, Acta Neurochir. (Berlin), 33:141-150.

Hansen, A. J., Gjedde, A., and Siemkowicz, E., 1980, Extracellular potas-
    sium and blood flow in the postischemic rat brain, Pflügers Arch.,
    389:1-7.

Harper, A. M., 1965, Physiology of cerebral blood flow, Br. J. Anaesth.,
    37:225-235.

Harper, A. M., and Bell, R. A., 1963, The effect of metabolic acidosis and
    alkalosis on the blood flow through the cerebral cortex, J. Neurol.
    Neurosurg. Psychiatr., 26:341-344.

Harper, A. M., Deshmukh, V. D., Rovan, J. O., and Jenett, B., 1972, The
    influence of sympathetic nervous activity on cerebral blood flow,
    Arch. Neurol., 27:1-6.

Harper, A. M., and Glass, H. I., 1965, Effect of alterations in the arteri-
    al carbon dioxide tension on the blood flow through the cerebral
    cortex at normal and low arterial blood pressure, J. Neurol. Neuro-
    surg. Psychiat., 28:449-452.

Harper, A. M., Jenett, B., Miller, D., and Rowan, J., eds., 1975, "Blood
    Flow and Metabolism in the Brain," Churchill Livingstone, Edinburgh.

Hartman, B. K., Zide, D., and Udenfriend, S., 1972, The use of dopamine
    β-hydroxylase as a marker for the central noradrenergic nervous sys-
    tem in rat brain, Proc. Natl. Acad. Sci., 69:2722-2726.

Hartshorne, D. J., and Gorecka, M., 1980, Biochemistry of the contractile
    proteins of smooth muscle, in: "Handbook of Physiology," Sec. 2:
    The Cardiovascular System; Vol. 2: Vascular Smooth Muscle, D. F.
    Bohr, A. P. Somlyo, and H. V. Sparks, eds., pp. 93-120, American
    Physiological Society, Bethesda, Maryland.

Hayakawa, T., and Waltz, A. G., 1975, Immediate effects of cerebral
    ischemia: evolution and resolution of neurological deficits after
    experimental occlusion of one middle cerebral artery in conscious
    cats, Stroke, 6:321-327.

Haynes, R. H., 1960, Physical basis of the dependence of blood viscosity
    on tube radius, Am. J. Physiol., 198:1193-1200.

Haynes, R. H., and Burton, A. C., 1959, Role of non-Newtonian behavior of
    blood in hemodynamics, Am. J. Physiol., 197:943-950.

Haynes, R. H., and Rodbard, S., 1962, The system of arteries and arterioles,
    in: "Blood Vessels and Lymphatics," D. Abramson, ed., pp. 25-40,
    Academic Press, New York.

Heiss, W. D., Hayakawa, T., and Waltz, A. G., 1976, Patterns of changes of
    blood flow and relationships to infarction in experimental cerebral
    ischemia, Stroke, 7:454-459.

Heistad, D. D., 1981, Summary of Symposium on Cerebral Blood Flow: Effect
    of Nerves and Neurotransmitters, J. Cereb. Blood Flow Metab., 1:447-
    450.

Heistad, D. D., Busija, D. W., and Marcus, M. L., 1981, Neural effects on
    cerebral vessels: alteration of pressure-flow relationship, Fed.
    Proc., 40:2317-2321.

Heistad, D. D., Marcus, M. L., and Abboud, F. M., 1978, Role of large
    arteries in regulation of cerebral blood flow in dogs, J. Clin.
    Invest., 62:761-767.

Heistad, D. D., Marcus, M. L., and Ehrhardt, I. C., 1976, Effect of stimu-
    lation of carotid chemoreceptors on total and regional cerebral blood
    flow, Circ. Res., 38:20-25.

Held, K., Gottstein, U., and Niedermayer, W., 1969, CBF in nonpulsatile
    perfusion, in: "Cerebral Blood Flow," M. Brock, C. Fieschi, D. H.
    Ingvar, N. A. Lassen, and K. Schürmann, eds., pp. 94-95, Springer-
    Verlag, Berlin-Heidelberg-New York.

Hering, H. E., 1937, "Carotissinusreflex," Steinkopff, Dresden.

Heuser, D., Astrup, J., Lassen, N. A., Nilsson, B., Norberg, K., and Sjesjö, B. K., 1977, Are H$^+$ and K$^+$ factors for the adjustment of cerebral blood flow to changes in functional state: a microelectrode study, in: "Cerebral Function, Metabolism and Circulation," D. H. Ingvar and N. A. Lassen, eds., pp. 216-217, Munksgaard, Copenhagen.

Heymans, C., and Neil, E., 1958, "Reflexogenic Areas of the Cardiovascular System," Churchill Livingstone, London.

Hill, L, 1896, "The Physiology and Pathology of the Cerebral Circulation," Churchill, London.

Himwich, W. A., Knapp, F. M., Wenglarz, R. A., Martin, J. D., and Clark, M. E., 1965, The circle of Willis as simulated by an engineering model, Arch. Neurol., 13:164-172.

Hirsch, H., and Schneider, M., 1968, Durchblutung und Sauerstoffaufnahme des Gehirns, in: "Handbuch der Neurochirurgie," H. Olivecrone and W. Tönnis, eds., Vol. 1, Sec. 2, pp. 434-552. Springer-Verlag, Berlin.

Hoff, J. T., MacKenzie, E. T., and Harper, A. M., 1975, Cerebrovascular responses to hypercapnia and hypoxia following VIIth cranial nerve section, in: "Blood Flow Metabolism in the Brain," A. M. Harper, B. Jenett, D. Miller, and J. Rowan, eds., pp. 2.37-2.38, Churchill Livingstone, Edinburgh.

Holmes, R. L., Newman, P. P., and Wolstencroft, J. H., 1958, The distribution of carotid and vertebral blood in the brain of the cat, J. Physiol. (London), 140:236-246.

Hossmann, K.-A., and Kleihues, P., 1973, Reversibility of ischemic brain damage, Arch. Neurol., 29:375-384.

Hossmann, K.-A., Sakaki, S., and Zimmermann, V., 1977, Cation activities in reversible ischemia of the cat brain, Stroke, 8:77-81.

Hürthle, K., 1889, Beiträge zur Hämodynamik. Dritte Abhandlung: Untersuchungen über die Innervation der Hirngefässe, Pflügers Arch., 44: 561-618.

Hutt, G., and Wick, H., 1954, Über Ringmuskelkonstraktion, Innenauskleidungsdicke und ihre gegenseitige Beeinflussung bei der Veränderung rörenförmiger Querschnitte, Pflügers Arch., 258:311-314.

Illig, L., 1955, Experimentelle Untersuchungen über die Entstehung der Stase, Virchows Arch., 326:501-562.

Ingvar, D. H., 1955, Extraneuronal influence upon the electrical activity of isolated cortex following stimulation of the reticular formation, Acta Physiol. Scand., 33:169-193.

Ingvar, D. H., 1958, Cortical state of excitability and cortical circulation, in: "Reticular Formation of the Brain," H. H. Jasper et al., eds., pp. 381-408, Little Brown, Boston.

Ingvar, D. H., 1975, Patterns of brain activity revealed by measurements of regional cerebral blood flow, in: "Brain Work," D. H. Ingvar and N. A. Lassen, eds., pp. 397-413, Munksgaard, Copenhagen.

Ingvar, D. H., and Lassen, N. A., eds., 1965, "Regional Cerebral Blood Flow," An International Symposium, Munksgaard, Copenhagen.

Ingvar, D. H., and Lassen, N. A., eds., 1977a, "Cerebral Function, Metabolism and Circulation," Munksgaard, Copenhagen.

Ingvar, D. H., and Lassen, N. A., 1977b, Measurement of regional cerebral blood flow, Int. J. Neurol., 11:107-117.

Ingvar, D. H., Lassen, N. A., Sjesjö, B. K., and Skinhoj, E., eds., 1968, "Cerebral Blood Flow and Cerebrospinal Fluid," Petersen, Copenhagen.

Ingvar, D. H., Lübbers, D. W., and Sjesjö, B. K., 1962, Normal and epileptic EEG patterns related to cortical oxygen tension in the cat, Acta Physiol. Scand., 55:210-224.

Ingvar, D. H., and Söderberg, U, 1956, A new method for measuring cerebral blood flow in relation to the electroencephalogram, Electroenceph. Clin. Neurophysiol., 8:403-412.

Isenberg, I., 1953, A note of the flow of blood in capillary tubes, Bull. Math. Biophys., 15:149-152.

Itakura, T., Yamamoto, K., Tohyama, M., and Shimizu, N., 1977, Central dual innervation of arterioles and capillaries of the brain, Stroke, 8:360-365.

Iwoyama, T., Furness, J. B., and Burnstock, G., 1970, Dual adrenergic and cholinergic innervation of the cerebral arteries of the rat. An ultrastructural study, Circ. Res., 26:635-646.

Jacobj, W., 1920, Beobachtungen am peripheren Gefässapparat unter lokaler Beeinflussung desselben durch pharmakoligische Agentian, Arch. Exp. Pathol. Pharmakol., 86:49-79.

Jenett, Sh., and Craigen, M. L., 1981, Pial arteriolar diameter during induction of hypoxia, J. Cereb. Blood Flow Metab., 1:Suppl. 1, S251-S252.

Johansson, B. B., 1976, Some factors influencing the damaging effect of acute arterial hypertension on cerebral vessels in rats," Clin. Sci. Mol. Med., 51:41-43.

Johansson, B., Li, Ch. L., Olsson, Y., and Klatzo, I., 1970, The effect of acute arterial hypertension on blood-brain barrier to protein tracers, Acta Neuropath. (Berlin), 16:117-124.

Johansson, B., and Mellander, S., 1975, Static and dynamic components in the vascular myogenic response to passive changes in length as revealed by electrical and mechanical recording from rat portal vein, Circ. Res., 36:76-83.

Johansson, B. B., and Nordberg, C., 1978, Cerebral vessels in spontaneously hypertensive rats, in: Pathology of Cerebral Microcirculation, Advances in Neurology, Vol. 20, "Pathology of Cerebral Microcirculation," J. Cervós-Navarro, E. Betz, G. Ebhardt, R. Ferszt, and R. Wüllenweber, eds., pp. 349-357, Raven Press, New York.

Johansson, B., and Somlyo, A. P., 1980, Electrophysiology and excitation-contraction coupling, in: "Handbook of Physiology," Sec. 2: The Cardiovascular System; Vol. 2: Vascular Smooth Muscle, D. F. Bohr, A. P. Somlyo, and H. V. Sparks, eds., pp. 301-323, American Physiological Society, Bethesda, Maryland.

Johnson, P. C., 1971, Red cell separation in the mesenteric capillary network, Am. J. Physiol., 221:99-104.

Johnson, P. C., 1978, "Peripheral Circulation," John Wiley and Sons, New York.

Johnson, P. C., 1980, The myogenic response, in: "Handbook of Physiology," Sec. 2: The Cardiovascular System; Vol. 2: Vascular Smooth Muscle, D. F. Bohr, A. P. Somlyo, and H. V. Sparks, eds., pp. 409-442, American Physiological Society, Bethesda, Maryland.

Johnson, P. C., Blaschke, J., Burton, K. S., and Dial, J. H., 1971, Influence of flow variations on capillary hematocrit in mesentery, Am. J. Physiol., 221:105-112.

Jokeleinen, P. T., Jokeleinen, G. I., and Coyle, P., 1982, Nonrandom distribution of rat pial arterial sphincters, in: "Cerebral Blood Flow. Effects of Nerves and Neurotransmitters," D. D. Heistad and M. L. Marcus, eds., pp. 107-116, Elsevier, New York.

Jones, A. W., 1980, Content and fluxes of electrolytes, in: "Handbook of Physiology." Sec. 2: Cardiovascular Physiology; Vol. 2: Vascular Smooth Muscle, D. F. Bohr, A. P. Somlyo, and H. V. Sparks, eds., pp. 253-299, American Physiological Society, Bethesda, Maryland.

Jones, J. V., Fitch, W., MacKenzie, E. T., Strandgaard, S., and Harper, A. M., 1976, Lower limit of cerebral blood flow autoregulation in experimental renovascular hypertension in the baboon, Circ. Res., 39:555-557.

Jones, W. T., 1851, On the state of the blood and the blood vessels in inflammation, Guy's Hosp. Rep., 7:1-124.

Kaasik, A. E., 1979a, Comments in discussion, in: "Regulation of Cerebral Circulation," G. I. Mchedlishvili, M. J. Purves, and A. G. B. Kovách, eds., p. 84, Akadémiai Kiadó, Budapest.

Kaasik, A. E., 1979b, Comments in discussion, in: "Regulation of Cerebral Circulation," G. I. Mchedlishvili, M. J. Purves, and A. G. B. Kovách, eds., pp. 200-201, Akadémiai Kiadó, Budapest.

Kahn, R. H., and Pollak, F., 1931, Die aktive Verengerung des Lumens der capillaren Blutgefässe, Pflügers Arch., 226:799-807.

Kaltenbrunner, G., 1826, Experimenta circa statum sanguinis et vosorum in inflammatione, Monachii.

Kanzow, E., and Krause, D., 1962, Vasomotorik der Hirnrinde und EEG-Aktivität wacher, frei beweglicher Katzen, Pflügers Arch., 274:447-458.

Kapp, J. P., Robertson, J. T., and White, R. P., 1976, Spasmogenic qualities of prostaglandin $F_{2\alpha}$ in the cat, J. Neurosurg., 44:173-175.

Kawamura, J., Meyer, J. S., Hiromoto, H., Aoyagi, M., and Hashi, K., 1974, Neurogenic control of cerebral blood flow in the baboon. Effect of alpha-adrenergic blockage with phenoxybenzamine on reactivity of changes in $PaCO_2$, Stroke, 5:747-758.

Kety, S. S., 1960, The cerebral circulation, in: "Handbook of Physiology," Sec. 1: Neurophysiology, H. W. McCoun, ed., Vol. 3, pp. 1751-1760, Williams and Wilkins, Washington, DC.

Kety, S. S., and Schmidt, C. F., 1948, The effects of altered arterial tension of carbon dioxide and oxygen on cerebral blood flow and cerebral oxygen consumption of normal young man, J. Clin. Invest., 27:484-452.

Klitzman, B., and Duling, B. R., 1979, Microvascular hematocrit and red cell flow in resting and contracting striated muscle, Am. J. Physiol., 237:H481-H490.

Klosovsky, B. N., 1951, "Blood Circulation in the Brain," Medgiz, Moscow.

Knisely, M. H., Block, E. H. Elior, T. S., and Werner, L., 1947, Sludged blood, Science, 106:431-440.

Kogure, K., Scheinberg, P., Reinmuth, O. M., Fujishima, M., and Busto, R., 1970, Mechanisms of cerebral vasodilation in hypoxia, J. Appl. Physiol., 29:223-229.

Kolossov, A., 1893, Über die Struktur des Pleuroperitoneae- und Gefässepithels (Endothels), Arch. Mikr. Anat., 42:318-383.

Koltover, A. N., Vereshchagin, N. V., Liubkovskaja, N. G., and Morgunov, V. A., 1975, "Pathological Anatomy of Disorders of the Cerebral Circulation," Meditsina, Moscow.

Kontos, H. A., Raper, A. J., and Patterson, J. L., 1977a, Analysis of vasoactivity of local pH, P_{CO_2}, and bicarbonate on pial vessels, Stroke, 8:358-360.

Kontos, H. A., Wei, E. P., Navari, R. M., Levasseur, Y. E., Rosenblum, W. I., and Patterson, Y. L., 1978, Responses of cerebral arteries and arterioles to acute hypotension and hypertension, Am. J. Physiol., 234:H371-H383.

Kontos, H. A., Wei, E. P., Paper, A. J., and Patterson, J. L., 1977b, Local mechanism of CO_2 action on cat pial arterioles, Stroke, 8:226-229.

Kosmarskaya, E. N., and Kapustina, E. V., 1953, Zones of collateral circulation in the brain, Byull. Eksp. Biol. Med., 35, No. 4: 78-83.

Kostiurin, S. D., 1880, On distribution of red blood cells in capillaries of the skin, Wratch, No. 23:375-379.

Kovách, A. G. B., Dóra, E., Szabo, L., and Urbanics, R., 1979, Effect of alpha receptor blockage on the autoregulatory vascular volume and redox state changes in the cat brain cortex, in: "Cerebral Blood Flow and Metabolism," F. Gotoh, H. Nagai, and Y. Tazaki, eds., pp. 104-105, Munksgaard, Copenhagen.

Kovách, A. G. B., Roheim, P. S., Iranyi, M., Scerhati, E., Gosztonyi, G., and Kovách, E., 1959, Circulation and metabolism in the head of the dog in ischemic shock, Acta Physiol. Acad. Sci. Hung., 15:217-229.

Kovalevsky, G. V., 1963, On functional morphology of arteries, Arch. Pathol. (Moscow), 45, No. 11:37-43.

Kramer, G. L., and Hardman, J. G., 1980, Cyclic nucleotides and blood vessel contraction, in: "Handbook of Physiology," Sec. 2: Cardiovascular System; Vol. 2: Vascular Smooth Muscle, D. F. Bohr, A. P. Somlyo, and H. V. Sparks, eds., pp. 179-199, American Physiological Society, Bethesda, Maryland.

Kreindler, A., 1975, "Cerebral Infarct and Cerebral Hemorrhages," Academic Press of Rumania, Bucharest.

Krogh, A., 1920, Studies on the capillarimotor mechanism. I. The reaction to stimuli and innervation of the blood vessels in the tongue of the frog, J. Physiol. (London), 53:399-419.

Krogh, A., 1921, Studies on the physiology of capillaries. II. The reactions to local stimuli of the blood vessels in the skin and the web of the frog, J. Physiol. (London), 55:412-422.

Krogh, A., 1922, "The Anatomy and Physiology of Capillaries," Yale Univ. Press, New Haven, Conn.

Krupp, P., 1966, "Cerebral Durchblutung und elektrische Hirnaktivität," S. Karger, Basel-New York.

Kuprianov, V. V., and Zhitsa, V. T., 1975, "Nervous Apparatus of Cerebral Blood Vessels," Shtiintsa, Kishinev.

Kursky, M. D., and Baksheev, N. S., 1974, "Biochemical Basis of the Mechanism of Serotonin Effect," Naukova Dumka, Kiev.

Kuschinsky, W., 1982, Role of hydrogen ions in regulation of cerebral blood flow and other regional flows, Adv. Microcirc., 11:1-19, Karger, Basel.

Kuschinsky, W., 1982-1983, Coupling between functional activity, metabolism and blood flow in the brain: state of the art, Microcirculation, 2:357-378.

Kuschinsky, W., Suda, S., and Sokoloff, L., 1981, Local cerebral glucose utilization and blood flow during metabolic acidosis, Am. J. Physiol., 241:H772-H777.

Kuschinsky, W., and Wahl, M., 1978, Local chemical and neurogenic regulation of cerebral vascular resistance, Physiol. Rev., 58:656-689.

Kuschinsky, W., and Wahl, M., 1979, Perivascular pH and pial arterial diameter during bicuculline-induced seizures in cats, Pflügers Arch., 382:81-85.

Kuschinsky, W., Wahl, M., Bosse, O., and Thurau, K., 1972, Perivascular potassium and pH as determinants of local pial arterial diameter in cats. A microapplication study, Circ. Res., 31:240-247.

Kuschinsky, W., Wahl, M., and Neiss, A., 1974, Evidence for cholinergic dilatatory receptors in pial arteries of cats. A microapplication study, Pflügers Arch., 347:199-208.

Lambertsen, C. J., Kough, R. H., Cooper, D. Y., Emmel, G. L., Loeschke, H. H., and Schmidt, C. F., 1953, Oxygen toxicity. Effect in man of oxygen inhalation at 1 and 3.5 atmospheres upon blood gas transport, cerebral circulation, and cerebral metabolism, J. Appl. Physiol., 5:471-486.

Lang, J., 1965, Mikroskopische Anatomie der Arterien, Angiologica, 2:225-282.

Langfitt, T. W., and Kassel, N., 1968, Cerebral vasodilatation produced by brainstem stimulation: neurogen control vs. autoregulation, Am. J. Physiol., 215:90-97.

Langfitt, T. W., McHenry, L. C., Reivich, M., and Wollman, H., eds., 1975, "Cerebral Circulation and Metabolism," Springer-Verlag, New York-Heidelberg-Berlin.

Lassen, N. A., 1959, Cerebral blood flow and oxygen consumption in man, Physiol. Rev., 39:183–238.

Lassen, N. A., 1964, Autoregulation of cerebral blood flow, Circ. Res., 15:Suppl. 1, pp. 201–204.

Lassen, N. A., 1966, The luxury-perfusion syndrome and its possible relation to acute metabolic acidosis localized within the brain, Lancet, 11:1113–1115.

Lassen, N. A., 1978, Brain, in: "Peripheral Circulation," P. C. Johnson, ed., pp. 337–358, John Wiley and Sons, New York.

Lavrentieva, N. B., Mchedlishvili, G. I., and Pletchkova, E. K., 1968, Distribution and activity of cholinesterase in the nervous structures of the pial arteries (a histochemical study), Byull. Eksp. Biol. Med., 64:No. 11, pp. 110–113.

Lawson, H. C., 1962, The volume of blood. A critical examination of methods for its measurement, in: "Handbook of Physiology," Sec. 2: Circulation, W. F. Hamilton, ed., Vol. 1, pp. 23–49, Williams and Wilkins, Baltimore.

Lazorthes, G., 1961, "Vescularisation et circulation cérébrale," Masson et Cie, Paris.

Lee, T. J. F., 1981, Nerve-muscle relationships in cerebral artery, Blood Vessels, 18:218.

Lee, T. J. F., Su, C., and Bevan, J. A., 1975, Nonsympathetic dilator innervation of cat cerebral arteries, Experiencia, 31:1424–1425.

Lee, T. J. F., Su, C., and Bevan, J. A., 1976, Neurogenic sympathetic vasoconstriction of the rabbit basilar artery, Circ. Res., 39:120–126.

Lende, R. A., 1960, Local spasm in cerebral arteries, J. Neurosurg., 17:90–103.

Leniger-Follert, E., and Hossmann, K.-A., 1979, Simultaneous measurements of microflow and evoked potentials in the somatomotor cortex of the cat brain during specific sensory activation, Pflügers Arch., 380:85–89.

Leniger-Follert, E., and Lübbers, D. W., 1976, Behaviour of microflow and local PO_2 of the brain cortex during and after direct electrical stimulation. A contribution to the problem of metabolic regulation of microcirculation in the brain, Pflügers Arch., 366:39–44.

Leniger-Follert, E., Lübbers, D. W., and Wrabitz, W., 1975, Regulation of local tissue PO_2 of the brain cortex at different arterial O_2 pressure, Pflügers Arch., 359:81–95.

Leniger-Follert, E., Urbanics, R., Harbig, K., and Lübbers, D. W., 1977, The behavior of local pH and NADH-fluorescence during and after direct activation of the brain cortex, in: "Cerebral Function, Metabolism and Circulation, D. Ingvar and N. Lassen, eds., pp. 214–215, Munksgaard, Copenhagen.

Lennox, W. G., and Gibbs, E. L., 1932, The blood flow in the brain and the leg of man and the changes induced by alterations of blood gases, J. Clin. Invest., 11:1155–1177.

Levtov, V. A., Regirer, S. A., and Shadrina, N. Kh., 1982, "Blood Rheology," Meditsina, Moscow.

Licata, R. H., Olson, D. R., and Wack, E. W., 1975, Cholinergic and adrenergic innervation of cerebral vessels, in: "Cerebral Circulation and Metabolism," T. W. Langfitt, H. L. C. McHenry, M. Revich, and H. Wollman, eds., pp. 466–469, Springer-Verlag, New York-Heidelberg-Berlin.

Lierse, W., 1963, Die Kapillardichte im Wirbeltiergehirn, Acta Anat., 54:1–31.

Lightfoot, E. N., 1974, "Transport Phenomena and Living Systems," John Wiley and Sons, New York.

Linder, A., and Alksne, J. F., 1978, Prevention of persistent cerebral smooth muscle contraction in response to whole blood, Stroke, 9:472–477.

Linton, R. A. F., Miller, R., and Cameron, I. R., 1975, The effect of hyper-
    capnia, hypoxia and carotid sinus nerve section on hypothalamic blood
    flow in anesthetized rabbits, in: "Blood Flow and Metabolism in the
    Brain," A. M. Harper, B. Jenett, D. Miller, and J. Rowan, eds., pp.
    2.32-2.34, Churchill Livingstone, Edinburgh.

Lipowsky, H. H., Kovalcheck, S., and Zweifach, B. W., 1978. The distribu-
    tion of blood rheological parameters in the microvasculature of rat
    mesentary, Circ. Res., 43:738-749.

Lipowsky, H. H., Rofe, S., Tannenbaum, L., Firell, J. C., Usami, S., and
    Chien, S., 1981, Microvessel hematocrit. Distribution of bifurca-
    tions, Microvasc. Res., 21:249-250.

Lipowsky, H. H., Usami, Sh., and Chien, Sh., 1980, *In vivo* measurements of
    "apparent viscosity" and microvessel hematocrit in the mesentery of
    the cat, Microvasc. Res., 19:297-319.

Lister, J., 1857-1858, On the early stages of inflammation, Edinburgh Med.
    J., 3:656-660; Physiol. Trans. R. Soc., London, 148:645-649.

Lübbers, D. W., 1968, The oxygen pressure field of the brain and its sig-
    nificance for the normal and critical oxygen supply to the brain, in:
    "Oxygen Transport in Blood and Tissue," D. W. Lübbers, U. C. Luft,
    G. Tews, and E. Wilzleb, eds., pp. 124-139, George Thieme Verlag,
    Stuttgart.

Lübbers, D. W., 1972, Physiology der Gehirndurchblutung, in: "Der
    Hirnkreisluf," H. Gänshirt, ed., pp. 214-260, George Thieme Verlag,
    Stuttgart.

Lübbers, D. W., Hauck, G., Weigelt, H., and Addicks, K., 1979, Contractile
    properties of frog capillaries tested by electrical stimulation, in:
    "Microcirculation in Inflammation," G. Hauck and J. W. Irwin, eds.,
    Bibl. Anat., No. 17:3-10, S. Karger, Basel.

Lugovoi, L. A., 1964, Circulation in individual areas of the cerebral
    cortex during photic and olfactory stimulation, Byull. Eksp. Biol. Med.,
    59:No. 10, 11-15.

Lundgren, B., Schultz, H., and Sjesjö, B. K., 1974, Changes in energy state
    and acid-base parameters of the rat brain during complete compression
    ischemia, Brain Res., 73:277-289.

Luse, A. A., 1962, Ultrastructure of the brain and its relation to trans-
    port of metabolites, in: "Ultrastructure and Metabolism of the Ner-
    vous System," pp. 1-26, Baltimore, Md.

Mabe, H., 1978, The role of sympathetic nerve and vasoactive amines in ex-
    perimental cerebral vasospasm, Neurol. Surg., 6:555-561.

MacKenzie, E. T., Farrar, J. K., Fitch, W., Graham, D. I., Gregory, P. C.,
    and Harper, A. M., 1979, Effects of hemorrhagic hypotension on the
    cerebral circulation. I. Cerebral blood flow and pial arteriolar
    caliber, Stroke, 10:711-718.

MacKenzie, E. T., McGeorge, A. P., Graham, D. I., Fitch, W., Edvinsson,
    L., and Harper, A. M., 1977, Breakthrough of cerebral autoregulation
    and the sympathetic nervous system, in: "Cerebral Function, Metabo-
    lism and Circulation," D. H. Ingvar and N. A. Lassen, eds., pp. 68-69,
    Munksgaard, Copenhagen.

Madow, B., and Bloch, E. H., 1956, The effect of erythrocyte aggregation
    on the rheology of blood, Angiology, 7:1-15.

Magendie, F., 1838, Leçons sur les Phénomènes Physiques de la Vie, Vol. 3,
    Brussels.

Mall, J. P., 1888, Die Blut- und Lymphwege im Dünndarm des Hundes. Königl.
    Sächs. Gesellsch. der Wissensch. Abhandlungen der math. physikal.
    Klasse, Leipzig, 14:153-161.

Mamisashvili, V. A., 1979, The participation of myogenic responses of vas-
    cular effectors in cerebral blood flow control with changes in sys-
    temic arterial pressure, in: "Regulation of Cerebral Circulation,"
    G. I. Mchedlishvili, M. J. Purves, and A. G. B. Kovách, eds., pp. 33-
    38, Akadémiai Kiadó, Budapest.

Mamisashvili, V. A., Babunashvili, M. K., and Mchedlishvili, G. I., 1975,
    The optimality criteria of functional behavior of larger and smaller
    pial arteries in regulation of the brain blood supply, Fiziol. Zh.
    SSSR, 62:1501-1506.
Mamisashvili, V. A., Babunashvili, M. K., and Mchedlishvili, G. I., 1977,
    Distribution of flow velocities and segmental resistances in the pial
    arterial system, in: "Brain Blood Supply," G. I. Mchedlishvili,
    A. G. B. Kovách, and I. Nyáry, eds., pp. 69-78, Akadémiai Kiadó,
    Budapest.
Mamisashvili, V. A., and Baratashvili, I. K., 1980, In vivo study of
    erythrocyte orientation in microvessels and effects on it of various
    factors, Fiziol. Zh. SSSR, 66:1466-1472.
Mamisashvili, V. A., Baratashvili, I. K., and Lominadze, D. G., 1982,
    Velocity profile in microvessels dependent upon red cell velocity and
    concentration, Fiziol. Zh. SSSR, 68:1673-1679.
Mamisashvili, V. A., Baratashvili, I. K., and Lominadze, D. G., 1984,
    Formation of velocity profile in microvessels, Proc. Georgian Acad.
    Sci., Biol. Ser., 10:197-203.
Mamisashvili, V. A., Mchedlishvili, G. I., Ormotsadze, L. G., and Laskhish-
    vili, G. O., 1983, On the mechanism of "autoregulation" of cerebral
    blood flow: the role of neurogenic and myogenic vascular responses,
    Fiziol. Zh. SSSR, 69: 391-396.
Marcus, M. L., and Heistad, D. D., 1979, Effects of sympathetic nerves on
    cerebral blood flow in awake dogs, Am. J. Physiol., 236:H549-H553.
Marin, J., Salaices, M., Rivilla, F., Burgos, J., and Marco, E. J., 1980,
    Bilateral innervation of the cerebral arteries by the superior cervi-
    cal ganglion in cats, J. Neurosurg., 53:88-91.
Martin, E. G., Wooley, E. C., and Miller, M., 1932, Capillary counts in
    resting and active muscles, Am. J. Physiol., 100:407-416.
Matteis, F., Mariotti, L., and Castellani, R., 1955, L'aggregazione eritro-
    citaria intravasculare "sludged blood" nella malattia reumatica,
    Giorg. Malatt. e Parass., 7:135-142.
Mayer, S., 1902, Die Muskularisierung der Capillaren Blutgefässe: Nach-
    weis der anatomischen Substanz ihrer Contractilität, Anat. Anz., 21:
    442.
Mayorova, N. F., Teplov, S. M., and Ugriumov, V. M., 1974, Features of the
    functional hyperemia of human brain and its correlation with EEG, in:
    "Third Tbilisi Symposium on Brain Blood Supply," pp. 22-23, Tbilisi.
McDonald, D. A., and Potter, J. M., 1951, The distribution of blood in the
    brain, J. Physiol. (London), 114:356-371.
Mchedlishvili, G. I., 1951, On hemodynamics of capillary circulation,
    Fiziol. Zh. SSSR, 36:304-311.
Mchedlishvili, G. I., 1952, On inflammatory changes of capillary circula-
    tion, in: Collection of Works Dedicated to 60th Anniversary of
    Scientific and Pedagogic Activity of V. V. Voronin," pp. 149-161,
    Georgian Acad. Sci. Publishers, Tbilisi.
Mchedlishvili, G. I., 1953, Investigations of mechanism of capillary
    stasis, in: Transactions of the Institute of Physiology, Georgian
    Academy of Sciences, 9:279-292, Georgian Acad. Sci. Publishers,
    Tbilisi.
Mchedlishvili, G. I., 1956a, On distribution of erythrocytes in the organ-
    isms' vascular system, Arkh. Patol. (Moscow), 17:No. 5, 88-89.
Mchedlishvili, G. I., 1956b, A method of studying capillary circulation in
    the cerebral cortex, in: Problems of the Modern Physiology of the
    Nervous and Muscle Systems, pp. 549-554, Georgian Academy of Sci.
    Publishers, Tbilisi.
Mchedlishvili, G. I., 1957, Mechanisms of changes of the capillary circu-
    lation, Usp. Sovrem. Biol. (Moscow), 43:82-96.

Mchedlishvili, G. I., 1958, "Capillary Circulation," Georgian Acad. Sci.
    Publishers, Tbilisi.
Mchedlishvili, G. I., 1959a, Role of the internal carotid and vertebral
    arteries in regulation of the cerebral circulation, Fiziol. Zh. SSSR,
    45:1221-1228.
Mchedlishvili, G. I., 1959b, Investigations into the localization of "clos-
    ing mechanisms" on regional brain arteries (internal carotid and ver-
    tebral arteries), Dokl. Akad. Nauk SSSR, 124:1371-1374.
Mchedlishvili, G. I., 1960a, The action of adrenalin on the regional arter-
    ies of the brain, Bull. Exp. Biol. Med., 49:No. 5, 10-15.
Mchedlishvili, G. I., 1960b, On the independence of mechanisms regulating
    the lumen of regional arteries of brain (the internal carotid and
    vertebral arteries) and of pial arteries, Byull. Eksp. Biol. Med., 49:
    No. 6, 21-25.
Mchedlishvili, G. I., 1960c, Changes in cerebral circulation during re-
    suscitation by intra-arterial blood transfusion, Patol. Fiziol. Eksp.
    Ter., 4:No. 4, 14-20.
Mchedlishvili, G. I., 1960d, Physiological mechanisms of cerebral circula-
    tion in terminal states, Fiziol. Zh. SSSR, 46:1210-1217.
Mchedlishvili, G. I., 1962, "Chest-head" preparation for investigation of
    cerebral circulation, Byull. Eksp. Biol. Med., 53:No. 2, 123-125.
Mchedlishvili, G. I., 1963, Mechanisms of regulation of the cerebral cir-
    culation. 2. Functional differences between various parts of the
    brain arterial system. Trans. Inst. Physiol., Georgian Acad. Sci.,
    13:147-160, Tbilisi.
Mchedlishvili, G. I., 1964, Vascular mechanisms pertaining to the in-
    trinsic regulation of the cerebral circulation, Circulation, 30:597-
    610.
Mchedlishvili, G. I., 1968, "Functional Behavior of Vascular Mechanisms of
    the Brain," Nauka, Leningrad.
Mchedlishvili, G. I., ed., 1969a, "Correlation of Blood Supply with Me-
    tabolism and Function," Proceedings of an International Symposium
    held in Tbilisi. Metsniereba Publishers, Tbilisi.
Mchedlishvili, G. I., 1969b, The conjectural role of the Fahraeus-Lindqvist
    rheological phenomenon in some microcirculatory events, in: 5th
    European Conference on Microcirculation, Gothenburg, 1968, Bibl.
    Anat., No. 10, H. Harders, ed., pp. 66-73, S. Karger, Basel.
Mchedlishvili, G. I., 1970, Distribution of blood and its constituents in
    microcirculation system, News of USSR Acad. Med. Sci., No. 11:48-57.
Mchedlishvili, G. I., 1972, "Vascular Mechanisms of the Brain," Plenum
    Press, New York.
Mchedlishvili, G., 1973, Pathophysiological mechanisms of spasm of the
    cerebral arteries, in: "Cerebral Vascular Disease," 6th International
    Conference, Salzburg, 1972, J. S. Meyer, H. Lechner, M. Reivich, and
    O. Eichhorn, eds., pp. 173-176, George Thieme Publishers, Stuttgart.
Mchedlishvili, G. I., 1974, Pathogenesis of vasospasm, Patol. Fiziol.
    Exper. Ter., No. 2:6-15.
Mchedlishvili, G. I., 1977a, "The Cerebral Arterial Spasm," Metsniereba
    Press, Tbilisi.
Mchedlishvili, G. I., 1977b, The systems approach in planning of research.
    An example with a complex biomedical problem, Vestn. Akad. Nauk SSSR,
    No. 5:89-93.
Mchedlishvili, G. I., 1980a, Physiological mechanisms controlling cerebral
    blood flow, Stroke, 11:140-248.
Mchedlishvili, G. I., ed., 1980b, "Regulation of Cerebral Circulation,"
    Proceedings of the 4th Tbilisi Symposium on Cerebral Circulation,
    April 19-21, 1978, Metsniereba Publishers, Tbilisi.
Mchedlishvili, G. I., 1981a, The nature of cerebral vasospasm, Blood
    Vessels, 18:311-320.

Mchedlishvili, G. I., 1981b, On the physiological mechanisms of regulation
    of cerebral blood flow, in: "Advances of Physiological Sciences,"
    Vol. 9: Cardiovascular Physiology, Neural Control Mechanisms, A. G. B.
    Kovách, P. Sandór, and M. Kollai, eds., pp. 109–118, Pergamon Press-
    Akadémiai Kiadó, Budapest.
Mchedlishvili, G. I., 1982, A systems approach to the organization of bio-
    medical research, IRCS Med. Sci., 10:590–591.
Mchedlishvili, G. I., and Akhobadze, V. A., 1961, The cerebral arterial
    system in brain injury and during traumatic edema, Physiol. Bohemo-
    slov., 10:S-14.
Mchedlishvili, G. I., Akhobadze, V. A., and Ormotsadze, L. G., 1962,
    Dynamics of cerebrovascular disorders and their compensation during
    temporary occlusion of the aorta, Patol. Fiziol. Eksp. Ter., 6:No. 3,
    17–23.
Mchedlishvili, G. I., Akhobadze, V. A., and Ormotsadze, L. G., 1973, Com-
    pensation of cerebral circulation during temporary occlusion of the
    cranial (superior) vena cava, Fed. Proc., 22:197–201.
Mchedlishvili, G. I., Antia, R. V., and Nikolaishvili, L. S., 1974,
    Dynamics of some metabolic changes in the cerebral cortex during
    ischemia and early postischemic periods, Neuropatol. Pol., 12:625–
    633.
Mchedlishvili, G. I., and Baramidze, D. G., 1965, Functional behavior of
    small arteries of the cerebral cortex, Dokl. Akad. Nauk SSSR, 163:
    529–532.
Mchedlishvili, G. I., and Baramidze, D. G., 1971, Functional behavior of
    the precortical arteries under conditions of experimental hypo- and
    hypertension, Byull. Eksp. Biol. Med., 72:No. 10, 14–16.
Mchedlishvili, G. I., and Baramidze, D. G., 1984, Physiological mechanisms
    regulating the microcirculation in the brain cortex, Fiziol. Zh.
    SSSR, 70:1473–1483.
Mchedlishvili, G. I., Baramidze, D. G., and Gordeladze, Z. T., 1984, Dis-
    tribution of pial arterial dilatatory responses to microapplication
    of strychnine to brain surface, Fiziol. Zh. SSSR, 70:667–672.
Mchedlishvili, G. I., Baramidze, D. G., and Nikolaishvili, L. S., 1967,
    Functional behavior of the pial and cortical arteries in conditions
    of increased metabolic demand from the cerebral cortex, Nature, 213:
    506–507.
Mchedlishvili, G. I., Baramidze, D. G., Nikolaishvili, L. S., Antia, R. V.,
    and Gordeladze, Z. T., 1978, On the control of microcirculation in
    the cerebral cortex during and following ischemia, Biochem. Exp.
    Biol., 14:285–297.
Mchedlishvili, G. I., Baramidze, D. G., Nikolaishvili, L. S., and
    Mamisashvili, V. A., 1974–1975, Vascular mechanisms responsible for
    microcirculation of the cerebral cortex, Biochem. Exp. Biol., 11:113–
    129.
Mchedlishvili, G. I., Baramidze, D. G., Nikolaishvili, L. S., and Ormo-
    tsadze, L. G., 1969, Function of the vascular mechanisms of brain in
    regulation of adequate blood supply to cerebral cortex, in: "Cor-
    relation of Blood Supply with Metabolism and Function," Proceedings
    of an International Symposium, G. I. Mchedlishvili, ed., pp. 85–100,
    Metsniereba Press, Tbilisi.
Mchedlishvili, G. I., Borodulya, A. V., and Ormotsadze, L. G., 1972, Ef-
    ferent adrenergic innervation and its role in development of spasm
    of internal carotid artery, Zh. Neiropatol. Psikhiat. (Moscow), 72:1172–
    1176.
Mchedlishvili, G. I., and Devdariani, M. G., 1964, Intrinsic mechanism
    determining the collateral circulation in the brain, Patol. Fiziol.
    Eksp. Ter., 8:No. 3, 20–29.
Mchedlishvili, G. I., and Gabashvili, V. M., 1965, Investigation of the
    genesis of pathological constriction and spasm of the internal ca-
    rotid arteries, Patol. Fiziol. Eksp. Ter., 9:No. 6, 9–14.

Mchedlishvili, G. I., Garbuliński, T., and Gosk, A., 1962, Researches of function of the internal carotid arteries, Acta Physiol. Polonica, 13:695–704.

Mchedlishvili, G. I., Garfunkel, M. L., Ormotsadze, L. G., Nikolaishvili, L. S., and Antia, R. V., 1972, Cerebral circulation under conditions of heterotransfusion shock, Patol. Fiziol. Eksp. Ter., No. 6:25–31.

Mchedlishvili, G. I., Ingvar, D. H., Baramidze, D. G., and Eckberg, R., 1970, Blood flow and vascular behavior in the cerebral cortex related to strychnine-induced spike activity, Exp. Neurol., 26:411–423.

Mchedlishvili, G. I., Kapuściński, A., and Nikolaishvili, L., 1976, Mechanisms of postischemic brain edema: contribution of circulatory factors, Stroke, 7:410–416.

Mchedlishvili, G. I., Kaufman, O. Ya, Ormotsadze, L. G., and Borodulya, V. A., 1971, Functional-morphological studies of the spasm of internal carotid artery, Krovoobrashchenie, 4:No. 4, 3–8.

Mchedlishvili, G. I., Kometiani, P. A., and Ormotsadze, L. G., 1970–1971, On the mechanism of spasm of the internal carotid artery, Biochem. Sper. Biol., 9:233–240.

Mchedlishvili, G. I., Kometiani, P. A., and Ormotsadze, L. G., 1971, Involvement of calcium ions in the formation of vascular tone and in the serotonin vasoconstrictory effect on internal carotid artery, Bull. Exp. Biol. Med., 71:No. 6, 3–5.

Mchedlishvili, G. I., Kometiani, P. A., and Ormotsadze, L. G., 1972, Disturbance in membrane function of vascular smooth muscles as a possible cause of spasm of the internal carotid artery, Byull. Eksp. Biol. Med., 74:No. 9, 19–21.

Mchedlishvili, G. I., Kovách, A. G. B., and Nyáry, I., eds., 1977, "Brain Blood Supply," Proceedings of the 3rd Tbilisi Symposium on Cerebral Circulation, Akadémiai Kiadó, Budapest.

Mchedlishvili, G., and Kuridze, N., 1984, The modular organization of pial arterial system in phylogeny, J. Cereb. Blood Flow Metab., 4:391–396.

Mchedlishvili, G. I., and Mamisashvili, V. A., 1974, Static and dynamic characteristics of factors responsible for resistance in the pial arteries controlling microcirculation of the cerebral cortex, Byull. Eksp. Biol. Med., 77:No. 4, 11–14.

Mchedlishvili, G. I., and Mamisashvili, V. A., 1981, Might the pure myogenic reactions of vascular effectors be responsible for cerebral blood flow "autoregulation"? J. Cereb. Blood Flow Metab., 1:Suppl. 1, S441–S442.

Mchedlishvili, G. I., Mitagvaria, N. P., and Ormotsadze, L. G., 1971, Computation of the resistance in larger and smaller arteries of the brain with a mathematical model, Fiziol. Zh. SSSR, 57:575–583.

Mchedlishvili, G. I., Mitagvaria, N. P., and Ormotsadze, L. G., 1973, Vascular mechanisms controlling a constant blood supply to the brain ("autoregulation"), Stroke, 4:742–750.

Mchedlishvili, G., Mossakowski, M., Itkis, M., Sikharulidze, N., and Januszewski, S., 1974, Cerebral blood volume changes during the development of brain edema, in: "Recent Progress in Study and Therapy of Brain Edema," K. G. Go and A. Baethman, eds., pp. 137–150, Plenum Press, New York.

Mchedlishvili, G. I., and Nikolaishvili, L. S., 1964, The nervous mechanism of nutritive reactions of the pial arteries supplying blood to cerebral cortex, Dokl. Akad. Nauk SSSR, 156:968–971.

Mchedlishvili, G. I., and Nikolaishvili, L. S., 1966, Studies of physiological mechanisms of blood supply correlation with functional state of brain cortex, Fiziol. Zh. SSSR, 52:380–386.

Mchedlishvili, G. I., and Nikolaishvili, L. S., 1967, Zum nervösen Mechanismus der funktionellen Dilatation der Piaarterien, Pflügers Arch., 296:14–20.

Mchedlishvili, G. I., and Nikolaishvili, L. S., 1970, Evidence for a cholinergic nervous mechanism mediating the autoregulatory dilatation of
the cerebral blood vessels, Pflügers Arch., 315:27-37.

Mchedlishvili, G. I., Nikolaishvili, L. S., and Antia, R. V., 1974, Cerebral blood flow and arterial behavior during ischemia and early postischemic periods, Neuropatol. Pol., 12:551-562.

Mchedlishvili, G. I., Nikolaishvili, L. S., and Antia, R. V., 1976, Are
the pial arterial responses dependent on the direct effect of intravascular pressure and extravascular and intravascular PO_2, PCO_2, and
pH? Microvasc. Res., 10:298-311.

Mchedlishvili, G. I., Nikolaishvili, L. S., Antia, R. V., Mitagvaria,
N. P., and Baramidze, D. G., 1971, The physiological mechanism of
dilatation of the pial arteries under conditions of decreased systemic arterial pressure, Fiziol. Zh. SSSR, 57:240-246.

Mchedlishvili, G. I., and Ormotsadze, L. G., 1962, Investigations of reflex effects from venous sinuses on regional arteries of the brain,
Byull. Eksp. Biol. Med., 53:No. 2, 9-13.

Mchedlishvili, G. I., and Ormotsadze, L. G., 1963, A hemodynamic regulating mechanism compensating for decreased blood supply to the cerebral
cortex, Physiol. Bohemoslov., 12:100-105.

Mchedlishvili, G. I., and Ormotsadze, L. G., 1970, A new modification of
resistography of the *in situ* isolated internal carotid artery for investigation of the vascular spasm, Patol. Fiziol. Exp. Ter., No. 3:
72-74.

Mchedlishvili, G., and Ormotsadze, L., 1979, Responses of internal carotid
artery to different endogenous vasoconstrictor substances, Blood Vessels, 16:126-134.

Mchedlishvili, G. I., and Ormotsadze, L. G., 1980, Relationship between
the internal carotid artery tone and cyclic AMP, Byull. Eksp. Biol.
Med., 90:393-395.

Mchedlishvili, G. I., and Ormotsadze, L. G., 1981, The effect of ethyl
apovincaminate on vasospasm of the circulatory isolated internal carotid artery in dogs, Arzneim-Forsch./Drug. Res., 31(1):No. 3, 414-
418.

Mchedlishvili, G. I., Ormotsadze, L. G., and Amashukeli, G. V., 1967a,
Resistography of the isolated internal carotid artery, Byull. Eksp.
Biol. Med., 64:No. 10, 3-6.

Mchedlishvili, G. I., Ormotsadze, L. G., and Kometiani, P. A., 1971,
Serotonin effect on the *in situ* isolated internal carotid artery,
Patol. Fiziol. Eksp. Ter., No. 5:21-24.

Mchedlishvili, G. I., Ormotsadze, L. G., and Labadze, T. S., 1977, Damping of pulsatile fluctuations of arterial pressure in the internal
carotid arteries, Fiziol. Zh. SSSR, 63:1302-1311.

Mchedlishvili, G. I., Ormotsadze, L. G., Mitagvaria, N. P., and Antia,
R. V., 1973, Resistance in large and small arteries of the brain in
spasmodic activity, Byull. Eksp. Biol. Med., 75:No. 3, 27-29.

Mchedlishvili, G. I., Ormotsadze, L. G., Nikolaishvili, L. S., and Baramidze, D. G., 1967b, Reaction of different parts of the cerebral vascular system in asphyxia, Exp. Neurol., 18:239-252.

Mchedlishvili, G. I., Ormotsadze, L. G., Nikolaishvili, L. S., and Baramidze, D. G., 1975, Peculiarities of functional behavior of different brain arteries, Fiziol. Zh. SSSR, 61:1478-1485.

Mchedlishvili, G. I., Ormotsadze, L. G., Samveljan, V. M., and Amashukeli,
G. V., 1969, Cholinergic and adrenergic structures in the walls of
internal carotid arteries, Dokl. Akad. Nauk SSSR, 184:999-1002.

Mchedlishvili, G. I., Purves, M. J., and Kovách, A. G. B., eds., 1979,
"Regulation of Cerebral Circulation," Proceedings of 4th Tbilisi
Symposium on Cerebral Circulation, Akadémiai Kiadó, Budapest.

Mchedlishvili, G. I., Sikharulidze, N. V., Itkus, M. L., and Janushewski,
S., 1980, Cerebral venous pressure, its relation to systemic venous
pressure and brain edema development, Byull. Eksp. Biol. Med., 89:14-16.

Mchedlishvili, G., and Varazashvili, M., 1980, Concentration of red cells in blood distributed to the brain and hind legs, IRCS Med. Sci., 8: 423.

Mchedlishvili, G., and Varazashvili, M., 1981a, Red cell/plasma ratio in blood flowing in microvascular beds under control and ischemic conditions, Microvasc. Res., 21:302-307.

Mchedlishvili, G., and Varazashvili, M., 1981b, Hematocrit in blood distributed to the brain: effect of velocity changes in carotid artery, IRCS Med. Sci., 9:943-944.

Mchedlishvili, G. I., and Varazashvili, M. N., 1982a, Effect of blood flow velocity in the carotid artery on hematocrit of the blood distributed to the brain, Byull. Eksp. Biol. Med., 93:No. 5, 12-14.

Mchedlishvili, G., and Varazashvili, M., 1982b, Flow conditions of red cells and plasma in microvascular bifurcation, Biorheology, 19:613-620.

Meldrum, B. S., and Nilsson, B., 1976, Cerebral blood flow and metabolic rate early and late in prolonged epileptic seizures induced in rats by bicuculline, Brain, 99:523-542.

Mellander, S., Grände, P.-O.,and Borgström, P., 1980, Static and dynamic components in the myogenic vascular response, in: "Vascular Neuroeffector Mechanisms," J. A. Bevan, T. Godfraind, R. A. Maxwell, and P. M. Vanhouette, eds., pp. 199-206, Raven Press, New York.

Mellander, S., and Johansson, B., 1968, Control of resistance, exchange and capacitance vessels in the peripheral circulation, Pharmacol. Rev., 20:117-196.

Meyer, J. S., 1958, Circulatory changes following occlusion of the middle cerebral artery and their relation to function, J. Neurosurg., 15: 653-673.

Meyer, J. S., 1968, The nature of high oxygen tension in bordering zones of cerebral ischemia, in: International Symposium on CSF and CBF, Scand. J. Lab. Clin. Invest., Suppl. 102, XVI:A.

Meyer, J. S., and Denny-Brown, D., 1955, Studies of cerebral circulation in brain injury. I. Validity of combined local cerebral electropolarography, thermometry and steady potentials as an indicator of local circulatory and functional changes, Electroenceph. Clin. Neurophysiol., 7:511-528.

Meyer, J. S., and Gotoh, F., 1961, Interaction of cerebral hemodynamics and metabolism, Neurology, 11:46-65.

Meyer, J. S., Gotoh, F., Ebihara, Sh., and Tomita, M., 1965, Effects of anoxia on cerebral metabolism and electrolytes in man, Neurology, 15:892-901.

Meyer, J. S., Gotoh, F., and Tazaki, Y., 1961, CO_2 narcosis, an experimental study, Neurology, 11:524-537.

Meyer, J. S., Gotoh, F., Tazaki, Y., Hamaguchi, K., Ishikawa, S., Nonailhat, F., and Symon, L., 1962, Regional cerebral blood flow and metabolism in vivo. Effects of anoxia, hypoglycemia, ischemia, acidosis, alkalosis, and alterations of blood PCO_2, Arch. Neurol., 7:560-581.

Meyer, J. S., Nomura, F., Sakamoto, K., and Kondo, A., 1969, The effect of stimulation of brainstem reticular formation on cerebral blood flow and oxygen consumption, Electroenceph. Clin. Neurophysiol., 26:125-132.

Meyer, J. S., Ott, E. O., Aoyagi, M., Kawamura, Y., Tagashira, Y., Matsuda, M., and Achari, A. N., 1977, Double cholinergic and adrenergic functional control of cerebral blood flow, in: "Brain Blood Supply," G. I. Mchedlishvili, A. G. B. Kovách, and I. Nyáry, eds., pp. 119-131, Akadémiai Kiadó, Budapest.

Meyer, J. S., Shimizu, K., Okamoto, Sh., Koto, A., Ohuchi, T., Sari, A., and Ericsson, A. D., 1972, Effects of alpha adrenergic blockage on autoregulation and chemical vasomotor control of CBF in stroke, Stroke, 4:187-200.

Meyer, J. S., Teraura, T., and Sakamoto, K., 1971, Central neurogenic control of cerebral blood flow, Neurology, 21:247-262.

Meyer, J. S., Yoshida, K., and Sakamoto, K., 1967, Autonomic control of
cerebral blood flow measured by electromagnetic flowmeters, Neurology,
17:638-649.

Mikhailov, S. S., 1963, Reflex reactions of the blood pressure and respiration to stimulation of the cavernous venous sinus, Fiziol. Zh. SSSR,
49:822-829.

Molinary, G. F., and Laurent, J. P., 1976, A classification of experimental models of brain ischemia, Stroke, 7:14-17.

Molnár, L., and Szántó, J., 1964, The effect of electrical stimulation of
the bulbar vasomotor center on the cerebral blood flow, Q. J. Exp.
Physiol., 49:184-193.

Monro, P. A. G., 1979, The regulation of cortical cerebral blood flow and
its possible control by the neuroglia, Microvasc. Res., 17:2, S, 93.

Morawetz, R. B., DeGirolami, U., Ojemann, R. G., Marcoux, F. W., and
Crowell, R. M., 1978, Cerebral blood flow determined by hydrogen
clearance during middle cerebral artery occlusion in unanesthetized
monkeys, Stroke, 9:143-149.

Morgan, H., White, R. P., Penine, M., and Robertson, J. T., 1972, Prostaglandins and experimental cerebral vasospasm, Surg. Forum., 23:447-
448.

Moskalenko, Yu., Cooper, R., Crow, H., and Walter, W. G., 1964, Variation
in blood volume and oxygen availability in human brain, Nature, 202:
159-161.

Moskalenko, Yu. E., Demchenko, I. T., Krivchenko, A. I., Burov, S. V., and
Deriy, A. N., 1975, About structural and functional organization of
regulatory control of local cerebral circulation, Fiziol. Zh. SSSR,
61:1468-1492.

Moskalenko, Yu. E., and Filanovskaia, T. P., 1967, On changes in pulsatile
blood flow in arteries of the cranial base, Fiziol. Zh. SSSR, 53:1387-
1392.

Moskalenko, Yu. E., Weinstein, G. B., Demchenko, I. T., Kislyakov, Yu. Ya.,
and Krivchenko, A. I., 1980, "Biophysical Aspects of Cerebral Circulation," Pergamon Press, Oxford.

Mossakowski, M., Mchedlishvili, G. I., and Januszewski, S., 1980, Excessive volume of blood in the brain in edema, Vopr. Neirokhirurg., No.
3:38-43.

Motavkin, P. A., and Chertok, V. M., 1980, "Histophysiology of Vascular
Mechanisms of Brain Circulation," Meditsina, Moscow.

Motavkin, P. A., and Dovbish, T. V., 1970, Cholinergic neural apparatus
of blood vessels in pia mater and brain, Byull. Eksp. Biol. Med., 70:
No. 7, 113-116.

Motavkin, P. A., Markina-Palashchenko, L. D., and Bozhko, G. C., 1981,
"Comparative Morphology of Vascular Mechanisms of Cerebral Circulation in Vertebrates," Nauka, Moscow.

Motavkin, P. A., and Osipova, L. P., 1973, Cholinergic innervation of the
human brain arteries, Z. Mikr. Anat. Forsch., 87:365-378.

Müller, J., 1837, "Handbuch der Physiologie des Menschen," III Auflage,
1:Buch 1, Coblenz.

Mutsuga, N., Schuette, W. H., and Lewis, D. V., 1976, The contribution of
local blood flow to the rapid clearance of potassium from the cortical extracellular space, Brain Res., 116:431-436.

Myers, R. E., and Intaglietta, M., 1976, Brain microvascular hemodynamic
responses to induced seizures, Stroke, 7:83-88.

Nadareishvili, K. Sh., 1962, Fluctuations in tone of regional arteries of
the brain synchronic with respiration, in: "Current Problems in
Morphology, Physiology, and Pathology," Dedicated to V. V. Voronin,
G. Mchedlishvili, ed., pp. 135-142, Metsniereba, Tbilisi.

Nadareishvili, K. Sh., 1963, Direct reactions of the cardiovascular system
of animals to the external action of ionizing radiation, in: Trans.
Inst. Physiol., Georgian Acad. Sci., 13:219-237.

Nagel, A., 1934, Die mechanischen Eigenschaften der Kapillarwand und ihre
Beziehungen zum Bindegewebslager, Z. Mikr. Anat. Forsch., 21:376-387.

Nakai, M., Iadocola, C., Tucker, L. W., Ruggerio, D. A., and Reis, D. J.,
1981, Evidence for an intrinsic cerebrovascular system in brain represented in fastigial nucleus of cerebellum, J. Cereb. Blood Flow
Metab., 1:Suppl. 1, S301-S302.

Nash, G. B., and Meiselman, H. J., 1981, Red cell aging: changes in deformability and other possible determinants of *in vivo* survival,
Microcirculation 1:255-284.

Natus, M., 1910, Beiträge zur Lehre von der Stase nach Versuchen am
Pankreas des lebenden Kaninchen, Virchows Arch., 199:1-82.

Needleman, P., and Isakson, P. C., 1980, Intrinsic prostaglandin biosynthesis in blood vessels, in: "Handbook of Physiology," Sec. 2: The
Cardiovascular System; Vol. 2: Vascular Smooth Muscle, D. F. Bohr,
A. P. Somlyo, and H. V. Sparks, eds., pp. 613-633, American Physiological Society, Bethesda, Maryland.

Nelson, E., and Rennels, M., 1970, Neuromuscular contacts in intracranial
arteries of the cat, Science, 167:301-302.

Nemoto, E. M., and Frinak, S., 1981, Brain tissue pH after global brain
ischemia and barbiturate loading in rats, Stroke, 12:77-81.

Nesterov, A. I., 1929,"Studies of Blood Capillaries and the Capillaroscopy
as Method of Their Investigation under Normal and Pathological Conditions," Tomsk.

Nielsen, K. C., and Owman, Ch., 1967, Adrenergic innervation of pial arteries related to the circle of Willis in the cat, Brain Res., 6:773-776.

Nielsen, K. C., and Owman, Ch., 1971, Contractile response and amine receptor mechanisms in isolated middle cerebral artery of the cat,
Brain Res., 27:33-42.

Nilsson, B., Norberg, K., Nordström, C. H., and Sjesjö, B. K., 1975, Influ-
ence of hypoxia and hypercapnia on CBF in rats, in: "Blood Flow and
Metabolism in the Brain," M. Harper, B. Jenett, D. Miller, and J.
Rowan, eds., pp. 9.19-9.23, Churchill Livingstone, Edinburgh-London-
New York.

Nilsson, B., Rehncrona, S., and Sjesjö, B. K., 1978, Coupling of cerebral
metabolism and blood flow in epileptic seizures, hypoxia and hypoglycemia, in: "Cerebral Vascular Smooth Muscle and Its Control,"
M. J. Purves, ed., pp. 199-212, Elsevier, Amsterdam.

Noell, W., and Schneider, M., 1942, Über die Durchblutung und die Sauer-
stoffversorgung des Gehirns im akuten Sauerstoffmangel. III. Mit.
Die arterio-venöse Sauerstoff- und Kohlensäuredifferenz., Pflügers.
Arch., 246:207-249.

Noell, W., and Schneider, M., 1944, Über die Durchblutung und die Sauerstoffversorgung des Gehirns. IV Mit. Die Rolle der Kohlensäure,
Pflügers Arch., 247:514-527.

Novack, P., Shenkin, H. A., Bortin, L., Goluboff, B., and Soffe, A. H.,
1953, The effects of carbon dioxide inhalation upon the cerebral
blood flow and cerebral oxygen consumption in vascular disease, J.
Clin. Invest., 32:696-702.

Olesen, J., 1974, "Cerebral Blood Flow. Methods for Measurement, Regulation, Effects of Drugs, and Changes in Disease," Munksgaard, Copenhagen.

Opdyke, D. F., 1946, Circulatory effects of partial cerebral ischemia,
Am. J. Physiol., 146:467-477.

Opitz, E., and Schneider, M., 1950, Über die Sauerstoffversorgung des
Gehirns und den Mechanismus der Mangelwirkungen, Ergebn. Physiol.,
46:126-260.

Orlov, R. S., 1979a, Direct responses of smooth muscle of cerebral arter-
    ies to stretch, in: "Regulation of Cerebral Circulation," G. I.
    Mchedlishvili, M. J. Purves, and A. G. B. Korvách, eds., pp. 27-32,
    Akadémiai Kiadó, Budapest.
Orlov, R. S., 1979b, Comments in discussion, in: "Regulation of Cerebral
    Circulation," G. I. Mchedlishvili, M. J. Purves, and A. G. B.
    Kovách, eds., pp. 202-203, Akadémiai Kiadó, Budapest.
Orlov, R. S., Azin, A. L., Brazgovski, V. A., Ignatenko, A. S., and Plech-
    anov, I. P., 1975, The mechanism of activation of smooth muscle con-
    striction of cerebral vessels, Fiziol. Zh. SSSR, 61:1458-1465.
Orlov, R. S., Azin, A. L., Brazgovsky, V. A., Ignatenko, A. S., and Plech-
    anov, I. P., 1977, Smooth muscle contraction mechanisms in the brain
    arterial and venous vessels, in: "Brain Blood Supply," G. I. Mched-
    lishvili, A. G. B. Kovách, and I. Nyáry, eds., pp. 245-253,
    Akadémiai Kiadó, Budapest.
Orlov, R. S., Isakov, B. Ja., Ketkin, A. T., and Plekhanov, I. P., 1971,
    "Regulatory Mechanisms of Cells of Smooth Muscles and Myocardium,"
    Nauka, Leningrad.
Orlov, R. S., Plekhanov, I. P., and Azin, A. L., 1972, Investigation into
    contractile responses of smooth muscle cells of cerebral vessels,
    Fiziol. Zh. SSSR, 58:79-82.
Orlov, R. S., and Priklonskaya, E. G., 1980, Contractile characteristics
    of venous smooth muscles of the head, Fiziol. Zh. SSSR, 66:727-732.
Ormotsadze, L. G., 1969, Elucidation of the closing mechanisms of the
    major arteries of the amphibians' brain, Bull. Georgian Acad. Sci.,
    55:685-688.
Ormotsadze, L. G., Samvelian, V. M., Nikolaishvili, L. S., and Mchedlish-
    vili, G. I., 1969, The effect of serotonin on internal carotid and
    pial arteries, Krovoobrashchenie, 2:No. 4, 16-19.
Ott, E. O., Abraham, J., Meyer, J. S., Achari, A. N., Chee, A. N. C., and
    Mathew, N. T., 1975, Disordered cholinergic neurotransmission and
    dysautoregulation after cerebral infarction, Stroke, 6:172-180.
Owman, Ch. and Edvinsson, L., eds., 1977, "Neurogenic Control of the
    Brain Circulation," Pergamon Press, Oxford.
Owman, Ch., and Edvinsson, L., 1979, Heterogeneous sympathomimetic flow
    response in various brain regions, in: "Cerebral Blood Flow and
    Metabolism," F. Gotoh, H. Nagai, and Y. Tazaki, eds., pp. 100-101,
    Munksgaard, Copenhagen.
Owman, Ch., Edvinsson, L., and Nielsen, K. C., 1974, Autonomic neurore-
    ceptor mechanisms in brain vessels, Blood Vessels, 11:2-31.
Owman, Ch., Falck, B., and Mchedlishvili, G. I., 1965, Adrenergic struc-
    tures of pial arteries and their relation with the cerebral cortex,
    Byull. Eksp. Biol. Med., 59:No. 6, 98-101; Fed. Proc., 25:612-614.
Palmer, A. A., 1959, A study of blood flow in minute vessels of the pan-
    creatic region of the rat with reference to intermittent corpuscular
    flow in individual capillaries, Q. J. Exp. Physiol., 44:149-159.
Pannier, J. L., Demeester, G., and Leusen, I., 1974, The influence of non-
    respiratory alkalosis on cerebral blood flow in cats, Stroke, 5:324-
    329.
Pappenheimer, J. R., and Kinter, W. B., 1956, Hematocrit ratio of blood
    within mammalian kidney and its significance for renal hemodynamics,
    Am. J. Physiol., 185:337-390.
Patterson, J. L., Heyman, A., Batley, L. L., and Ferguson, R. W., 1955,
    Threshold of response of cerebral vessel of man to increase in blood
    carbon dioxide, J. Clin. Invest., 34:1857-1864.
Pawlik, G., Rackl, A., and Bing, R. J., 1981, Quantitative capillary to-
    pography and blood flow in the cerebral cortex of cats: an *in vivo*
    microscopic study, Brain Res., 208:35-58.

Pearce, W. J., and Bevan, J. A., 1981, Sympathetic stimulation, cerebral blood flow, and the role of extracerebral venoconstriction, in: Adv. Physiol. Sci., Vol. 9: "Cardiovascular Physiology, Neural Control Mechanisms," A. G. B. Kovách, P. Sándor, and M. Kollai, eds., pp. 269-278, Pergamon Press-Akadémiai Kiadó, Budapest.

Pearce, W. J., Scremin, O. U., Sonnenschein, R. R., and Rubinstein, E. H., 1981, The electroencephalogram, blood flow, and oxygen uptake in rabbit cerebrum, J. Cereb. Blood Flow Metab., 1:419-428.

Pease, D. C., and Schultz, R. L., 1962, Circulation to the brain and spinal cord. Submicroscopical anatomy, in: "Blood Vessels and Lymphatics," D. I. Abramson, ed., pp. 233-239, New York.

Peerless, S. J., and Kendall, M. J., 1975, Experimental cerebral vasospasm, in: "Cerebral Vascular Disease," J. P. Whisnant and B. A. Sandok, eds., pp. 49-58, Grune and Stratton, New York-San Francisco-London.

Pfeifer, R. A., 1940, "Die angioarchitektonische areale Gliederung der Grosshirnrinde auf Grund vollkommener Gefassinjektionspraparate vom Gehirn des Nacacus rhesus dargestellt," Leipzig.

Pickard, J. D., 1973, The mechanism of action of prostaglandin $F_{2\alpha}$ on cerebral blood flow in the baboon, J. Physiol. (London), 234:46P-47P.

Pinard, E., Purves, M. J., Seylaz, J., and Vasquez, J. V., 1979, The cholinergic pathways to cerebral blood vessels. II. Physiologic Studies, Pflügers Arch., 379:165-172.

Pletchkova, E. K., Mchedlishvili, G. I., Lavrentieva, N. B., and Nikolaishvili, L. S., 1969, On the cholinergic mechanism responsible for functional dilatation of the arteries supplying the cerebral cortex, in: "Correlation of Blood Supply with Metabolism and Function," Proceedings of an International Symposium, G. Mchedlishvili, ed., pp. 172-184, Metsniereba Press, Tbilisi.

Plum, F., 1978, Introduction: a multiple factor theory for control of cerebral vascular smooth muscle, in: "Cerebral Vascular Smooth Muscle and Its Control," M. J. Purves, ed., pp. 3-7, Elsevier, Amsterdam.

Ponte, J., and Purves, M. J., 1974, Role of the carotid body chemoreceptors and carotid sinus baroreceptors in the control of cerebral blood vessels, J. Physiol. (London), 237:315-323.

Pool, J. L., 1957, Vasocardiac effects of the circle of Willis, Arch. Neurol. Psychiat., 78:355-368.

Pries, A. R., Gaehtgens, P., and Kanzow, G., 1981, Microvascular distribution of blood volume flow and hematocrit as related to oxygen delivery, in: Adv. Physiol. Sci., Vol. 25: "Oxygen Transport to Tissue," A. G. B. Kovách, E. Dora, M. Kessler, and I. A. Silver, eds., pp. 291-300, Pergamon Press-Akadémiai Kiadó, Budapest.

Pulsinelli, W. A., and Brierley, J. B., 1979, A new model of bilateral hemispheric ischemia in the unanesthetized rat, Stroke, 10:267-272.

Purves, M. J., 1972, "The Physiology of the Cerebral Circulation," Cambridge Univ. Press, Cambridge.

Purves, M. J., 1979a, The neural control of cerebral blood vessels, in: "Regulation of Cerebral Circulation," G. I. Mchedlishvili, M. J. Purves, and A. G. B. Kovách, eds., pp. 109-112, Akadémiai Kiadó, Budapest.

Purves, M. J., 1979b, Summarizing remarks on mechanisms which regulate an adequate blood supply to brain tissue, in: "Regulation of Cerebral Circulation," G. I. Mchedlishvili, M. J. Purves, and A. G. B. Kovách, eds., pp. 164-165, Akadémiai Kiadó, Budapest.

Quint, S. R., Scremin, O. U., Sonnenschein, R. R., and Rubinstein, E. H., 1980, Enhancement of cerebrovascular effect of CO_2 by hypoxia, Stroke, 11:286-289.

Raichle, M. E., Grubb, R. L., Gado, M. H., Eichling, D. O., and Ter-Pogossian, M. M., 1976, Correlation between regional cerebral blood flow and oxidative metabolism, Arch. Neurol., 33:523-526.

Raichle, M. E., Grubb, R. L., and Ter-Pogossian, M. M., eds., 1981, "Tenth International Symposium on Cerebral Blood Flow and Metabolism," Raven Press, New York.

Raichle, M. E., Hartman, B. K., Eichling, J. O., and Sharpe, L. G., 1975, Central adrenergic regulation of cerebral blood flow and vascular permeability, Proc. Natl. Acad. Sci. USA, 72:3726-3730.

Rapela, C. E., Green, H. D., and Denison, A. B., 1967, Baroreceptor reflexes and autoregulation of cerebral blood flow in the dog, Circ. Res., 21:559-568.

Raper, A. J., Kontos, H. A., and Patterson, J. L., 1971, Response of pial precapillary vessels to changes of arterial carbon dioxide tension, Circ. Res., 28:518-523.

Rasmussen, H., and Tenenhouse, H., 1968, Cyclic adenosine monophosphate: Ca^{++} and membranes, Proc. Natl. Acad. Sci. USA, 59:1364-1370.

Raynor, R. B., and McMurtry, J. G., 1963, Prevention of serotonin-produced cerebral vasospasm, J. Neurosurg., 20:94-96.

Raynor, R. B., McMurtry, J. G., and Pool, J. L., 1961, Cerebrovascular effects of topically applied serotonin in the cat, Neurology, 11:190-195.

Raynor, R. B., and Ross, G., 1960, Arteriography and vasospasm. The effect of intracranial contrast media on vasospasm, J. Neurosurg., 17:1055-1061.

Recklinghausen, F., 1883, "Handbuch der allgemeinen Pathologie des Kreislaufs und Ernährung," Stuttgart.

Rehncrona, S., Nordstrom, C.-H., Sjesjö, B. K., and Westerberg, E., 1977, Adenosine in rat cerebral cortex during hypoxia and bicuculline-induced seizures, in: "Cerebral Function, Metabolism, and Circulation," D. H. Ingvar and N. A. Lassen, eds., pp. 220-221, Munksgaard, Copenhagen.

Reivich, M., 1964, Arterial PCO_2 and cerebral hemodynamics, Am. J. Physiol., 206:25-35.

Reivich, M., Marshall, W. J. S., and Kessel, N., 1969, Loss of autoregulation produced by cerebral trauma, in: "Cerebral Blood Flow," M. Brock, C. Fieschi, D. H. Ingvar, N. A. Lassen, and K. Schürmann, eds., pp. 205-208, Springer-Verlag, Berlin, Heidelberg-New York.

Reivich, M., Sokoloff, L., Kennedy, C., and Des Rosiers, M., 1975, An autoradiographic method for the measurement of local glucose metabolism in the brain, in: "Brain Work," D. H. Ingvar and N. A. Lassen, eds., pp. 377-384, Munksgaard, Copenhagen.

Rhodin, J. A. G., 1962, Fine structure of vascular walls in mammals with special reference to smooth muscle component, Physiol. Rev., 45:(Suppl. 5), 48-87.

Rhodin, J. A. G., 1980, Architecture of the vessel wall, in: "Handbook of Physiology," Sec. 2: The Cardiovascular System, D. F. Bohr, A. P. Somlyo, and H. V. Sparks, eds., pp. 1-31, American Physiological Society, Bethesda, Maryland.

Ricker, G., and Regendanz, P., 1921, Beiträge zur Kenntniss der örtlichen Kreislaufsstörung, Virchows. Arch., 231:1-184.

Riggs, H. E., and Griffiths, J. O., 1938, Anomalies of the circle of Willis in persons with nervous and mental diseases, Arch. Neurol. Psychiat., 39:1353-1354.

Rogers, J. B., 1935, Observations *in vivo* on the capillaries in the greater omentum of the cat, Anat. Rec., 63:193-198.

Romer, A. S., 1956, The Vertebrate Body, 2nd edn., W. B. Saunders Company, Philadelphia.

Rosen, R., 1967, "Optimality Principles in Biology," Butterworth, London.

Rosenblum, W. I., 1972, Ratio of red cell velocities near the vessel wall to velocities at the vessel center in cerebral microcirculation, and an apparent effect of blood viscosity on this ratio, Microvasc.Res., 4:98-101.

Ross Russel, R. W., ed., 1971, "Brain and Blood Flow," Pitman, London.

Rothenberg, S. F., and Corday, E., 1961, Primary and traumatic cerebral angiospasm, in: "Cerebral Anoxia and Electroencephalogram," J. S. Meyer and H. Gastaut, eds., pp. 130-133, C. C. Thomas, Springfield, Illinois.

Rouget, Ch., 1873, Mémoire sur le développement, la structure et les proprietés physiologiques des capillaires sanguins et lympatiques, Arch. Physiol. Norm. Pathol., 5:603-663.

Rouget, Ch., 1874, Note sur le développement de la tunique contractile des vaisseaux, Compt. Rend. Acad. Sci., 79:559-562.

Rouget, Ch., 1879, Sur la contractilité des capillaires sangousins, Compt. Rend. Acad. Sci., 88:916-918.

Rovere, A. A., Scremin, O. U., Reresi, M. R., et al., 1973, Cholinergic mechanism in the cerebrovascular action of carbon dioxide, Stroke, 4:969-972.

Roy, C. S., and Brown, J. G., 1879, The blood pressure and its variations in the arterioles, capillaries, and smaller veins, J. Physiol. (London), 2:323-360.

Roy, C. S., and Sherrington, C. S., 1890, The regulation of the blood supply of the brain, J. Physiol. (London), 11:85-121.

Rushmer, R. F., 1961, "Cardiovascular Dynamics," W. B. Saunders, Philadelphia.

Sadoshima, S., Fujishima, M., Tamaki, K., Nakatomi, Y., Ishitsuka, T., Ogata, J., and Omae, T., 1980, Response of cortical and pial arteries to changes of arterial CO_2 tension in rats: a morphometric study, Brain Res., 189:115-120.

Sagawa, K., and Guyton, A. C., 1961, Pressure-flow relationships in isolated canine cerebral circulation, Am. J. Physiol., 200:711-714.

Salanga, V. D., and Waltz, A. G., 1973, Regional cerebral blood flow during stimulation of seventh cranial nerve, Stroke, 4:213-217.

Sandison, J. C., 1932, Contraction of blood vessels and observation on the circulation in the transparent chamber in the rabbit's ear, Anat. Rec., 54:105-127.

Saratikov, A. S., Belopasov, V. V., and Plotnikov, M. B., 1979, "Experimental and Clinical Pharmacology of Cerebral Circulation," Tomsk University Publishers, Tomsk.

Sausa Pereira, J. M. M., 1979, Histological, histochemical, and microsurgical research on anatomophysiological basis of neurogenic control of cerebral blood flow, in: "Cerebral Blood Flow and Metabolism," F. Gotoh, H. Nagai, and Y. Tazaki, eds., pp. 94-95, Munksgaard, Copenhagen.

Scharrer, E., 1962, "Brain Function and the Evolution of Cerebral Vascularization," The American Museum of Natural History, New York.

Scheinberg, P., and Joyne, H. W., 1952, Factors influencing cerebral blood flow and metabolism, Circulation, 5:225-236.

Schmid-Schönbein, H., 1976, Mircorheology of erythrocytes, blood viscosity, and the distribution of blood flow in the microcirculation, in: "International Review of Physiology," Cardiovascular Physiology II, Vol. 9, A. C. Guyton and A. W. Cowley, eds., pp. 1-62, University Park Press, Baltimore.

Schmid-Schönbein, H., 1977, Microrheology of erythrocytes and thrombocytes, blood viscosity, and the distribution of blood flow in the microcirculation, in: "Handbuch der allgemeinen Patholgie," Band 3, Teil 7: Microcirculation, H. Meessen, ed., pp. 289-384, Springer-Verlag, Berlin-Heidelberg-New York.

Schmid-Schönbein, H., 1981, Hemorheology and the experimental basis of classical humoral pathology, Clin. Hemorheol., 1:179-195.

Schmid-Schönbein, H., and Riegel, H., 1981, Why hemodilution in low flow states? Bibliotheca haemat., No. 47:99-121, Karger, Basel.

Schmid-Schönbein, H., Riegel, H., and Fischer, T., 1980a, Blood fluidity as a consequence of red cell fluidity: flow properties of blood and flow behavior of blood in vascular diseases, Angiology, 31:301-319.

Schmid-Schönbein, H., Skalak, R., Usami, S., and Chien, S., 1980b, Cell distribution in capillary networks, Microvasc. Res., 19:18-44.

Schmid-Schönbein, H., Wells, R. E., and Goldstone, J., 1969, Influence of deformability of human red cells upon blood viscosity, Circ. Res., 25:131-145.

Schmid-Schönbein, G. W., and Zweifach, B. W., 1975, RBC velocity profiles in arterioles and venules of the rabbit omentum, Microvasc. Res., 10: 153-164.

Schmidt, C. F., 1950, "The Cerebral Circulation in Health and Disease," C. C. Thomas, Springfield, Illinois.

Schneider, M., 1957, The metabolism of the brain in ischemia and hyperthermia, in: "Metabolism of the Nervous System," D. Richter, ed., pp. 238-244, Pergamon Press, London-New York.

Schneider, W., Wahl, M., Kuschinsky, W., and Thurau, K., 1977, The use of microelectrodes for measurement of local H^+ activity in the cortical subarachnoid space of cats, Pflügers Arch., 372:103-107.

Schuler, F., 1854, Beiträge zur Lehre von der Stase in der Schwimmhaut der Frösche. Verhandl. Phys.-Med. Gesellschaft in Würzburg, 4:248-253.

Schultz, A., 1866, Zur Lehre von der Blutbewegung im Innern des Schädels. St. Petersburg Med. Z., 11:122-124.

Scremin, O. U., Rubinstein, E. H., and Sonnenschein, R. R., 1977, Evidence for a cholinergic neurogenic component in the cerebral vasodilatation to hypercapnia in the rabbit, Fed. Proc., 36:568.

Scremin, O. U., Sonnenschein, R. R., and Rubinstein, E. H., 1982, Cholinergic cerebral vasodilatation in the rabbit: absence of concomitant metabolic activation, J. Cereb. Blood Flow Metab., 2:241-247.

Seidel, Ch. L., and Bohr, D. F., 1971, Calcium and vascular smooth muscle contraction, Circ. Res., 28-29:Suppl. 2, 88-95.

Serota, H. M., and Gerard, R. W., 1938, Localized thermal changes in the cat's brain, J. Neurophysiol., 1:115-124.

Serscombe, R., Lacombe, P., Quibineau, P., Mamo, H., Pinard, E., Reynier-Rebuffel, A.-M., and Seylaz, J., 1979, Is there an active mechanism limiting the influence of the sympathetic system on the cerebral vascular bed? Evidence for vasomotor escape from sympathetic stimulation in the rabbit, Brain Res., 164:81-102.

Shalit, M. N., Reinmuth, O. M., Shymojyo, S., and Sheinberg, P., 1967, Carbon dioxide and cerebral circulatory control. II. The intravascular effect, Arch. Neurol., 17:337-341.

Simeone, F. A., Vinale, P. E., Alderman, J. L., and Irwin, J. D., 1979, Role of adrenergic nerves in blood-induced cerebral vasospasm," Stroke, 10:375-380.

Sjesjö, B. K., 1978, "Brain Energy Metabolism," John Wiley and Sons, New York.

Sjesjö, B. K., Berntman, L., and Rehncrona, S., 1979, Effect of hypoxia on blood flow and metabolic flux in the brain, in: "Cerebral Hypoxia and Its Consequences," Advances in Neurology, S. Fahn, J. N. Davis, and L. P. Rowland, eds., Vol. 26, pp. 267-283, Raven Press, New York.

Sjesjö, B. K., and Thews, G., 1962, Ein Verfahren zur Bestimmung der CO_2 Diffusionskoeffizienten im Gehirngewebe, Pflügers Arch., 276:192-210.

Sjöstrand, T., 1935, "On the Principles for the Distribution of the Blood in the Peripheral Vascular System," Berlin.

Skinhoj, E., and Paulson, O. H., 1969, Carbon dioxide and cerebral circulatory control. Evidence of a nonfocal site of action of carbon dioxide on cerebral circulation, Arch. Neurol., 20:249-252.

Söderberg, U., and Weckman, N., 1959, Changes in cerebral blood supply caused by changes in the pressure drop along arteries to the brain of the cat, Experientia, 15:346-348.

Sokoloff, L., 1959, The action of drugs on the cerebral circulation, Pharmacol. Rev., 11:1-85.

Sokoloff, L., 1960, Metabolism of the central nervous system *in vivo*, in: "Handbook of Physiology," Sec. 1, Neurophysiology, H. W. McGoun, ed., Vol. 3, pp. 1843-1864, Williams and Wilkins, Washington, DC.

Sokoloff, L., 1961, Local cerebral circulation at rest and during altered cerebral activity induced by anesthesia or visual stimulation, in: "Regional Neurochemistry," S. S. Kety and J. Elkes, eds., pp. 107-117, Pergamon Press, Oxford.

Sokolova, I. A., Blinkov, S. M., and Radionov, I. M., 1981, Rarefaction of capillary network in the brain of rats with induced DOCa-saline and renal hypertension, Microvasc. Res., 22:125-126.

Somlyo, A. P., 1979, Vascular smooth muscle contraction, in: Cerebrovascular Diseases," T. R. Price and E. Nelson, eds., pp. 273-281, Raven Press, New York.

Somlyo, A. P., and Somlyo, A. V., 1968, Vascular smooth muscle: normal structure, pathology, biochemistry, and biophysics, Pharmacol. Rev., 20:197-292.

Somlyo, A. V., Vinall, P., and Somlyo, A. P., 1971, Excitation-contraction coupling and electrical events in two types of vascular smooth muscle, Microvasc. Res., 1:354-373.

Sparks, H. V., 1964, Effect of quick stretch on isolated vascular smooth muscle, Circ. Res., 15:(Suppl. 1), 254-260.

Sparks, H. V., 1980, Effect of local metabolic factors on vascular smooth muscle, in: "Handbook of Physiology," Sec. 2: The Cardiovascular System; Vol. 2: Vascular Smooth Muscle, D. F. Bohr, A. P. Somlyo, and H. V. Sparks, eds., pp. 475-513, American Physiological Society, Bethesda, Maryland.

Spector, W. S., ed., 1956, "Handbook of Biological Data," W. B. Saunders, Philadelphia.

Stehbens, W. E., 1961, Discussion on vascular flow and turbulence, Neurology, 11:66-67.

Steinbock, P., Kendall, M. J., Clarke, R. J., and Peerless, S. J., 1976, The reactivity of canine cerebral arteries to O_2 and CO_2 *in vitro*, Can. J. Neurol. Sci., 3:255-262.

Stone, H. L., and Raichle, M. E., 1975, The effect of sympathetic denervation on cerebral CO_2 sensitivity, Stroke, 5:13-18.

Strandgaard, S., MacKenzie, E. T., Jones, J. V., and Harper, A. M., 1976, Studies on the cerebral circulation of the baboon in acutely induced hypertension, Stroke, 7:287-290.

Stricker, S., 1877, Untersuchungen über die Contractilität der Capillaren. Sitzungsber. Akad. Wissensch., 74:III, Abt., 313-332.

Stroica, E., Meyer, J. S., Kawamura, Y., Hiromoto, H., Hashi, K., Aoyagi, M., and Pascu, Y., 1973, Central neurogenic control of cerebral circulation. Effects of intravertebral injection of pyrithioxin on cerebral blood flow and metabolism, Neurology, 23:687-698.

Strong, C. D., and Bohr, D. F., 1967, Effects of prostaglandins E_1, E_2, A_1, and $F_{1\alpha}$ on isolated vascular smooth muscle, Am. J. Physiol., 213: 725-733.

Sundt, T. M., and Waltz, A. C., 1971, Cerebral ischemia and reactive hyperemia. Studies of cortical blood flow and microcirculation before, during, and after temporary occlusion of middle cerebral artery of squirrel monkeys, Circ. Res., 28:426-433.

Svanes, K., and Zweifach, B. W., 1968, Variations in small blood vessel
    hematocrits produced in hypothermic rats by microocclusion, Microvasc.
    Res., 1:210-220.

Symon, L., 1967, An experimental study of traumatic cerebral vascular
    spasm, J. Neurol. Neurosurg. Psychiat., 30:497-505.

Symon, L., 1969, The concept of intracerebral steal, in: Int. Anesth.
    Clin. Cereb. Circ., 7:597-615.

Symon, L., 1971, Vasospasm and aneurism, in: "Cerebral Vascular Diseases,"
    Seventh Conference, pp. 232-240, Grune and Stratton, New York.

Symon, L., 1973, Vasospasm, in: "Recent Progress in Neurological Surgery,"
    Proceedings of the Symposia of the Fifth International Congress of
    Neurological Surgery, October 7-13, 1973, pp. 176-182, Excerpta
    Medica, Amsterdam.

Symon, L., Branston, N. M., and Strong, A. J., 1976, Autoregulation in
    acute focal ischemia. An experimental study, Stroke, 7:547-554.

Symon, L., Held, K., and Dorsch, N. W. C., 1971-1972, On the myogenic
    nature of autoregulatory mechanism in the cerebral circulation, in:
    "European Neurology," H. E. Kaeser, ed., Vol. 6, pp. 11-18, S. Karger,
    Basel-München-New York.

Tannenberg, J., and Fischer-Wasels, B., 1927, Die lokalen Kreislaufsstör-
    ungen. Die Stase, in: "Bethe's Handbuch der Normalen und patholo-
    lishen Physiologie, Vol. 7, pp. 1626-1643, Berlin.

Tarchanoff, J., 1874, Beobachtungen über contractile Elemente in den
    Blut- und Lymphcapillaren, Pflügers Arch., 9:407-416.

Tarkanoff, J., 1875, Du rôle des vaisseaux capillaires dans la circulation,
    Compte Rend. Soc. Biol., 1:Ser. 6, 331-333.

Ter-Grigorian, A. A., 1962, Structure of tunica media of intraosseal part
    of the human internal carotid artery in aspects of aging, in: "Proc.
    of Erevan Medical Institute," No. 12, pp. 109-113, Erevan.

Thoma, R., 1893, "Untersuchungen über die Histogenese und Histomechanik
    des Gefässsystems," Stuttgart.

Thoma, R., 1910, Die Viscosität des Blutes und seine Strömung im Arterien-
    system. Dtsch. Arch. Klin. Med., 99:565-636.

Thorsen, G., and Hint, H., 1950, "Aggregation, Sedimentation, and Intra-
    vascular Sludging of Erthyrocytes," Norstedt and Söner, Stockholm.

Thuránszky, K., 1956, Über die Rolle der extra- und intraokularer Faktoren
    in der Regulation des Blutkreislaufs der Retina, Acta Physiol. Acad.
    Sci. Hung., Suppl. 9, pp. 44-46.

Thuránszky, K., 1957, "Der Blutkreislauf der Netzhaut," Budapest.

Tilton, R. G. ,Kilo, Ch., Williamson, J. R., and Murch, D. W., 1979, Dif-
    ference in pericyte contractile function in rat cardiac and skeletal
    muscle microvasculature, Microvasc. Res., 18:336-352.

Tkachenko, B. I., 1964, Reflex changes in the cerebral circulation to
    stimulation of the coronary vessels, Fiziol. Zh. SSSR, 50:487-495.

Tkachenko, B. I., 1979, "Venous Blood Circulation," Meditsina, Leningrad.

Toda, N., 1979, Acetylcholine-induced relaxation in isolated dog cerebral
    arteries, J. Pharmacol. Exp. Ther., 209:352-358.

Toda, N., and Fujita, L., 1973, Responsiveness of isolated cerebral and
    peripheral arteries to serotonin, norepinephrine, and transmural
    electrical stimulation, Circ. Res., 33:98-104.

Toidze, Sh. S., Ormotsadze, L. G., and Mchedlishvili, G. I., 1983,
    Anatomical basis for resistance and damping functions of internal
    carotid arteries, in: Proceedings of Georgian Acad. Sci., Biol.
    Series, Vol. 9, pp. 27-33.

Tomita, M., Gotoh, F., Sato, T., Tanahashi, N., Tanaka, K., and Kobari,
    M., 1982, The vertebral arterial system in rhesus monkeys is less ef-
    ficient in autoregulation of blood flow than the internal carotid
    arterial system, in: "Cerebral Vascular Disease, 4," Proceedings of
    11th Int. Salzburg Conference, J. S. Meyer, H. Lechner, M. Reivich,
    and E. O. Ott, eds., pp. 48-52, Excerpta Medica, Amsterdam.

Torack, R. M., and Barrnett, R. J., 1964, The fine structural localization of nucleoside phosphatase activity in the blood-brain barrier, Neuropath. Exp. Neurol., 23:46-59.

Traystman, R. J., and Fitzgerald, R., 1981, Cerebrovascular response to hypoxia in baroreceptor- and chemoreceptor-denervated dogs, Am. J. Physiol., 241 (Heart Circ. Physiol., Vol. 10):H724-H731.

Traystman, R. J., Fitzgerald, R. S., and Loscutoff, S. C., 1978, Cerebral circulatory responses to arterial hypoxia in normal and chemodenervated dogs, Circ. Res., 42:649-657.

Ulrich, K., Auer, L. M., and Kuschinsky, W., 1981, Cat pial venoconstriction by topical microapplication of norepinephrine, J. Cereb. Blood Flow Metab., 2:109-111.

Urbanics, R., Leniger-Follert, E., and Lübbers, D. W., 1978, Time course of extracellular H^+ and K^+ activities during and after direct electrical stimulation of the brain cortex, Pflügers Arch., 378:47-53.

Vamada, S., and Burton, A. C., 1954, Effect of reduced tissue pressure on blood flow in the fingers; the veni-vasomotor reflex, J. Appl. Physiol., 6:501-505.

Van Citters, R. L., Wagner, B. M., and Rushmer, R. F., 1962, Structural changes of arterial walls during vasoconstriction, Cor et Vasa, 4:175-180.

Vasadze, G. Sh., 1960, Pathogenesis of severe traumatic and burn shock, in: "Shock and Terminal States," pp. 93-102, Meditsina, Leningrad.

Vasin, N. Ya., 1959, Reflexes from the longitudinal sinus of the dura mater arising during sinusography, Fiziol. Zh. SSSR, 45:1201-1207.

Vimtrup, Bj., 1922, Beiträge zur Anatomie der Capillaren. I. Über contraktile Elementen in der Gafässwand der Blut-capillaren, Z. Anat. Entwgesch., 65:150-184.

Vinall, P. E., and Simeone, F. A., 1982, *In vitro* myogenic autoregulation in cerebral blood vessels, in: "Cerebral Blood Flow. Effect of Nerves and Neurotransmitters," D. D. Heistad and M. L. Marcus, eds., pp. 16-18, Elsevier, New York.

Voronin, V. V., 1897, "Investigations of Inflammation," Moscow.

Voronin, V. V., 1947, "Handbook of Pathological Physiology," Part 1, Gruzmedgiz, Tbilisi.

Voronin, V. V., 1959, "Inflammation," 2nd revised and updated edition, Georgian Academy of Sciences Publishers, Tbilisi.

Wackenheim, A., Babin, B., Nuhlmann, M., Helot, N., Kehr, P., Megret, M., Ben Amor, N., Serbano, S., and Beysang, R., 1972, Arterial spasms. Neuroradiology, 3:193-198.

Wahl, M., and Kuschinsky, W., 1976, The dilatatory action of adenosine on pial arteries of cats and its inhibition by theophylline, Pflügers Arch., 362:55-59.

Wahl, M., and Kuschinsky, W., 1977, Influence of H^+ and K^+ on adenosine-induced dilatation of pial arteries of cats, Blood Vessels, 14:285-293.

Wahl, M., and Kuschinsky, W., 1979, Unimportance of perivascular H^+ and K^+ activities for the adjustment of pial arterial diameter during changes of arterial blood pressure in cats, Pflügers Arch., 382:203-208.

Wahl, M., Kuschinsky, W., Bosse, O., Olesen, J., Lassen, N. A., Ingvar, D. H., and Thurau, K., 1971-1972, Adrenergic control of cerebral vascular resistance. A micropuncture study, in: "Cerebral Blood Flow and Intracranial Pressure," Eur. Neurol., 6:185-189.

Wahlström, B. A., 1973, A study on the action of noradrenaline on ionic content and sodium, potassium, and chloride effluxes in the rat portal vein, Acta Physiol. Scand., 89:522-530.

Waltz, A. G., 1969, Red venous blood: occurrence and significance in ischemic and nonischemic cerebral cortex, J. Neurosurg., 31:141-148.

Waltz, A. G., 1970, Effect of PaCO$_2$ on blood flow and microvasculature of ischemic and nonischemic cerebral cortex, Stroke, 1:27–37.

Waltz, A. G., Sundt, T. M., and Owen, Ch. A., 1966, Effect of middle cerebral artery occlusion on cortical blood flow in animals, Neurology, 16:1185–1190.

Watts, C., 1977, Reserpine and cerebral vasospasm, Stroke, 8:112–114.

Waugh, W. H., 1964, Circulatory autoregulation in the fully isolated kidney and in the humorally supported, isolated kidney, Circ. Res., 15: Suppl. 1, 156–169.

Wayland, H., 1965, Rheology in microcirculation, in: "Second European Conference on Microcirculation. Bibl. Anat.," Vol. 5, pp. 2–22, Karger, Basel–New York.

Weber, H., 1852, Experimente über die Stase an der Froschschwimmhaut. Arch. Anat., Physiol. u. Wiss. Med., pp. 36–371.

Webster, 1981, "New Collegiate Dictionary," C. and C. Merriam Company, Springfield, Illinois.

Wei, E. P., Kontos, H. A., and Patterson, J. L., 1980, Dependence of pial arteriolar response to hypercapnia on vessel size, Am. J. Physiol., 238:H697–H703.

Weinstein, G. B., 1970, "Dynamics of the Intercranial Pressure during Action of Transversal Overloads," Thesis, Leningrad.

White, R. P., Hagen, A. A., Morgan, H., Dawson, W. N., and Robertson, J. T., 1975, Experimental study on the genesis of cerebral vasospasm, Stroke, 6:52–57.

White, R. P., Huang, S.-P., Hager, A. A., and Robertson, I. T., 1979, Experimental assessment of phenoxybenzamine in cerebral vasospasm, J. Neurosurg., 50:158–163.

Whitmore, R. L., 1968, "Rheology of the Circulation," Pergamon Press, Oxford.

Whittacker, S. R. F., and Winton, F. R., 1933, The apparent viscosity of blood flowing in the isolated hindlimb of the dog, and its variation with corpuscular concentration, J. Physiol. (London), 78:339–369.

Winn, H. R., Rubio, R., and Berne, R. M., 1979, Brain adenosine production during 60 seconds of ischemia, Circ. Res., 45:486–492.

Winn, H. R., Welsh, J. E., Rubio, R., and Berne, R. M., 1980, Changes in brain adenosine during bicuculline-induced seizures in rats, Effect of hypoxia and altered systemic blood pressure, Circ. Res., 47:568–577.

Yamamoto, Y. L., Feindel, E., Wolfe, L. S., Katch, H., and Hodge, C. P., 1972, Experimental vasoconstriction of cerebral arteries by prostaglandins, J. Neurosurg., 37:385–397.

Zervas, N. T., Kuwayama, A., Rosoff, Ch. B., and Salzman, E. W., 1973, Cerebral arterial spasm, Arch. Neurol., 28:400–404.

Zeuthen, T., Dóra, E., Silver, I. A., Chance, B., and Kovách, A. G. B., 1979, Mechanism of the cerebrocortical vasodilatation during anoxia, Acta Physiol. Hung., 54:305–318.

Zweifach, B. W., 1934, A micro-manipulative study of blood capillaries, Anat. Res., 59:83–108.

Zweifach, B. W., 1939, The character and distribution of blood capillaries, Anat. Res., 73:475–495.

Zweifach, B. W., 1940a, The structural basis of permeability and other functions of blood capillaries, Cold Spring Harbor Symp. Quant. Biol., 8:216–223.

Zweifach, B. W., 1940b, The distribution of blood perfusates in capillary circulation, Am. J. Physiol., 130:512–520.

Zweifach, B. W., and Kossman, Ch., 1937, Micromanipulation of small blood vessels in the mouse, Am. J.Physiol., 120:23–35.

Zweifach, B. W., Lowenstein, B. E., and Chambers, R., 1944, Responses of blood capillaries to acute hemorrhage in the rat, Am. J. Physiol., 142:80–93.

Index

Acetylcholine
  effect on cerebral arteries,
    166
Adenosine
  effect on cerebral arteries,
    157–158
Adequate blood supply to brain
    tissue
  evidence for, 96–101
  regulation of, 102–113, 122–174
Adrenaline: *see* Catecholamines
Adrenergic nerves
  of major brain arteries, 74–77
  of pial arteries, 159–165
Anastomoses
  of circle of Willis, physiolog-
    ical significance of, 15
  of pial arterial system, 130–
    135, 137–139
Angiotensin: *see* Hypertensin
Antidiuretic hormone: *see*
    Vasopressin
Aortic arch
  hemodynamic effect on red cell
    and plasma distribution
    to brain, 287
Arterial blood pressure
  damping in brain major
    arteries, 14, 53–55
  effect on cerebral blood flow,
    43–57
  in circle of Willis, 52–55
Arterial anastomoses: *see*
    Anastomoses
Arterial hyperemia (*see also*
    Hyperemia in the brain)
  changes of microcirculation
    265–266, 281–283

Arterial hypertension
  effect on cerebral blood flow,
    44–49
Arterial hypotension
  effect on cerebral blood flow,
    44–49
Arterial walls
  anatomy and function, 10–11
Arterioles
  as regulators of cerebral
    blood flow, 34, 42
Arteriovenous pressure difference
  effect on cerebral blood flow,
    43–49
  effect on distribution of blood
    flow in capillary net-
    works, 263–267
Asphyxia
  behavior of brain major arteries
    during, 65–66
  behavior of intracerebral
    (parenchymal) arteries
    during, 110, 119–120
  behavior of pial arteries
    during, 118–119
  effect on cerebral blood flow,
    121
Autoregulation of cerebral blood
    flow: *see* Cerebral blood
    flow, regulation of con-
    stancy, Cerebral blood
    pressure, regulation of
    constancy
Automatic control: *see* Regulation
    of cerebral blood flow

Baroreceptors (*see also* Stretch
    receptors)

Baroreceptors (cont.)
  in carotid sinus and cerebral
       arteries, 89
  involvement in regulation of
       constant cerebral blood
       pressure and flow, 88–90
Blood flow patterns
  in largest microvessels, 244–245
  in smallest microvessels, 245–247
  in transient microvessels, 247–
       250
Blood flow velocity
  effect on red cell and plasma
       distribution in vascular
       bifurcations, 282–289
  in microvessels, 247–249, 265–267
Blood fluidity
  distrubances in microvessels,
       249–252, 253–256, 291–293
  factors determining, 237–242,
       249–252
Blood pressure: see Arterial
       pressure
Blood stasis
  disturbing microcirculation,
       250–252, 253–256
Blood viscosity
  disturbances in microvessels,
       249–252, 253–256, 265,
       291–293
  factors determining, 237–242
Blood volume in cerebral
       vasculature: see Cerebral
       blood volume
Brain activity
  linkage with local cerebral
       blood flow, 96–104
Brain tissue blood supply: see
       Cerebral microcirculation

Calcium ions
  involvement in development of
       cerebral vasospasm,
       221–226
  involvement in development of
       pathological dilatation,
       221–222, 226–227
Capillaries
  active and nonactive, 232–233,
       267–274, 290
  blood flow distribution in,
       263–267
  blood flow velocity in, 232,
       233–234
  blood pressure in, 232, 234–
       236, 263–267, 273

Capillaries (cont.)
  of brain, 11–12
  contractility (mobility) of
       walls of, 271–274
  diameter of, 245–247, 268–269,
       271, 273
  main capillaries and net
       capillaries, 260–263
  plasmatic capillaries, 269–271,
       274, 290
Carbon dioxide in cerebral blood
       and tissue
  coupling with cerebral blood
       flow, 117
  effect on cerebral arteries,
       149–152
  regulation of constancy of,
       113–114
    neurogenic mechanism of,
       166–169
    vascular effectors of, 117–
       121
Catecholamines (Adrenaline,
       Epinephrine, Noradrenaline,
       Norepinephrine)
  effect on cerebral arteries,
       165–166
  involvement in development of
       cerebral vasospasm,
       202–203, 205–210
Cerebral arterial bed
  integral consideration of, 9–10
Cerebral arterial walls
  anatomy, 10–11
Cerebral blood flow
  dependence on systemic cirucla-
       tion, 44–45, 47–49
  general consideration of, 1–3
  regulation of constancy of,
       45–46
    disturbance of, 47–49
    evidence for, 45–46
    feedback of, 88–92
    mechanism of, 46–47, 88–92
    myogenic vs. neurogenic
       mechanisms of, 81–88
    vascular effectors of, 49–56
Cerebral blood pressure
  regulation of constancy
    disturbance of, 47–49
    evidence for, 45–46
    feedback of, 88–92
    mechanism of, 46–47, 88–92
    myogenic vs. neurogenic
       mechanisms of, 81–88
    vascular effectors of, 49–56

Cerebral blood volume
  active regulation of constancy
      of, 56-71
    disturbances related to
      increase of, 69-71
    during asphyxia, 65-66
    during postischemic hyperemia,
      66-67
    during venous blood stagna-
      tion, 60-61, 65
    during widespread functional
      hyperemia, 67
    feedback of, 92-94
    neurogenic mechanism of, 92-94
    vascular effectors of, 60-61,
      64-69
  biophysical factors maintaining
      constancy of, 56-58
  distribution among arteries,
      capillaries, and veins,
      57
Cerebral microcirculation
  coupling with local activity,
      99-101
  coupling with metabolic rate
      of tissue, 96-99
  principal physiological
      parameters of, 231-233
  regulation of, 102-104
    feedback of, 148-174
    humoral mechanisms of, 148-154
    neurogenic mechanism of,
      159-174
    vascular effectors of, 104-113
Cerebral parenchymal arteries
  anatomy of walls of, 108
  functional behavior during
      regulation of constant
      P_{O_2} and P_{CO_2} in cerebral
      tissue, 119-120
  functional behavior during
      regulation of microcir-
      culation, 108-112
  role in regulation of cerebral
      blood flow, 174
Cerebral vasospasm: see Vasospasm
Cerebral veins
  structure and function, 12-14
Cerebrovascular resistance
  notion of and effect on cerebral
      blood flow, 6, 14-15, 44,
      47, 103
Chemoreceptors
  of carotid sinus, 167-168
  of cerebral veins, 117, 167-168
Cholinergic nerves
  of brain major arteries, 75-77
  of pial arteries, 159-165

Circle of Willis: see Anastomoses,
      Arterial blood pressure
Circulation
  relationship of central
      (systemic) and peripheral,
      3-9
Collateral blood supply: see
      Vasospasm, compensatory
      events accompanying
Compensation for
  changes of O_2 and CO_2 contents
      in cerebral blood and
      tissue, 25, 113-122,
      149-154, 159-169
  deficient blood supply to
      cerebral tissue, 24-25,
      98-113, 122-148, 154-166,
      169-174
  elevated systemic arterial
      pressure, 25, 43-56, 81-92
  excessive blood volume in
      cerebral vasculature, 25,
      56-71, 92-94

Density
  of cerebral capillary networks,
      260, 267-274
  of pial arterial vessels,
      131-135
  of radial arteries feeding
      cerebral cortex, 129-130,
      259
Disturbances of cerebral blood
      flow
  related to brain perfusion
      pressure, 47-49
  related to cerebral vasospasm,
      176-178
  related to increased cerebral
      blood volume 69-71
  related to pathological dila-
      tation, 178

Effectors of cerebral blood flow
      regulation: see Vascular
      effectors of regulation
Efficiency requirements
  of cerebral blood flow regula-
      tion, 36-38
Electrolytes: see Hydrogen ions,
      Potassium ions
Epinephrine: see Catecholamines
Erythrocytes: see Red blood cells

Flow conditions
  in microvessels, 242-249
  following vasomotor disorders,
      291-293

Hematocrit (*see also* Red cell:
       plasma ratio in flowing
       blood)
   effect on blood rheological
       properties in micro-
       vessels, 241–242
   local changes related to blood
       flow velocity, 280–286
Hormones: *see* Adrenaline,
       Vasopressin
Humoral mechanisms
   of adequate blood supply
       regulation to cerebral
       tissue, 154–159
   of carbon dioxide and oxygen
       effect on cerebral blood
       vessels, 149–154
Hydrogen ions
   involvement in functional and
       postischemic vasodila-
       tation, 154–155
   involvement in producing
       pathological vasodila-
       tation in the brain,
       214–215
   involvement in vasomotor effect
       of carbon dioxide, 150–
       152
Hyperemia in the brain
   functional type of
       behavior of intracerebral
           (parenchymal) arteries
           during, 108–111
       behavior of pial arteries
           during, 104
       humoral mechanism of the
           cerebral vasodilatation
           during, 154–159, 174
       involvement of brain major
           arteries, 67
       neurogenic mechanism of the
           cerebral vasodilatation
           during, 169–174
   postischemic (reactive) type of
       behavior of brain major
           arteries during, 66–67
       behavior of intracerebral
           (parenchymal) arteries
           during, 110
       behavior of pial arteries
           during, 105–106
       humoral mechanism of the
           cerebral vasodilatation
           during, 154–159, 174
       neurogenic mechanism of the
           cerebral vasodilatation
           during, 169–174

Hypertensin
   involvement in development of
       cerebral vasospasm, 205–210
Hypertension: *see* Arterial
       hypertension
Hypotension: *see* Arterial
       hypotension

Ischemia in the brain
   caused by cerebral vasospasm,
       176–178
   collateral blood supply during,
       228–229
   microcirculation during, 266–
       267, 280–283, 288, 290–293

Main capillaries
   effect on distribution of
       blood in capillary
       networks, 263–267
   structural and functional
       peculiarities of, 260–263
Major arteries of the brain
   anatomical and functional
       peculiarities of, 71–73, 77
   as effectors of regulation of
       cerebral blood flow,
       52–56, 64–69
   methods of study of functional
       behavior of, 61–63
   myogenic responses of, 81–88
   neurogenic control of, 74–79,
       84–94
   responses of vasoconstrictor
       drugs, 77–80
   as site of vasospasm, 181–184
Microcirculation: *see* Cerebral
       microcirculation,
       Microvascular bed,
       Microvessels
Microvascular bed (*see also*
       Microvessels)
   distribution of blood in,
       263–267
   functional arrangement of,
       256–260
Microvessels
   driving force of blood flow in,
       234–236
   factors determining blood flow
       rate in, 233–234
   flow conditions of red cells
       in, 242–249
   fluidity of blood in, 237–242
   resistance to blood flow in,
       236–237
   viscosity of blood in, 237–242

Myogenic responses of cerebral
    arteries
  in regulation of cerebral blood
      pressure and flow, 81-88

Neural centers: *see* Vasomotor
    centers
Neural regulation
  of adequate blood supply to
      cerebral tissue, 169-174
  of constancy of cerebral blood
      pressure and flow, 84-92
  of constancy of cerebral blood
      volume, 93-94
  of constancy of oxygen and
      carbon dioxide content
      in cerebral blood and
      tissue, 166-169
Noradrenaline: *see* Catecholamines
Norepinephrine: *see* Catecholamines

Oxygen in cerebral blood and
    tissue
  coupling with cerebral blood
      flow, 114-117
  effect on cerebral arteries,
      152-154
  regulation of constancy of,
      113-114
    neurogenic mechanism of,
        166-169
    vascular effectors of,
        117-122
  transport of, dependent on
      changes of red cell:
      plasma ratio in micro-
      vessels, 274-291

Pathological vascular responses:
      see Pathological
      vasodilatation, Vasospasm
Pathological vasodilatation
  basic processes in vascular
      walls causing, 194-195
  compensatory events
      accompanying, 230
  criteria of, 186-187
  effect of endogenous substances
      on development of, 213-216
  essence of, 192-194
  involvement of vascular smooth
      muscle intravascular
      processes in development
      of, 221-222, 226-227
  involvement of vascular smooth
      muscle plasma membranes
      in development of, 220-221

Pathological vasodilatation (cont.)
  involvement of vasoactive sub-
      stances in development
      of, 213-216
  localization of, 187-188
  mechanical factors involved in
      development of, 193-194,
      212-213
  notion of, 176-178, 184-186
Perfusion pressure for brain:
      see Arteriovenous
      pressure difference
Peripheral resistance: *see*
      Cerebrovascular resistance
Pial arterial bed
  arrangement of, 122-141
  basic structural units of,
      129-135
  functional heterogeneity of
      vasomotor responses,
      143-144
  interarterial anastomoses in,
      137-139
  neurogenic control of, 159-166
  significance of bifurcations
      of, 124-129
  specific vascular portions of,
      135-141
Pial arteries
  role in regulation of cerebral
      microcirculation, 144-148,
      174
  as vascular effectors of re-
      gulation of adequate
      microcirculation, 104-106
  as vascular effectors of re-
      gulation of constant O_2
      and CO_2 in brain tissue,
      118-119
  vasomotor responses of, 141-148,
      158-159
Pitressin: *see* Vasopressin
Plasma skimming
  in arterial bifurcations,
      280, 289
Postischemic hyperemia: *see*
      Hyperemia in the brain,
      postischemic type
Potassium ions
  involvement in functional and
      postischemic vasodilata-
      tion, 155-157
  involvement in vascular muscle
      cell plasma membrane
      depolarization causing
      development of cerebral
      vasospasm, 218-220

Precapillary sphincters
  role in blood flow distribution
      in capillary networks,
      263-264
  role in occurrence of plasmatic
      capillaries, 274
  structure and functional
      behavior of, 260
Precortical arteries
  nerve supply of, 162-163
  structure and functional
      behavior of, 136-137,
      143-148
Pressure of blood (*see also*
      Arterial pressure)
  in peripheral vessels, relation-
      ship with wall tension
      and vessel radius, 191-
      192, 212-213, 273
Pressure-flow relationship
  for cerebral blood flow, 43-49
Prostaglandins
  involvement in development of
      cerebral vasospasm,
      203-204, 205-210

Reactive hyperemia: *see* Hyperemia
      in the brain, postischemic
      (reactive) type
Receptors in cerebral vessel
      walls: *see* Baroreceptors,
      Chemoreceptors, Stretch
      receptors
Red blood cells
  aggregation of, effect on blood
      fluidity in microvessels,
      251, 253-256, 292
  behavior of, in microvessels,
      244-249
  concentration, effect on blood
      fluidity in microvessels,
      237, 241-242
  deformability of, effect on
      blood fluidity in
      capillaries, 242, 292
  sedimentation of, relation to
      their aggregation, 252-253
Red cell:plasma ratio in flowing
      blood (*see also*
      Hematocrit)
  changes in blood vessels, 274-291
  in large and minute vessels,
      276-279
  mechanisms of changes of, 282-289
  methods of estimating, 275-276
  relationship to blood flow rate,
      280-286

Red cell:plasma ratio in flowing
      blood (cont.)
  role in transformation of active
      capillaries into inactive
      forms, 269-271
  significance for rate of
      microcirculation, 280-
      282, 286-287, 289-291
Regulation of cerebral blood flow
  coordination systems of, 29-31
  efficiency requirements of,
      36-38
  general consideration of, 18-22
  historical sketch of, 17-18
  humoral mechanism of, 149-159
  myogenic mechanism of, 81-88
  neurogenic mechanism of, 73-80,
      84-94, 159-174
  in small areas of cerebral
      tissue: *see* Cerebral
      microcirculation
  systems analysis of the problem
      of, 39-41
  triggering mechanisms of, 26-29
  types of, 22-26
  vascular effectors of, 20,
      34-36, 42-43, 49-55,
      104-113
  vasomotor mechanisms of, 31-34,
      73-92, 149-174
Regulation of constant O_2 and CO_2
      contents
  in cerebral blood and tissue,
      113-117
Regulation effectors of cerebral
      blood flow: *see* Vascular
      effectors of regulation
Resistance in cerebral blood
      vessels: *see* Cerebro-
      vascular resistance
Rheological properties of blood:
      see Microvessels,
      fluidity of blood in,
      viscosity of blood in

Serotonin
  effect on cerebral arteries,
      197-200
  involvement in development of
      cerebral vasospasm, 201-
      202, 205-210
Sphincters
  at offshoots of capillary
      branches: *see* Precapillary
      sphincters
  at pial arterial offshoots,
      135-136, 143-148

Stretch receptors (*see also*
      Baroreceptors)
   in cerebral veins, 93–94
   involvement in regulation of
      constant cerebral blood
      volume, 28, 93–94
Sympathetic nerves
   involvement in regulation of
      adequate blood supply to
      cerebral tissue, 173
   involvement in regulation of
      constant cerebral blood
      pressure and flow, 91–92
Systems analysis
   of the problem of pathological
      behavior of cerebral
      arteries, 188–189
   of the problem of regulation of
      cerebral circulation,
      39–41

Vascular closure
   of arteries during vasospasm,
      191–192
   of blood capillaries, 271–274
Vascular effectors of regulation
   of adequate blood supply to
      cerebral tissue, 104–113
   of constant cerebral blood
      pressure and flow,
      49–56, 71–73
   of constant cerebral blood
      volume, 60–73
   of constant oxygen and carbon
      dioxide tension in
      cerebral blood and
      tissue, 117–122
Vascular mechanisms of the brain
   notion, 34–36, 42–43
Vascular obstruction: *see*
      Vasospasm
Vascular smooth muscle (*see also*
      Vasospasm)
   depolarization and repolariza-
      tion of muscle cell
      plasma membranes, involve-
      ment in contraction and
      relaxation of, 216–221
   effect of vasoactive substances
      on, 149–159, 196–210,
      213–216
   intracellular calcium transport,
      involvement of contraction
      and relaxation of, 221–226
   involvement of contractile
      machinery in, 226–227

Vasoconstriction of cerebral
      arteries (*see also*
      Vasospasm)
   caused by endogenous vasoactive
      substances, 196–210
   physiological and pathological
      178
Vasodilatation of cerebral
      arteries (*see also*
      Pathological vasodilata-
      tion)
   caused by endogenous vasodilator
      substances, 149–159, 213–
      216
   causing functional hyperemia in
      the brain, 104
   causing postischemic (reactive)
      hyperemia in the brain,
      105–106
   physiological and pathological
      vasodilatation, 178
Vasomotion, 264
Vasomotor centers
   regulating cerebral circulation,
      90–91, 165, 173
Vasomotor control: *see* Neurogenic
      regulation
Vasomotor nerves: *see* Neurogenic
      regulation, Sympathetic
      nerves
Vasoparalysis: *see* Pathological
      vasodilatation
Vasopressin
   involvement in development of
      cerebral vasospasm, 204,
      205–210
Vasospasm
   basic processes in vascular
      walls causing, 194–195
   characteristics and criteria
      of, 178–180
   compensatory events accompany-
      ing, 227–229
   disturbances in "calcium pumps"
      in smooth muscle cells
      responsible for develop-
      ment of, 221–226
   effect of endogenous vasocon-
      strictor substances on
      development of, 196–210
   essence of, 189–192
   historical sketch of, 180–181
   involvement of contractile
      proteins of vascular
      smooth muscle in develop-
      ment of, 226–227

Vasospasm (cont.)
  involvement of vascular smooth
        muscle plasma membranes
        in development of, 216–220
  localization of, 181–184
  mechanical factors involved in
        development of, 191–192
  neurogenic effects in develop-
        ment of, 210–212
  notion of, 176–178
  systems analysis of the problem
        of, 188–189
Veins
  structure and function of
        cerebral veins, 12–13
Velocity of blood flow: see
        Blood flow velocity
Venous blood pressure in the
        brain
  relationship with systemic
        venous pressure, 58–59

Venous blood stagnation in the
        brain
  behavior of major arteries
        during, 60–69
  microcirculation during, 235–
        236, 267
  physiological mechanism
        eliminating, 60–69
Viscosity of blood: see Blood
        viscosity
Volumetric equilibrium of blood,
        cerebrospinal fluid, and
        brain tissue within the
        skull
  the Monro-Kellie doctrine, its
        influence on the concepts
        of cerebral blood flow
        regulation, 17–18
  regulation of constant blood
        volume within the skull,
        56–69